Contents

Acknowledgements

Reviewers of the UK edition

Anne Baileff, RN, RM, BSc(Hons), MSc
Consultant Nurse in Unscheduled Care
Southampton City PCT

James M. Bowen, BTechEMC, MTechEMC
Senior Lecturer in Paramedic Sciences
Department of School of Health and Emergency Professions
University of Hertfordshire

Simon Brook, RN, BA(Hons), MSc, PGCEA
Consultant Nurse in Unscheduled Care
Southampton City Primary Care Trust

Neal Cook, RN, BSc, MSc, PD Dlp, PGCert, IFPA
Lecturer in Nursing and Academic Coordinator
School of Nursing
University of Ulster

Pat Deeny, RN, RNT, BSc, Adv Dip E
Senior Lecturer
School of Nursing
University of Ulster

Janet C. Flournoy, RSCN, CPNP, MSN
Lecturer
University of Southampton

Sue Green, RN, BSc(Hons), MMedSci, PhD, PGCert
Senior Lecturer
School of Health Sciences
University of Southampton

Bridget Malkin, RGN, BSc, MA (Ed)
Senior Lecturer
Clinical Skills Division
Department of Nursing and Women's Health
Birmingham City University

Cheryl Phillips, RGN, MSc, PGCE
Senior Lecturer
Faculty of Health
Sport & Science
University of Glamorgan

Catherine Powell, PhD, BNSc(Hons), RGN, RSCN, RHV
Consultant Nurse Safeguarding Children
Portsmouth City Teaching PCT

Carmel Sheppard, RGN, BSc(Hons), MSc, DBMS
Consultant Nurse Breast Care
Portsmouth Hospitals NHS Trust

Andy Williams, MA, BA(Hons), RMN, RGN, FAETC
Lecturer in Mental Health
School of Health Sciences
University of Southampton

The UK adaptor would like to offer her particular thanks to Simon Brook, Janet Flournoy and Gill Taylor, whose considerable generosity in terms of their time and expertise has been invaluable in the completion of this project.

Foreword

I am delighted to introduce you to this first UK edition of *Assessment Made Incredibly Easy!* I believe that the skills covered in this book are fundamental to the delivery of excellent healthcare, and can help you to make a real difference to the quality of care which your patients receive.

Traditionally in the UK, many of the skills covered in this book were mainly carried out by doctors. Other professions focused on assessment skills related to particular body systems, or on assessing the activities of living. But much has changed in recent years, and there is a growing 'blurring of the boundaries' between the different healthcare professions. This means that many of the skills which are covered in this book have relevance across several different healthcare professions and roles, and can help you to undertake a more holistic health assessment of your patients.

Some of you will be learning these skills as part of your initial training and registration as a healthcare professional. Others will have been qualified for a while, perhaps for many years, and will be learning these skills to enable you to advance your practice, or move into a new field of practice, or to help you be more autonomous in the care that you deliver. Whatever the reason, I very much hope that you will find this book a helpful aid to your learning.

It is important to remember that no book can cover everything. This book, like all the Incredibly Easy! texts, is designed to be used alongside key textbooks and journal articles which will offer you greater detail on the subjects covered. In this case, these will include your preferred anatomy and physiology text, and your preferred health assessment text. What this book aims to do is to help you understand these texts more easily and apply theory to practice. It also offers a valuable revision aid that will help as you prepare for your examinations, or further down the line when you need something to jog your memory about a skill you haven't practised for a while.

In order to help you, the book is divided into two main sections. Part I emphasises the core knowledge and skills which you need before you undertake any health assessment, and Part II guides you through the assessment of the different body systems. Throughout the book, numerous illustrations and photographs will help you to hone your clinical assessment skills. In addition, text-specific logos highlight critical information:

Memory Jogger helps you to remember important points.

Bridging the Gap explains cultural variables which may influence the health assessment.

 Peak Technique illustrates and describes the best ways to perform specific physical examination techniques.

 Ages and Stages pinpoint age-related variations in assessment findings.

 Interpretation Stations provide guidelines for interpreting assessment findings quickly and easily.

It is important to remember that becoming competent at some of the assessment skills described in this book will take months or even years of practise. So take things one step at a time. As you learn the skills, take every opportunity (with your patients' consent) to practise them. Tell others in your workplace or placement about the skills you are learning, and ask them to help you, watch you and give you feedback. The more normal heart sounds you listen to, for example, the better you will get at spotting the abnormalities. Indeed, it makes sense to have recognition of the difference between 'normal' and 'abnormal' as your first goal when learning many of these assessment skills (and you will probably also be surprised at just how many variations of 'normal' there are!). Remember, in the early stages, you will often be able to do little more than refer someone whom you suspect has an abnormality to a more senior or specialist practitioner for further assessment.

As you progress you will become more confident in your assessment findings, and will begin to understand many of the different abnormalities which you are identifying. On some occasions you will have a good idea of what is wrong with the patient, and the care they need. On other occasions you will require further information in the form of investigations such as blood tests, X-rays and so on. As you move onto these other skills you will need further information, and you will find that skills such as specialist screening tests (for example, cervical screening), ordering and interpreting investigations, pathophysiology and diagnostic decision-making each have texts of their own. But *Assessment Made Incredibly Easy!* will help to give you a firm foundation on which to build these other skills – the crucially important first two steps of history-taking and physical examination.

Helen Rushforth, PhD, BA, RGN, RSCN
Senior Lecturer and Award Leader
MSc Advanced Clinical Practice
School of Health Sciences
University of Southampton, UK

Contributors and consultants to the US edition

Deborah A. Andris, RN,CS, MSN, APNP
Nurse Practitioner
Bariatric Surgery Program
Medical College of Wisconsin
Milwaukee

Jemma Bailey-Kunte, APRN-BC, MS, FNP
Clinical Lecturer
Binghamton (N.Y.) University
Nurse Practitioner
Lourdes Hospital
Binghamton

Cheryl A. Bean, APRN, BC, DSN, ANP, AOCN
Associate Professor
Indiana University School of Nursing
Indianapolis

Natalie Burkhalter, RN, MSN, ACNP, CS, FNP
Associate Professor
Texas A&M International University
Laredo

Shelba Durston, RN, MSN, CCRN
Nursing Instructor
San Joaquin Delta College
Stockton, Calif.
Staff Nurse
San Joaquin General Hospital
French Camp, Calif.

Tamara D. Espejo, RN, MS
Registered Nurse and Clinical Educator
Aurora Behavioral Healthcare-Charter Oak
Covina, Calif.

Michelle L. Foley, RN,C, MA
Director of Nursing Education
Charles E. Gregory School of Nursing

Raritan Bay Medical Center
Perth Amboy, N.J.

Catherine B. Holland, RN, PHD, ANP, APRN,BC, CNS
Associate Professor
Southeastern Louisiana University
Baton Rouge

Julia Anne Isen, RN, MS, FNP-C
Nurse Practitioner – Internal Medicine
Veterans Administration Medical Center
San Francisco
Assistant Clinical Professor
School of Nursing
University of California at San Francisco

Nancy Banfield Johnson, RN, MSN, ANP (inactive)
Nurse-Manager
Kendal at Ithaca (N.Y.)

Gary R. Jones, MSN, CNS, FNP
ARNP, Disease Management Program
Mercy Health Center
Fort Scott, Kansas

Vanessa C. Kramasz, RN, MSN, FNP-C
Nursing Faculty & Family Nurse
  Practitioner
Gateway Technical College
Kenosha, Wis.

Priscilla A. Lee, MN, FNP
Instructor in Nursing
Moorpark (Calif.) College

Susan Luck, RN, MS, CCN
Director of Nutrition
Biodoron Immunology Center
Hollywood, Fla.

Ann S. McQueen, RNC, MSN, CRNP
Family Nurse Practitioner
Healthlink Medical Center
Southampton, Pa.

Dale O'Donnell, RN, BSN
Administrator Community Surgery Center
Community Hospital
Munster, Ind.

William J. Pawlyshyn, RN, MS, MN, APRN, BC
Nurse Practitioner Consultant
New England Geriatrics
West Springfield, Mass.

Catherine Pence, RN, MSN, CCRN
Assistant Professor
Good Samaritan College of Nursing
Cincinnati

Abby Plambeck, RN, BSN
Freelance Writer
Milwaukee, Wis.

Theresa Pulvano, RN, BSN
Nursing Educator
Ocean County Vocational Technical School
Lakehurst, N.J.

Monica Narvaez Ramirez, RN, MSN
Faculty
University of the Incarnate Word
San Antonio, Tex.

Regina Reed, MSN, FNP
Associate Professor
Washington State Community College
Marrietta, Ohio

Part I

Beginning the assessment

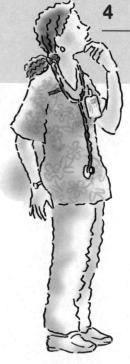

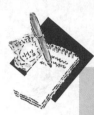

Just the facts

In this chapter, you'll learn:

♦ reasons for performing a health history
♦ techniques for communicating effectively during a health history assessment
♦ essential steps in a complete health history
♦ questions specific to each step of a health history.

A look at health assessment

Knowing how to complete an accurate health assessment initially involves two components, taking a health history and performing a physical examination. It is these two key steps that are the focus of this book. These techniques help to establish a list of possible problems and health needs that the patient might have, and inform decisions about what investigations, if any, to request or suggest. The findings from the history, physical examination and investigations are then used to make a diagnosis and/or to identify a healthcare need. Finally, the information is used to develop a treatment plan or a plan of care, which is then implemented and evaluated.

Legal aspects

It is firstly important that you are aware of the legal and professional regulations underpinning the role and skills you are undertaking or learning. To do this you will need to refer to your professional code of conduct and any other regulations or guidelines regarding the scope and boundaries of your professional practice. As you learn new skills you must always ensure that you are practising with appropriate supervision, and that there are clear agreements in place regarding how your achievement of competence will be determined. If you are a pre-registration student you also need to ensure that you are practising in accordance with policy set out by your university, and to the standards for pre-registration students set out by the body that will award your professional qualification.

Blurring boundaries in healthcare

Historically, different healthcare practitioners conducted separate elements of the health assessment with different purposes in mind. This often led to both repetition and omission. However, in recent years professional boundaries have started to blur, making it increasingly likely that you will be asked to collect data from your patient that will inform not only your own patient care but also that of other members of the multidisciplinary healthcare team. It is therefore important when you carry out an assessment that you are clear regarding its purpose.

Patient diagnosis?

The other factor to be aware of is that patients also increasingly view healthcare very differently. In particular, widespread access to the internet means that people often come to visit a health practitioner having already established a well-formed (and *sometimes* correct!) idea of what they think they have wrong with them.

Objective and subjective assessment

Any assessment involves collecting two kinds of data; objective and subjective. The term objective data refers to verifiable data obtained through observation, such as data gained from the physical examination and any investigations. For instance, a red, swollen arm in a patient who's complaining of arm pain is an example of data that can be seen and verified by someone other than the patient. So are observations of respirations, pulse rate and temperature. Subjective data, in contrast, can't be verified by anyone other than the patient; being gathered solely from the patient's own account – for example, 'My head hurts' or 'I have trouble sleeping at night.'

Exploring past and present

You'll therefore use a health history to gather subjective data about the patient and explore past and present problems. The history is a crucial part of the assessment process – it is sometimes said that 80% of the information that contributes to a diagnosis comes from the history (Epstein *et al.* 2003). But it is also about much more than just achieving a medical diagnosis. A good health history gives a holistic picture of the person; physically, psychologically, socially, emotionally and spiritually.

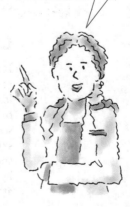

Here's a way to remember the two types of data: you 'observe' objective data, whereas only the 'subject' provides subjective data.

The comprehensive health history

Health histories vary from case to case according to their purpose. The most complete is referred to as the 'comprehensive health history', and includes all of the elements described later in the chapter. This type of history is the one most likely to give a picture of the whole patient. It is especially useful in situations such as:
- where reaching a diagnosis is difficult or complex
- where the patient has a range of different health problems
- prior to major treatment or surgery
- when a patient is newly enrolling with a healthcare provider, such as joining a new general practice.

It is regarded as the 'gold standard' in history taking, and is arguably under-used in many settings, often due to time constraints. But a well-conducted comprehensive health history may well be invaluable in recognising a previously unidentified health problem or unmet need.

Getting straight to the point

Other approaches to history taking are more selective. In some situations, a selective approach, if performed safely, may be more appropriate. This is often described as a 'focused health history', and most commonly involves the examiner asking selected questions directed by the presenting problem or need. Examples of situations where this approach may be appropriate include:
- emergency situations, where it is necessary to gain a brief history and move on to rapid physical examination (with the likelihood of returning to a more comprehensive history later) (See *Assessing a severely ill patient*, page 29)
- minor illness or injury, where information relating directly to the presenting problem and its management may be all that is required
- pre-operative assessment, where the focus is on history relating to past surgery, and the respiratory and cardiovascular systems, in order to ensure safe anaesthesia
- follow-up or ongoing assessment, where the patient is well known to the examiner and thus the examiner builds their history taking on previously established information
- nutritional assessment (discussed fully in Chapter 3)
- mental health assessment (discussed fully in Chapter 4).

It takes a lot of practise to make wise judgements about what to ask and what not to ask, so if in doubt it is better to ask rather than not. For example, if a patient has broken their arm, it may not seem relevant to explore all aspects of their family history or past medical history. Yet some factors, such as a history of previous fractures or a family history of osteoporosis, would be relevant. Guidance in the specific chapters, together with experience, will help you make these judgements.

Skills for getting the scoop

Keep in mind that the accuracy and completeness of your patient's answers largely depend on your skill as an interviewer. Therefore, before you start asking questions, review the following communication guidelines.

Beginning the interview

To make the most of your patient interview, before you begin you'll need to create an environment in which the patient feels comfortable. During the interview, you'll want to use various communication strategies to make sure you communicate effectively. You may find it helpful to look at the SOLER model (Egan 2001), which is designed to promote effective listening. (See *SOLER*, below.)

Settling in

Consider the following guidelines when selecting a location for the interview.
• Choose a quiet, private, well-lit interview setting if you can. If not, consider use of screens and curtains to create 'psychological privacy', but remember you can still be heard. Such a setting makes it easier for you and your patient to interact and helps the patient feel more at ease.

Memory jogger

SOLER

The mnemonic SOLER, proposed by Egan (2001) as part of his work on the 'Skilled Helper', can help you conduct a better interview with the patient by enabling you to think about how to listen effectively. He suggests:

S – **Sit squarely** facing the patient (although he notes that some people prefer to create a slight angle between the two seating positions)

O – **Open** posture

L – **Lean** towards the patient (as appropriate)

E – **Eye contact** – maintain appropriately

R – **Relaxed** approach.

• Make sure that the patient is comfortable, and ideally seated at the same height as you. As you will see in the Egan SOLER model, some people suggest sitting squarely facing the patient, about 1 to 1.5 metres (m) away, whilst others suggest that sitting at a 45 to 90 degree angle may be more comfortable, enabling the patient to look at you or away as he/she prefers. Try both ways and see which works best for you. Alternatively, if the patient is in bed, find a seat of an appropriate height so you neither tower over the patient nor sit too low. Adjust the bed height if necessary. Avoid standing whilst the patient is sitting.

• Try to avoid creating a barrier between you and the patient with a bed table or desk – if you need to lean on something to make notes, put a table to one side of you, or position chairs at the side and end of a desk so a barrier is avoided.

> Take a moment to set the stage. A supportive encouraging approach will make your patient much more forthcoming and will enable you to provide optimal care.

Watch what you say

• It is important to start by setting the scene and managing the patient's expectations for the interview. Introduce yourself and explain that the purpose is to identify key problems and gather information to aid in planning care. Remember also to seek their consent to take their history.

• Reassure the patient that information will be kept confidential within the healthcare team. (Although note exceptions in cases where you may have to share information with other professionals outside the healthcare team – see *Safeguarding children and vulnerable adults*, page 23.)

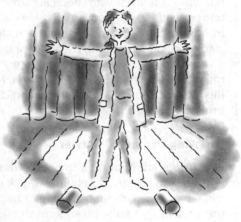

• Tell the patient how long the interview will last and ask what he/she expects from the interview.

• Use touch sparingly and appropriately. Many people aren't comfortable with strangers touching them, although sometimes touch may be appropriate, particularly if a patient is distressed.

• Assess the patient to see if language or communication barriers exist, and consider whether an interpreter is necessary. (See *Overcoming interview obstacles*, page 8.) Note that older patients in particular are often hard of hearing. Hearing-aid induction loop facilities are now available in some settings.

• Speak clearly, using easy-to-understand language. Avoid using medical terms and jargon.

• Establish with the patient how they like to be addressed. Do they prefer 'Mr Jones' or 'Jim'. Avoid using terms of endearment, such as 'dear', but also note that many patients are put off by terms like 'Sir' or 'Madam'. Treating the patient with respect encourages them to trust you and provide more accurate and complete information.

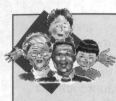

Bridging the gap

Overcoming interview obstacles

With a little creativity, you can overcome barriers to interviewing. You should find that there are both national (country specific) and local (healthcare setting specific) policies and guidelines regarding services for vulnerable patient groups. You need to be aware of these and use them to guide your practice – ask a colleague if you are unsure.

Interpreter information

If you and the patient don't both speak the same language, you will require an interpreter to help you take the patient's history. A trained medical interpreter – one who is familiar with medical terminology, knows interpreting techniques and understands the patient's rights – would be ideal. Be sure to ask the interpreter to translate the patient's speech verbatim and to capture not only what is said but also any clues regarding meaning or emotion.

Inevitably it is sometimes necessary to use one of the patient's adult family members or friends as an interpreter. Negotiate ground rules carefully, as this violates the patient's right to confidentiality; a trained interpreter is always preferable if one is available.

Breaking the sound barrier

Is your patient hearing impaired? Make sure any hearing aid is working properly and they can hear you clearly. Check if a hearing-aid induction loop system is available. Try to choose as quiet a place as possible to conduct the interview. If the patient lip reads, make sure the light is bright enough for them to see your lips move. Then face them and speak slowly and clearly. If the patient uses sign language, it is possible you may be able to access a sign language interpreter.

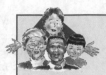

Bridging the gap

Overcoming cultural barriers

To promote a good relationship with your patients, remember that their cultural behaviours and beliefs may differ from your own. For example, eye contact within some cultures can be seen as aggressive or disrespectful. Be aware of these differences and respond appropriately.

Communicate effectively

Realise that you and the patient communicate non-verbally as well as verbally. Being aware of these forms of communication will aid you in the interview process.

Non-verbal communication strategies

To make the most of non-verbal communication, follow these guidelines.

• Listen attentively and make eye contact frequently. (See *Overcoming cultural barriers*, above and *SOLER*, page 6.)

- Use reassuring gestures, such as nodding your head, to encourage the patient to keep talking.
- Watch for non-verbal clues that indicate the patient is uncomfortable or unsure about how to answer a question. For example, they might lower their voice or glance around uneasily.
- Be aware of your own non-verbal behaviours that might cause the patient to stop talking or become defensive. For example, if you cross your arms, you might appear closed off. If you glance at your watch, you might appear to be bored or rushed, which could keep the patient from answering questions completely.
- Observe the patient closely to see if they understand each question. If they don't appear to understand, repeat the question using different words or familiar examples. For instance, instead of asking 'Do you have any problems passing urine?', ask 'Do you have any problems with your waterworks?' If in doubt, ask them whether they understand the question you are asking.

Verbal communication strategies

Verbal communication strategies include open-ended and closed questions, as well as employing such techniques as silence, facilitation, confirmation, reflection, clarification, summary and conclusion.

An open . . .

Asking open-ended questions such as 'How did you fall?' lets the patient respond more freely. The response may provide answers to many other questions. For instance, a male patient might tell you that he has previously fallen, that he was unsteady on his feet before he fell and that he fell just before eating dinner. Armed with this information, you might begin to draw very different conclusions about the care required when compared with another patient with a similar injury who tripped over the cat (although it's still important to check issues like vision, for example, in this instance). Note that a common mistake when asking this initial question is interrupting too soon – if you do this you might miss vital information, so try to wait until the patient finishes speaking.

. . . and shut case

You will also need to ask some closed questions. These are used to establish specific things you need to know or clarify, or to refocus the conversation. A closed question might be 'You said you had fallen before, tell me how many times you have fallen?' or 'When you have fallen previously, was that also shortly before a meal?'

Silence is golden

Another technique is to allow moments of silence during the interview. Besides encouraging the patient to continue talking, silence also gives you a chance to assess their ability to organise thoughts. You may find this technique difficult (most people are uncomfortable with silence), but the more often you use it, the more comfortable you'll become.

Give 'em a boost

Using such phrases as 'please continue', 'go on', and even 'uh-huh' encourages the patient to continue with the story. Known as facilitation, this technique shows the patient that you're interested in what's being said.

Confirmation conversation

Confirmation helps ensure that you and the patient are on the same track. For example, you might say 'If I understand you correctly you have a burning pain in the middle of your stomach, and it gets worse just after you eat.' The patient might then confirm what you have said, or clarify any misconception. For example, 'It's sort of in the middle but perhaps a bit more to the left hand side.'

Clear skies

When information is vague or confusing, use the technique of clarification. For example, if your patient says 'I can't stand this,' you might respond 'What can't you stand?' or 'What do you mean by "I can't stand this"?' Doing so gives the patient an opportunity to explain the statement.

Put the landing gear down . . .

Get in the habit of restating the information the patient gives you. Known as summarisation, this technique ensures that the information you've collected is accurate and complete. Summarisation can signal that the interview is about to end, although in a longer interview you might summarise at more than one point. For example, you might summarise after you have established the presenting complaint, and before you ask other questions. Summarisation helps to ensure you have understood the patient correctly and have a shared understanding of the problem/situation.

. . . and come in for a safe landing

Signal to the patient when you're ready to conclude the interview. Known as conclusion, this signal gives the patient opportunity to gather his/her thoughts and make any pertinent final statements. You can do this by saying 'I think I have asked you everything I need to know right now. Is there anything you would like to add?'

Maintaining a professional attitude

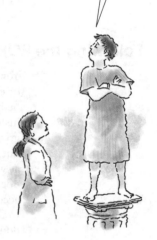

What about the assessment process makes you uncomfortable?

Don't let your personal opinions interfere with your assessment. Maintain a professional, non-judgemental approach, and offer any advice sensitively and in the context of what you have learned about the person's health, lifestyle and willingness to change. For example, gently saying 'Have you ever considered giving up smoking?' offers the patient sensitivity and choice, whereas 'Oh dear!' or 'I think you're going to have to do something about that' will immediately put the patient on the defensive and they might not answer subsequent questions honestly.

Also, avoid leading questions such as 'You don't do drugs, do you?' or 'You don't have any chest pain?' as the patient is more likely to simply agree. Remember that there are some things the patient will almost certainly tell you (their main reason for coming to the appointment, for example), but what else they tell you is very much dependent on how you ask the questions.

Make a note of it

Practitioners are often anxious about documentation when they are learning to take a history. It is difficult for any textbook to cover this topic in detail because local practice varies so much, but there are some important principles to consider.

As you plan your interview, you will need to make some decisions about note taking. Notes can be made as you go along, at the end of the interview or a combination of both. It is also good practice as you discuss confidentiality to reassure the patient who will have access to the notes you make.

When do I write it down?

The more you write as you go, the better the accuracy. But, if you are looking down and writing, you lose eye contact and visual cues, and may also disrupt the flow of the conversation. On the other hand, if you wait to write down everything at the end, you might forget something. So there is no 'right way'. You might like to try it both ways and see what works for you.

Many people find in reality they do a combination of the two approaches; making brief notes as they go along and then completing the write up more fully at the end. And if, as you write up at the end, you find you have forgotten something and need to go back and ask further questions, it's not a problem. Just reassure the patient you are trying to get a complete and accurate picture.

Following the FORMula . . .

You may well find your healthcare setting uses 'proformas' – paper or electronic forms that you fill in when taking a history. These can be helpful and stop you forgetting things, but can also limit your history by not including an important question for that patient. A good proforma should be a helpful tool to guide your interviewing, but should not limit the interview. It should allow space for open as well as closed questions to be asked and for answers to be documented, and also enable you to be flexible in your approach according to an individual patient's needs. If the forms you are asked to use seem to be hindering rather than helping your history taking, don't be afraid to suggest ways they might be adapted.

. . . or starting from scratch

In contrast, some settings still expect notes to be written 'from scratch' on blank sheets. If this is the case, structure your rough note taking and write up using the headings below. Initially you will probably need to carry the list in your pocket, but as you become more experienced it will become automatic. (See *Documenting your findings* in Chapter 2, page 57.)

Getting it right

Either way, in order to help your learning, look through other patient notes in your healthcare setting and discuss them with more experienced practitioners. Also ask for feedback on notes you have documented, so you can continue to develop your learning. It is often said that novice practitioners write too much, whereas experienced practitioners at times perhaps write too little. Getting the balance right takes a lot of experience. For more detail on documentation see further discussion under *Documenting your findings* in Chapter 2 (page 57) and refer to the policy of your professional body regarding record keeping.

Taking the health history

You've just learned how to ask questions. Now it's time to learn the right questions to ask when taking a comprehensive health history.

Asking the right questions

A complete health history requires information from each of the following categories. Note the precise headings and order vary from one text to the next, so feel free to be flexible, provided that all the information listed is covered in a logical manner with the biographical data and presenting complaint first:

- biographical data (establishing or confirming)
- presenting complaint (sometimes called chief complaint) including the history (detail) of the presenting complaint
- past medical history including allergies and medication
- exposure to hazards – alcohol, smoking, recreational drugs and occupational hazards
- family history
- social history
- lifestyle issues/activities of living
- review of systems.

Biographical data

Before you begin, it helps to read any referral letters or recent previous notes that are available, although in a 'walk in' setting this won't always be the case. Then start the health history by obtaining or verifying biographical information from the patient. Do this first so you know you have the correct patient, and also so you don't forget about this information after you become involved in details of the patient's health. Ask or check the patient's full name, address, telephone number, date of birth, marital status, religion, nationality, next of kin (including contact details) and general practitioner.

Take a hint

Your patient's answers to these initial questions can provide important clues about health status, particularly understanding and

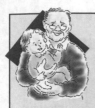

Ages and stages

Advanced directives, age of consent and mental capacity

On occasions you will encounter situations that mean you need specific guidance regarding the legal situation surrounding a patient's request or the way in which a care situation should be managed. This includes:

- Patients who make a particular request regarding how their care is managed in certain situations (sometimes called 'Living Wills' or Advanced Directives)
- Patients aged under 18 who wish to give/withhold consent for procedures, or who disagree with the wishes of their parents
- Patients whose mental capacity may not be sufficient for them to make informed judgements about their treatment or care.

It is beyond the scope of this book to offer detailed advice regarding how to manage specific situations. It is also important to remember that legislation differs between the countries of the UK on some matters (e.g. giving and/or withholding of consent by 16 and 17-year-olds), and is also likely to be frequently updated. It is thus vital that such situations are carefully discussed by the multidisciplinary team and current national/local policy is followed. The following reference sources may be helpful in these respects: Dimond (2007, 2008, 2009), Patient UK (2006, 2007a), DH (2007), Scottish Parliament (2006).

memory. Asking the patient their address rather than showing it to them for verification, for example, is a good idea. If they don't recall it spontaneously you will need to explore the problem further (as well as find someone who can provide or verify the information). Document the source of the information (for example, a parent if the patient is a child), as well as whether an interpreter is necessary. But even if another person needs to be present, always address as much to the patient as you possibly can; for example, a school-age child won't be able to answer all the questions but can answer many of them.

Presenting complaint

Try to pinpoint why the patient is seeking healthcare, or their presenting complaint. Ask a very open question such as 'How can I help you today?' Let the patient speak and try not to interrupt. Most patients will tell you the problem in the first 1 to 2 minutes if you let them speak (Snadden *et al.* 2005). Document the key problem in the patient's exact words if you can, to avoid misinterpretation.

Document information using the patient's own words.

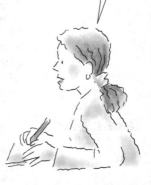

Alphabet soup

In order to establish the history of the presenting complaint, such as how and when the symptoms developed, as well as more detail regarding the exact nature of the problem, there are some helpful mnemonics that you can use. These help to ensure that you don't omit pertinent data. The two most popular are the PQRSTU mnemonic and the OLD CART mnemonic, which both provide a systematic approach to obtaining information. (See *What's the story?*, page 16.) Try both and see which one works best for you.

Pain particulars

Both these mnemonics are particularly helpful for comprehensively assessing pain, which is very common as either a presenting complaint in its own right, or as a key related symptom. Note recommendations in both for the patient to rate their pain from 1 to 10, with 1 being no pain and 10 the worst imaginable. This helps to give you some quantifiable measure of their pain, alongside their description of how it feels. Assessment of pain in children who are too young to use this scale requires different tools. A variety of behavioural scales exist to help assess pain in infants, whilst for older children there are simplified pictorial representations of the adult 1 to 10 scale, using faces or colour. A good summary of the assessment of children's pain can be found in Twycross and Smith (2006).

Red flags

As you gather information about the presenting complaint it is important to look for 'red flags'. These are things the patient says that alert you to the likelihood of a serious health concern. For example, if a 50-year-old patient tells you he has had a pain in his chest for the past 3 hours, you will want to ask a series of questions to help you establish the likelihood of this being a heart attack (myocardial infarction). Learning the pain radiates up into the patient's jaw and into his left arm would be a 'red flag' in this situation.

The history-taking sections of the system-specific chapters will offer further questions to help you establish the 'red flags', but developing sound underpinning knowledge of anatomy, physiology and pathophysiology is also very important in helping you to take and interpret a comprehensive history safely.

Once you are clear regarding the presenting complaint, check if the patient has any other current healthcare problems you need to know about, before going on to the past medical history. Use the mnemonic again if necessary.

Peak technique

What's the story?

There are a couple of very helpful mnemonics which can help you to ask appropriate questions. Using these means that you will gain a comprehensive picture of the problem, and even if you know very little about the complaint or the type of questions to ask, you will still gather relevant and useful information.

OLD CART (based on Seidel *et al.* 2003)

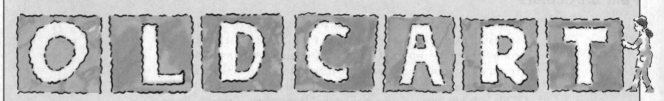

Onset	Location	Duration	Characteristics	Associated factors	Relieving/ aggravating factors	Treatment
• When did the symptom begin? • Was the onset sudden or gradual? • Does the symptom seem to be diminishing, intensifying or staying the same? • If relevant (for example, chest pain), what were you doing at the time?	• Where in the body does the symptom occur? • Does the symptom radiate (spread or extend) to any other areas of the body? If so, where?	• How often does the symptom occur? • How long does the symptom last?	Ask the patient to describe the symptom: • What does the symptom feel like, look like or sound like? • How severe is the symptom? How would you rate it on a scale of 1 to 10, with 10 being the most severe? • If it seems relevant, ask to what degree does the symptom affect normal activities?	• Do you have any other symptoms at the moment that seem as though they might be linked to this one?	• What if anything provokes the symptoms/ makes them worse (consider both actions and situations)? • What if anything relieves the symptoms/ makes them better?	• What treatments if any have you tried? • Have you tried anything else?

NB: If you choose this model, remember to ask at the end what the patient thinks the problem might be – the model doesn't explicitly cover this.

What's the story? *(continued)*

PQRSTU (based on Morton 1993)

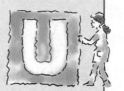

Provocative or palliative	Quality or quantity	Region or radiation	Severity	Timing	Understanding
Ask the patient: • What if anything provokes the symptoms/makes them worse? • What if anything (including treatments tried by the patient) relieves the symptoms/makes them better?	Ask the patient to describe the symptom: • What does the symptom feel like, look like or sound like? • If it seems relevant, ask to what degree does the symptom affect normal activities?	Ask the patient: • Where in the body does the symptom occur? • Does the symptom radiate (spread or extend) to any other areas of the body? If so, where? • Is the symptom associated with any other factors?	Ask the patient: • How severe is the symptom? How would you rate it on a scale of 1 to 10, with 10 being the most severe? • Does the symptom seem to be diminishing, intensifying or staying the same?	Ask the patient: • When did the symptom begin? • Was the onset sudden or gradual? • How often does the symptom occur? • How long does the symptom last?	Ask the patient: • Do you have any thoughts about what might have caused the symptom?

Past medical history

Once you have established the presenting complaint(s), ask the patient about past medical problems, or chronic health problems not already mentioned. Start initially with an open question such as 'Now I'd like to ask about your previous health. Tell me about any key health issues that you have had in the past?' You will probably then also find the following prompts useful to ensure everything has been covered, as patients often need cues to help them remember past health problems, particularly if they occurred some time ago:

• Have you ever been hospitalised? If so, when and why?
• Have you ever had surgery? If so, when and why?
• Have you ever had any serious illnesses, either in childhood or as an adult? If so, what and when?
• Do you know if you received all your childhood immunisations? Do you know when you last had a tetanus immunisation? Have you received any immunisations for foreign travel or other reasons in recent years?

For more information and an up-to-date immunisation schedule, see page 420 for the NHS immunisation schedule website.

Allergic response

It is essential to ask the patient if they are allergic to anything in the environment or to any drugs or foods. If so, what kind of allergic reaction do they have? Note how important this question is in *any* history, be it comprehensive or focused, and how it's also really important to describe the nature and severity of the allergic reaction.

Medication survey?

Then establish whether the patient is taking any medications, including:
- prescribed medication
- over-the-counter preparations, such as paracetamol
- herbal/health food type preparations such as vitamins or St John's Wort (hypericium).

Patients can easily overlook 'over the counter', herbal and homeopathic preparations if not prompted, yet St John's Wort, for example, interacts adversely with some other medications. For each drug ask 'how much do you take and how often do you take it?' It may also be appropriate to ask about other complementary therapies, such as acupuncture or use of a chiropractor.

Health hazards

It is then really important to explore the patient's exposure to hazards as this may affect prescriptions and treatment plans, as well as health promotion advice. Note an adolescent may be reluctant to tell you the truth in answer to these questions if a parent is present or they think they will get into trouble. So offer reassurances of confidentiality where this is possible, emphasise the importance of honest answers and create space where you can talk to the adolescent alone.

Smoking history

Ask the patient if they smoke cigarettes. If so, how many do they smoke each day, and for how long have they smoked? If not, have they ever smoked and how much? (See *Pack years*, page 19.) Also ask if anyone else in the household smokes, to explore exposure to passive smoking. Note that if a patient hesitates before saying 'no', it may be that they smoke another substance such as cannabis, for example, rather than nicotine, so explore carefully.

Alcohol alert

Does the patient drink alcohol? If so, what and how much? If they are unsure or unclear (for example, 'I drink a glass of wine a night'), it may be easier to find out how long a bottle of wine would last

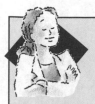

Peak technique

Pack years

The health hazards of smoking are considerable, and continue for years after a patient has given up smoking. The more they smoke or smoked, the greater the risk. Therefore being able to describe their smoking in 'pack years', as well as in terms of whether they still smoke or how long ago they gave up, can be really helpful.

Pack years are worked out as follows:

It is assumed a pack contains 20 cigarettes.

$$\frac{\text{Number of cigarettes smoked per day} \times \text{number of years smoked}}{20}$$

So if a patient has smoked 10 a day for 30 years:

$10 \times 30 = 300$ divided by $20 = 15$, therefore 15 pack years.

Whereas if a patient has smoked 30 a day for 40 years:

$30 \times 40 = 1200$ divided by $20 = 60$, therefore 60 pack years.

Useful tip: If the patient smokes 20 a day, the pack years will always be the same as the number of years they have smoked.

Or for an easy calculator see page 420 for the smoking pack years website.

them than trying to find out the size of the glass. (See *Units – they all add up*, page 20.)

Patients tend to under-report the amount they drink because of embarrassment, so bear this in mind. If you're having trouble getting what you believe are honest answers to such questions, you might try overestimating the amount. For example, you might say 'So would that be as much as five bottles of wine a week?' The patient's response might be, 'No, I would say three at the most.'

If you are concerned about the patient's alcohol consumption or feel you are not getting honest answers, try the CAGE scoring system to help you assess whether there is cause for concern. (See *CAGE*, page 21.)

Illicit drugs?

Ask the patient if they use any illicit drugs. If so, what and how often? Note you need to ask this question sensitively as some patients may be offended, but in terms of physical or mental health

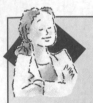

Peak technique

Units – they all add up

Over recent years, it seems people are drinking more alcohol. Not only that, but many wines and lagers are also much stronger than they used to be. This seems to have led the public to underestimate the amount of alcohol they drink, and therefore their risk. A recent UK health campaign, the 'Units – They All Add Up' campaign, set out to address this problem (see page 420 for the alcohol unit calculator website).

Working out how many units there are in a drink is simple if you know the percentage of alcohol it contains and how big the drink is. The number of units in a litre of any alcoholic drink is simply equal to the percentage alcohol it contains (this should be written on the bottle). The units in a bottle or glass can then be calculated by knowing the number of units in a litre and calculating the proportion of a litre contained in a glass or bottle – or by using the formula: units per litre divided by millilitres (ml) per bottle/glass × 100.

So, for example:

If a wine contains 12% alcohol, then:

- a litre (1000 ml) contains 12 units
- a standard 750 ml bottle contains 9 units (three-quarters of a litre)
- a large pub measure of 250 ml contains 3 units (one-third of a bottle).

If a premium bottled beer contains 5% alcohol, then:

- a litre contains 5 units
- a typical 330 ml bottle contains 1.6 units (approximately one-third of a litre).

If a bottle of spirit contains 40% alcohol, then:

- a litre contains 40 units
- a pub measure of 25 ml contains 1 unit (1/25th of a litre).

Interestingly, unlike wine and beer, the strength of spirits tends not to have changed in recent years, so a wine drinker may actually be more at risk than a spirit drinker in terms of units of alcohol consumed; in fact, someone drinking half a litre of gin a week is probably drinking less than someone having one large glass of wine a night!

implications, and drug or anaesthetic interactions, this information is really important. Note that you may need to try different terms (for example, 'street drugs', 'recreational drugs' or 'illegal drugs') or even give examples, to establish understanding.

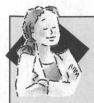

Peak technique

CAGE

The CAGE scoring system (Ewing 1984), used alongside data regarding the number of units of alcohol consumed in a day and in a week, is a useful starting point to determine whether someone's alcohol intake may be placing them at risk. The patient answering yes to two or more questions cannot lead you to conclude beyond doubt that there is a problem, but it definitely helps you to identify whether your concerns should be taken further.

C – Have you ever felt the need to **Cut down** on your drinking?
A – Have you ever felt **Annoyed** by comments or criticism about your drinking?
G – Have you ever felt **Guilty** about your drinking, or about something you said or did whilst you were drinking.
E – Have you ever felt the need for an **Eye opener** in the morning?

Occupational hazards

Ask the patient their occupation and explore any occupational hazards. Note that most occupations have some form of potential hazard (as well as the boss!). For example, consider the widespread use of computers, and potential risks such as back pain, neck pain, eyestrain or repetitive strain injury. Also remember previous occupations (for example, mining or farming) could have had longer-term effects on the patient's health.

Family history

Questioning the patient about their family's health is an important part of assessing their risk of having or getting certain diseases. It is helpful to explore the current and previous health of parents, siblings and children as a minimum. You might ask, for example, 'Are your mother and father living?' If not, sensitively ask what their cause of death was and how old they were. Also ask about any other health problems they had; for example, a mother may have died of a stroke but previously had breast cancer – if you just asked about the cause of death you would miss a disease with an important familial risk. If parents are alive ask about any major health problems they might have now or have had in the past. Then ask about siblings and children using similar questions.

Looking further afield

Exploring the health of other relatives, particularly grandparents, can also be useful in establishing strong familial traits. For example,

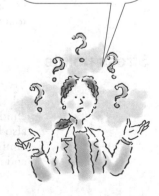

Want to know if a patient is at increased risk for certain illnesses? Ask about the family's health history.

if a patient's father has a heart condition, it is useful to know whether either of his parents also had a heart condition. Or if a mother had breast cancer, it is important to know whether one of her sisters or other close relatives also had the disease. Rather than listing various relatives, you might ask 'Are there any other family members who have also had breast cancer?'

Illness inventory

For the family as a whole, or individual members, you may find prompts of particular illnesses with strong familial links useful, including:

- diabetes
- epilepsy
- high blood pressure
- heart disease
- asthma
- cancer
- renal problems
- thyroid disease.

Note that it can be helpful to draw a family tree. Typically squares are used to indicate male family members, circles for females and lines crossing them out to show people who are no longer alive. The patient should be clearly indicated with an arrow, and different generations plotted on different horizontal lines. By each person you can write their age (or age at death), and any significant medical information.

Social history

Find out about the patient's social situation, such as who he/she lives with, housing, employment status/education, dependants, carer responsibilities (for example, older relatives) and hobbies/interests. How much and what you ask will depend on circumstances, but note the effect poor housing can have on family health, for example. Practical issues may also direct your questions; for example, it is useful to know whether the patient needs to climb stairs in the home following lower limb surgery.

Stress points

Try to consider potential sources of stress. For example, you might ask about 'work–life balance' or ask 'What do you do to relax?' For children, think about bullying or pressure at school. It may well also be appropriate to ask about emotional and social support from family and friends, or about practicalities such as the ease of travel to and from the hospital/surgery.

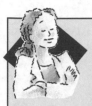

Peak technique

Safeguarding children and vulnerable adults: being alert to abuse

Abuse is a tricky subject. Anyone can be a victim of abuse: a child, a partner or a parent. Those who are particularly vulnerable include children, the elderly, people with learning differences and people with mental health concerns. Abuse can come in many forms: physical, psychological/emotional and sexual, as well as in the form of neglect. So, when taking a health history, be very alert to any indications that abuse might be taking place. This might be from something that the patient says, from an inconsistent or atypical account of how an injury occurred, a delayed presentation or as a result of observing physical signs such as bruising which are not readily or convincingly explained.

Even when you don't immediately suspect an abusive situation, be aware of reactions to certain questions. Is the patient, parent or carer defensive, hostile, confused or frightened? How do they interact with you and others? Do they seem withdrawn or frightened, or show other inappropriate behaviour? Is it proving difficult to see the patient on their own? Is there a history of missed appointments with health professionals? Keep these questions in mind when you perform your physical assessment. One of the most important factors in being alert to potential abuse is to 'think the unthinkable'; that way you'll keep an open mind and recognise abuse more readily.

If a patient tells you that they are experiencing abuse, or you suspect abuse, fundamental principles to follow include 'acknowledge, believe, support and signpost'. Share your concerns with an appropriate senior colleague. Actions taken will need to follow national and local policy, and will depend on the exact nature of the situation. However, patient welfare and the welfare of others at risk as a result of the abuse (for example, children in a domestic abuse situation involving the parents) are always paramount.

Further texts on the subject will be helpful – a very useful recent text looking at safeguarding children is Powell (2007). Healthcare organisations incorporate basic awareness training on safeguarding children and vulnerable adults as part of their mandatory training programmes.

Lifestyle issues

Exploring key lifestyle issues will help you to assess the patient holistically and offer health promotion advice, as well as identifying issues that may be affecting his/her current health.

Diet

Ask the patient about their diet, including any particular dietary restrictions. For example, those on a vegetarian diet may eat very healthily in lots of ways but be prone to anaemia. Check out knowledge of healthy eating, such as government advice to eat five portions of fruit and vegetables a day. Ask about any recent weight loss or gain, which can offer helpful clues in respect of your assessment of possible health problems. For example, unplanned weight loss can be a sign of cancer and unplanned weight gain could be caused by an underactive thyroid. If diet seems to be a key issue, get the patient to summarise for you what they eat in a typical day, or ask them to keep a food diary for a week to bring to their next appointment.

You seem a little tired. Are you having any difficulty sleeping?

Exercise and sleep

It can be helpful to explore the amount of exercise the patient takes, as this may offer opportunities for health promotion. Also ask how many hours the patient sleeps at night, what their sleep pattern is like and whether they feel rested after sleep. If there are any difficulties with sleep, establish if these are in the form of getting to sleep, or waking early and being unable to go back to sleep, as different sleep problems may offer clues to different health issues.

Work and leisure

If not already identified, ask about employment, voluntary work or education. Also explore hobbies and interests, especially if there are concerns about the patient's mental health. Someone with no hobbies and interests may be suffering with depression, but equally may just be extremely busy with family, study and/or work commitments.

Recent travel

Find out if the patient has recently travelled, particularly abroad. Consider if there are any links between this and the patient's symptoms. For example, are gastrointestinal problems linked with eating a different diet, or might leg pain be linked with a long flight?

Religious observances

Establish whether the patient has religious or other beliefs that affect diet, dress or health practices. Patients will feel reassured when you make it clear that you understand these points.

Review of systems

The last part of a comprehensive health history is a systematic review of the patient's body structures and systems. Although time consuming, this is an invaluable tool to cover any important issues you or the patient might have overlooked. Reassure the patient that it may seem repetitive, but will help create a complete picture of their healthcare needs. Note in a more seriously ill patient the review of systems is likely to be conducted later. (See *Assessing a severely ill patient*, page 29.)

Follow a process

It often helps to start with some general questions about overall health and well-being. From here you can move onto the skin, head and neck and then work your way down the body. This helps keep you from skipping any areas. The following section lists lots of questions you might ask; usually more than is possible in the time available. To begin with you will probably ask more than you need, but as you gain knowledge and experience you will make wise judgements based on the presenting problem and the history so far.

If you find a new problem use the PQRSTU or OLD CART mnemonic discussed earlier to explore it further, along with the system specific guidance given later in the book.

Keep it open to begin with

As you start asking about each new system, try to ask an initial open question first as indicated below (for example, 'do you have any problems with your mouth or throat?'). Leave the patient time to

Ages and stages

Communication challenges

An elderly patient might have sensory or memory impairment or a decreased attention span. If this is the case, you may need to rely on a family member for some or all of the health history, but do try to involve the patient as far as possible. Similarly, if the patient is a child try to avoid the temptation to address all questions to the parent(s). Depending on age and understanding, try to include the child as much as you possibly can, particularly when asking about symptoms such as pain, for example.

answer. Then move in with the 'closed question' prompts. If you ask the closed questions too early, you may lose valuable information to do with a specific problem that you haven't listed, and thus the patient may interpret a problem which they were going to mention to you as unimportant.

Ask specific questions

Here are some key questions to ask your patient about each body structure and system.

General well-being

How would you describe your energy levels compared with what is normal for you? What about your appetite? Also ask about weight loss or gain if not previously covered.

Skin survey

Do you have any problems with your skin? Do you have any problems with skin rashes or dry skin? Any other skin complaints such as eczema or psoriasis?

Head first

Do you have any problems with your head? Do you get headaches? Have you ever had a head injury?

Vision quest

Do you have any problems with your eyes? Do you have your eyes checked regularly, and if so when was your last eye examination? Do you wear glasses? Any other eye problems? You might then list specific problems as cues such as glaucoma, cataracts or blurred/double vision.

How long have you had poor hearing?

Your earrings? They're very nice.

An earful

Do you have any hearing problems or other problems with your ears? Do you have any loss of balance? Any ringing in your ears? Have you ever had ear surgery? If the patient is deaf/hard of hearing, ask about any hearing aids. You might also ask about any pain, swelling or discharge from the ears.

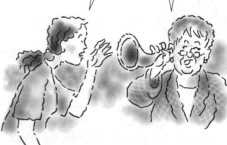

Nose knows

Do you have any problems with your nose? Do you ever have sinusitis or nosebleeds? Do you get frequent colds? Do you have any problems with your sense of smell? Any problems with blockages that cause breathing difficulties?

Mouth and throat run-through

Do you have any problems with your mouth or throat? Do you have regular mouth ulcers? Any dental problems? Do you have regular dental check ups? Do you have any difficulty swallowing? Also check if the patient has dentures, or any caps/crowns or loose teeth; this is especially relevant preoperatively or if the patient is seriously ill and might be intubated.

Neck check

Do you have any problems with your neck? Do you have swelling, soreness, lack of movement, stiffness or pain in your neck? Have you ever had an injury to your neck?

Respiratory research

Do you have any problems with your breathing? Do you have any shortness of breath on exertion or while resting/lying in bed? How many pillows do you use at night? (More than 2 may signify some orthopnoea – difficulty in breathing when lying down.) Does breathing cause any pain or wheezing? Do you have a persistent cough or ever cough up blood (haemoptysis)? Have you had any frequent or severe infections of the chest such as pneumonia? Have you ever had asthma?

Heart health hunt

Do you have any problems with your heart or circulation? Do you ever have any chest pain, palpitations or irregular heartbeat? Have you ever had an electrocardiogram? Do you have, or have you ever had, high blood pressure? Do you ever get swollen ankles? Do you ever get cold extremities or pain in your legs? Have you ever been diagnosed with anaemia? Do you bruise easily? Prior to major surgery, ask if they have ever had a blood transfusion, and if so were there any problems?

> Asking these questions will help you get to the root of the patient's problem.

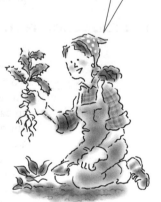

Breast test

Ask women 'Do you have any problems with your breasts? Have you ever had any abnormalities in your breasts? Are you aware of the changes to your breasts you should look out for? Have you ever had a mammogram? Age groups offering routine mammography vary across the countries of the UK, and are currently under review. Note any breast concerns related to new/changing symptoms need referral for further consultation/screening; you cannot reassure a woman that 'everything is OK' based on history/examination alone (see Chapter 10).

Remember too that breast problems, including cancer, also occasionally occur in men, so don't assume asking about breasts applies only to women.

Stomach symptom search

Do you have any problems with your stomach or digestion? Do you have frequent nausea, vomiting or indigestion? Any loss of appetite, heartburn, burping, abdominal pain or passing of wind? Do you have any problems with your bowels? Any changes from your normal pattern? Do you ever need to use laxatives? Is there ever any blood in your stool? You might also mention specific conditions such as haemorrhoids, hernias, gallbladder disease or liver disease.

Urinary interview

Do you have any problems passing urine? Do you ever have burning during urination, incontinence, urgency or difficulty passing urine? Do you get up during the night to urinate, and if so how many times? Have you ever noticed blood in your urine, or colour changes? Have you ever been treated for any renal problems such as kidney stones? Ask men carefully about changes in urinary flow, problems passing urine or dribbling.

Reproduction review

Ask for women about menstruation, including any problems with excessive bleeding, bleeding between periods or excessive pain. If women are postmenopausal, or going through the menopause, are there any problems associated with this? Also ask about cervical smears, including date of last smear, outcome and any previous abnormal smears. Ages and frequency of smear testing vary slightly across the four countries of the UK – see Chapter 12.

Ask for detail about pregnancies if relevant, especially if a woman is of childbearing age, has young children or has a gynaecological presenting complaint. Remember infertility or miscarriage can be a painful subject so explore sensitively. You may well also need to ask about contraception in women of childbearing age.

Ask men, especially younger men, about monthly testicular self-examinations. Ask older men if they have ever had a prostate examination.

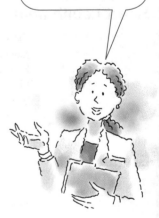

Don't forget to ask male patients about testicular self-examinations.

Sexual health?

Asking about sexual health again requires sensitivity as some patients find this embarrassing – maybe simply ask 'Do you have any problems or concerns with your sexual health?' You may have learned whether the patient has a partner from earlier in the history, but try to avoid assumptions regarding marital status or the gender of the partner.

Sometimes, such as with a possibility of sexually transmitted disease, you will need to ask directly about sexual practices, safe sex, single or multiple partners and the gender of partners. Aim to do so sensitively and non-judgementally.

Monitoring muscle

Do you have any problems with your joints? Do you have any difficulty walking, sitting or standing? Are you steady on your feet or do you lose your balance easily? Do you have arthritis, any back problems, muscle weakness or paralysis?

Nervous system scrutiny

Have you ever had any seizures or fits? Do you ever experience tremors, twitching, numbness, tingling or loss of sensation in a part

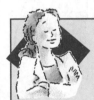

Peak technique

Assessing a severely ill patient

When caring for a severely ill patient, you need to use your skill and judgement to prioritise the assessment process. Firstly, always remember the fundamental assessment priorities of:

- airway
- breathing
- circulation
- disability
- environment,

before proceeding with other elements of the history or examination. For further guidance see Resuscitation Council UK (2006) in respect of adults and Mackway-Jones et al. (2005) in respect of children.

In respect of history taking, it may well be necessary to undertake a physical examination with only a brief history from the patient, relative or paramedic. As and when the patient is stable enough for you to proceed with the history, you will then need to judge how much information the patient can give you personally. If they are not well enough, or are only well enough to give brief information, then try to gain as much information as possible from other sources such as a partner or other family member, clearly documenting the source of the information in your notes.

of your body? Are you less able to get around than you think you should be?

Endocrine inquiry

Have you felt more tired than usual lately? Do you feel hungry or thirsty more often than usual? How well can you tolerate heat or cold? Do you have any problems with excessive sweating? Have you been losing hair or noticed any changes in texture of your hair, skin or nails?

Psychological survey

How would you describe your mood? Do you ever experience mood swings or memory loss? Do you ever feel particularly anxious, depressed or unable to concentrate? Are you feeling unusually stressed at the moment? Do you ever feel unable to cope?

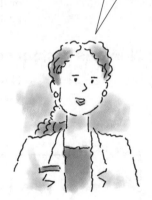

Throughout your initial assessment, be aware of the patient's emotional status. Keep in mind that stress levels and emotional well-being can affect all body systems.

Concluding the interview

Finally, it's important to bring the interview to a conclusion. Indicate that you have covered all you want to but remember to ask the patient whether 'There is anything else you would like to add?' You will be surprised, despite all the questions that you have asked, how often the patient mentions something else important at this point.

Next steps

You then need to give the patient a clear idea of what will happen next. It is likely you will want to carry out an examination or some observations, in which case you will probably explain what you would like to examine, what it will involve and seek their consent. Alternatively, you may wish to go and discuss their history with a colleague, or need to carry out or request some investigations. You may even have gathered enough information to be able to discuss a plan without needing further information. Whatever the circumstances, be sure to give the patient a clear idea regarding what will happen next.

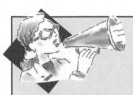

That's a wrap!

Health history review

Obtaining assessment data

- Collect subjective data (data that's obtained from the history and can be verified only by the patient).
- Collect objective data (data that's obtained and verified through the physical examination or investigations).

Patient interview

- Select a quiet, private setting and position yourself/the patient appropriately.
- Choose terms carefully and avoid using medical jargon.
- Use appropriate body language.
- Use open-ended and closed-ended questions as appropriate.
- Use silence effectively.
- Encourage responses.
- Confirm patient statements to avoid misunderstanding.
- Use clarification to eliminate misunderstandings.
- Summarise and conclude with 'Is there anything else?'

Components of a complete health history

- Biographical data (establishing or confirming)
- Presenting complaint (sometimes called chief complaint) and history (detail) of presenting complaint

- Past medical history including allergies and medication
- Exposure to hazards – alcohol, smoking, recreational drugs and occupational hazards
- Family history
- Social history
- Lifestyle issues/activities of living
- Review of systems.

Review of structures and systems

- General well-being
- Skin
- Head
- Eyes
- Ears
- Nose
- Mouth and throat
- Neck
- Respiratory
- Cardiovascular
- Breasts
- Gastrointestinal
- Urinary
- Reproductive
- Musculoskeletal
- Neurologic
- Endocrine
- Psychological.

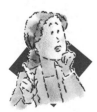

Quick quiz

1. How can I help you today?' is an example of:
   A. an open question.
   B. a closed question.
   C. a leading question.
   D. a forced choice question.

2. When obtaining a health history from a patient, ask first about:
   A. family history.
   B. presenting complaint.
   C. lifestyle issues.
   D. biographical data.

3. Silence is a communication technique used during an interview to:
   A. show respect.
   B. change the topic.
   C. encourage the patient to continue talking.
   D. clarify information.

4. Information is considered subjective if obtained from:
   A. the patient's verbal account.
   B. the results of investigations.
   C. the patient's records.
   D. the physical examination.

5. Which of the following is *not* a part of the CAGE scoring system for exploring alcohol intake?
   A. feeling the need to *cut down* on drinking.
   B. getting *annoyed* with comments about your drinking.
   C. feeling *guilty* about your drinking.
   D. feeling *embarrassed* about your drinking.

For answers see page 398.

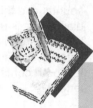

Just the facts

In this chapter, you'll learn:

♦ skills for performing an initial observation of the patient

♦ ways to prepare your patient for an assessment

♦ techniques for performing inspection, palpation, percussion and auscultation.

A look at physical assessment

Physical assessment is generally the vitally important second step in the assessment process, following your history. Your history will guide you regarding the nature of the physical assessment that you need to carry out. During the physical assessment you'll use a systematic approach to build on your history, using the key assessment skills of inspection, palpation, percussion and auscultation. As you proceed through the examination, you may well also have the opportunity to engage in some health promotion, for example regarding the value of exercise. More than anything else, successful assessment requires critical thinking. Don't just look at findings in isolation. Look at your findings as a whole and consider how one particular finding fits into the bigger picture.

Collecting the tools

Before starting a physical assessment, ensure the necessary tools are to hand. These will vary depending on the nature of the assessment that you are about to carry out, but will most commonly include a

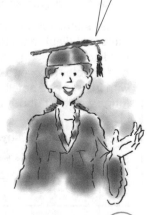

Performing a physical assessment gives me the opportunity to use critical thinking.

stethoscope, gloves and a pen torch. Neurological examinations, in particular, require additional equipment.

Two heads are better than one

You'll need a stethoscope with both a diaphragm and a bell to auscultate sounds of varying pitches. (See *Choosing the right stethoscope*, below.)

All the better to see you with . . .

You may well need a pen torch to illuminate the inside of the patient's nose and mouth, to evaluate pupillary reactions, to cast tangential (sideways) light on the neck to view jugular venous pressure or to more clearly see any 'lumps and bumps'.

Memory jogger

Remember that the bell of a stethoscope is used to hear low-pitched sounds and the diaphragm is used to hear high-pitched sounds. Bell and low both contain the letter **l**.

Choosing the right stethoscope

Use a stethoscope with a diaphragm and a bell. The diaphragm has a flat, thin, plastic surface that picks up high-pitched sounds such as breath sounds. The bell has a smaller, concave, open end that picks up low-pitched sounds, such as some abnormal heart sounds and some vascular sounds. A good quality stethoscope generally gives clearer sound.

Only one head . . .

Some stethoscopes appear to have a single head (just a diaphragm). These are cardiac (or cardiology) stethoscopes. The single head works as a bell with light pressure and a diaphragm with firm pressure.

. . . or two diaphragms . . .

Some stethoscopes seem to have a large and a small diaphragm. Don't mistake the small diaphragm for an unusual looking bell. These stethoscopes work like a cardiac stethoscope, but offer the choice of two sizes of end-piece. The larger one is able to cover a larger surface area, and the smaller end-piece is for use with infants and small children, or to assess small areas such as the apices of the lungs which sit under the hollow just above the clavicle.

. . . or just seems tiny.

Some stethoscopes have a head that looks much smaller than normal. These are paediatric stethoscopes, especially designed for use with infants and small children.

Beginning the examination

The first part of the physical assessment concerns forming your initial impressions of the patient and obtaining baseline data. In the acute or emergency care situation, always remember ABCDE (Resuscitation Council UK 2006) as the priority for any patient assessment. Initial assessment focuses sequentially on ABC – airway, breathing and circulation. Once these have been deemed stable, or have been stabilised, remaining elements of the assessment can proceed (Mackway-Jones *et al.* 2005). The next priority is then D (for disability), which includes assessing level of consciousness; the AVPU tool will be helpful here. (See *Interpreting level of consciousness and vital signs*, page 38.) Pupil reaction and blood glucose monitoring may also be indicated at this point; in some cases a full Glasgow Coma Score will be required. Finally E (for exposure) includes viewing the exposed body if required, and assessing temperature and skin condition/rashes.

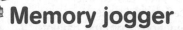

Memory jogger

The mnemonic SOME TEAMS might be a helpful checklist to remind you about some key points as you make your initial general observation of the patient.

Symmetry – Are face and body symmetrical?

Older or younger – Does the patient look notably older or younger than his/her given age?

Mental acuity – Is the patient alert, confused, agitated or inattentive?

Expression – Does the patient appear distressed, in pain or anxious?

Trunk – Does the patient seem a normal weight, thin or obese? Is the chest a normal shape?

Extremities – Are there any problems with the nails/hands. Are there any joint abnormalities or swelling?

Appearance – Is the patient clean and well groomed?

Movement – Are posture, gait and coordination seemingly normal?

Speech – Is speech relaxed, clear, strong, understandable and appropriate? Does it indicate any signs of stress?

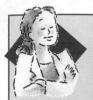

Peak technique

Tips for assessment success

Before starting the physical assessment, follow these guidelines:

- Eliminate as many distractions and disruptions as possible.
- Ask your patient to void (pass urine) before beginning the physical assessment. Take a urine specimen if indicated.
- Pay careful attention to hand hygiene both before and after patient contact. Be sure to follow local and national policy regarding hand washing and the use of alcohol hand rub.

- Have all the necessary equipment to hand and in working order.
- Ensure the stethoscope and any other reusable equipment has been cleaned.
- Make sure the examination room is well lit and warm, and that appropriate covers, drapes and/or gown are available to maintain privacy and dignity.
- Warm your hands and equipment before touching the patient.
- Be aware of your non-verbal communication and possible negative reactions from the patient.

Beyond this, the exact nature of your assessment will depend on the presenting complaint, and will be covered in more detail in the following chapters. But the following general principles will underpin any assessment.

Preparing the patient

If you haven't just taken the history, introduce yourself to the patient. Keep in mind that the patient is likely to be worried that you'll find a serious problem, and may also be worried about embarrassment or an invasion of privacy, because you're observing and touching sensitive, private and perhaps painful body areas. Ensure you follow national and local guidelines on the requirement for a chaperone.

No surprises

Before you start, briefly explain what you're planning to do and why, and how long it will take. This may help to decrease their anxiety. (See *Tips for assessment success*, above.) Always remember to seek verbal consent at the beginning, and repeatedly as you explain each new step of the assessment. A well-prepared patient who knows what to expect next won't be surprised or feel unexpected discomfort, so is likely to trust you more and cooperate better.

Professional balancing act

Put your patient at ease but know where to draw the line. Maintain professionalism during the examination. Humour, within appropriate boundaries, can help put the patient at ease. A good examiner strikes a balance between friendliness and professionalism. Aim to create a situation where patients feel at ease asking questions but also have confidence and trust in your abilities. Similarly, aim to be efficient and fluent in your examination, but without making the patient feel unduly 'rushed'. Achieving all this takes practise but will really help you and your patients.

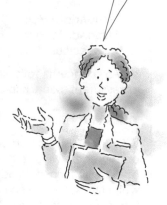

Explaining everything in advance will help the patient relax and ensure their cooperation.

Initial observation of the patient

As you introduce yourself to the patient and initiate the examination, continue to observe their behaviour, general demeanour and appearance. If you have taken the history yourself, you will already have started this important process, which can offer subtle clues about health. Exactly what points to consider will be informed to some extent by the history, but the general overview typically includes colour, nutritional status, body symmetry, posture and facial expression. (See *Memory jogger*, page 35.) Be alert to concerning signs such as pallor, cyanosis, shortness of breath, diaphoresis (sweating) or apparent pain/discomfort.

Get it down on paper

You might find it helpful to document your initial observations up to this point in a concise, short paragraph. For example, you might say 'Mr Jones is a very thin, pale gentleman who appears very anxious and short of breath, and who is struggling to speak in full sentences.'

Recording vital signs and statistics

Accurate measurements of your patient's vital signs provide crucial information about body functions. Even if these have been carried out by another practitioner it is important to reassess pulse and respiratory rate as a minimum, as you need to judge the quality (such as rhythm and depth) as well as rate, and be alert to any changes or deterioration. No matter whether you plan to write up your notes as you go along or later, chart or make a note of vital signs as you record them, as they are very easily forgotten.

Interpreting level of consciousness and vital signs

AVPU

A rapid determination of level of consciousness can be achieved using the AVPU scale. This scale is applicable to all age groups. The practitioner assesses the patient as fitting into one of four categories:

- **A**lert
- Responds to **V**oice
- Responds to **P**ain
- **U**nconscious.

Any concerns following this initial assessment should be followed up with a full Glasgow Coma Score assessment (see Chapter 14).

Track and trigger

NICE (2007b) recommends that a physiological 'track and trigger system' (in the form of a multiparameter or aggregate weighted scoring system) should be used to determine deterioration or to grade the risk of deterioration in all adult patients in acute hospital settings. A variety of different systems exist, with weighted systems such as an Early Warning Score (EWS) or a Modified Early Warning System (MEWS) being amongst the most commonly used. Such systems consider vital signs and other findings such as urine output and AVPU to determine deterioration or risk. Choice of tools and parameters vary from one setting to the next, so it is important to familiarise yourself with the tool(s) used in your care setting. Scoring systems are also being developed for use with children – Paediatric Early Warning Systems (PEWS). For more information on EWS, see Baines and Kanagasunduram (2008).

Accuracy

If you obtain an isolated abnormal value when monitoring vital signs, firstly look at the whole patient and other findings. If the value seems unexpected and the patient seems otherwise well, it may be appropriate to recheck the reading again, but don't automatically assume the reading is inaccurate. Electronic devices in particular MAY give inaccurate readings for a variety of reasons, but on the other hand patients with concerning abnormal findings may not look obviously unwell. Remember also that normal readings vary with the patient's age – for example, blood pressure increases as you get older. But don't make assumptions that such abnormal readings are 'normal in the elderly'; any such abnormalities should still be reported and explored further.

Individuality

Also remember that an abnormal value for one patient may be a normal value for another. Each patient has their own baseline values, which is what makes recording baseline vital signs so important wherever this is possible.

Repeat recordings

Afterwards, take or request measurements of vital signs at regular intervals, with frequency depending on the patient's condition. A series of readings invariably provides more valuable information than a single set.

MEWSing on the problem

If the patient is acutely unwell or deteriorating, repeat initial observations and AVPU scoring at frequent intervals. Consider findings in relation to a 'track and trigger system' such as an Early Warning Scoring system (EWS) or a Modified Early Warning Scoring system (MEWS), which uses vital signs and other findings to predict risk of deterioration. (See *Interpreting level of consciousness and vital signs*, page 38.)

Height and weight

Accurate weight is essential for calculating drug dosages, especially in children. Repeated weighing is often important in assessing fluid loss or gain. Weight and height are also important parameters for evaluating nutritional status – for full discussion of this see Chapter 3: Nutritional Assessment. If you aren't familiar with recording height and weight see *Measuring weight and height*, page 40, and for guidance on weighing and measuring children see *Obtaining paediatric height, weight and head circumference measurements*, page 41. Make sure weight is clearly documented on all key patient records, including any prescription chart.

Body temperature

Body temperature is routinely measured in degrees Celsius (°C), but note that many older patients in particular may still think in terms of degrees Fahrenheight. Average normal body temperature is 36.8°C in adults (McGee 2007), but a range from 35.8 to 37.3°C can be normal depending on individual differences and the route used for measurement (Jarvis 2008).

Routes to avoid

Traditional 'mercury' in glass thermometers have been replaced in recent years with other safer modes of assessment. Rectal temperature reading, once commonplace, has also been replaced with other safer and less embarrassing methods. Always be cautious about using any form of oral thermometer in patients who are confused or who have a reduced level of consciousness; if in doubt use a tympanic thermometer or the axilla.

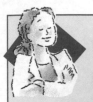

Peak technique

Measuring height and weight

Ask the patient to remove their shoes and to dress in a hospital gown or take off heavy clothing as appropriate. Then use these techniques to measure height and weight.

Measuring weight

Various types of scales are available to measure weight. Electronic sitting or standing scales, and manual sitting or standing balance beam scales are the most common types. Any scale should be calibrated regularly. It is essential that you know the correct procedure for using the scales available in your practice setting, so seek guidance if unsure. If you need to repeatedly weigh the same patient at regular intervals, always try to use the same set of scales and make sure the patient is wearing the same type of garments.

Weight is measured and documented in kilos, but electronic scales can usually translate weight into stones if patients would like this information.

For manual scales, conversion charts are available. In some settings (for example, renal units or intensive care units), scales which can weigh patients in bed may be available.

Measuring height

Height measuring devices are typically manual although some electronic devices now exist.

Ask the patient to step on/under the scale and turn his/her back to it. Note most are fixed to the wall; if you have a free-standing height measuring device make sure it is locked.

Ask the patient to face forwards so that their head is straight, to place their feet together and their heels as far back as they will go. Ensure that they are standing straight (you may need to offer support if the patient is frail or unsteady on their feet).

Now, if it's a manual height measuring device, lower the bar until the horizontal arm touches the top of his/her head. Read the height measurement from the height bar. For electronic devices, follow the manufacturer's instructions.

In some settings, for example emergency departments, devices exist that can be used to estimate height whilst patients are lying down. This may be important for calculation of some drug dosages.

Thermometers three

Other than in intensive care units (where pulmonary artery temperature monitoring is feasible) three types of thermometer are commonly used in practice (for indicators of when to use which thermometer, see *Monitoring body temperature*, page 42).

• Digital thermometers – give a digital reading from an oral or axillary position

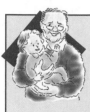

Ages and stages

Obtaining paediatric height, weight and head circumference measurements

The height and weight of an infant or young child are measured differently from those of an adult. In addition to obtaining height and weight, you may include head circumference in your measurements.

Measuring the height of an infant/toddler

Until a child is able to stand easily, measure height from the top of the head to the bottom of the heels while he or she is lying down. When measured in this fashion, height is commonly referred to as length. A fixed rule or tape measure can be used for this purpose. Because infants tend to flex and curl, make sure you hold the infant's head in the midline position, and then hold the knees together with your other hand, gently pressing them down toward the table until fully extended. Try to have a parent with you if possible, both to help position the infant and prevent distress.

Weight

Infants tend to be weighed regularly throughout the first year of life, so may find this less distressing. Infant scales may be of digital or manual balance beam design. The infant or child either sits or lies down in a 'bowl' or other enclosed area. To prevent injury, never turn away from a child on a scale or leave them unattended.

   You can usually use an adult scale to weigh children older than about 18 months to 2 years. If a child of any age is unwilling to sit or stand on the scale, then use an adult scale to weigh a parent or other adult alone, and then weigh the child and adult together. The child's weight can then be calculated by subtracting the smaller figure from the larger one.

Head circumference

Head circumference measurement reflects the growth of the cranium and its contents, and is an important indicator of hydrocephalus (excessive fluid around the brain) and other developmental abnormalities.

   It is recommended that head circumference is measured in all children up to 2 years of age. To measure a child's head circumference, place a clinically recommended (for example, a Lasso®) measuring tape around the child's head, ensuring the hairstyle (for example, ponytail) is not enlarging the circumference. Normally measure above the ears at the side, midway between the eyebrows and the forehead at the front, and over the occipital prominence at the back of the head. But if the head is unusually shaped measure at the widest point. (For further guidance, see UCL Institute of Child Health 2007.)

   Note this technique takes practise so always undertake it with supervision until you are confident. Poor technique can mean an inaccurate baseline is recorded and abnormal findings missed or exaggerated.

   Also note the importance of the anterior fontanelle in infants. Sometimes called the 'soft spot', this gap in the sutures between the bones of the cranium allows you to evaluate raised pressure (if it bulges) or dehydration (if it is depressed).

Monitoring body temperature

You can take your patient's temperature in three ways. The chart below describes each method. However there will be some variation in 'normal readings' depending on the route used.

Method	Indications for use
Oral (electronic or chemical dot)	• Adults and older children who are awake, alert, oriented and cooperative.
Axillary (armpit – electronic or chemical dot)	• Infants, young children, confused or unconscious patients • Chemical dot thermometer applicable in situations where infection risk is a particular concern, as fully disposable • Digital axilliary thermometer *only* acceptable route in infants under 4 weeks old (NICE 2007a)
Tympanic (ear)	• Adults and children, conscious and cooperative patients, and confused or unconscious patients • Accepted for use in infants aged 4 weeks or older by NICE (2007a)

• Tympanic thermometers – rapid temperature readings from the tympanic membrane (eardrum) when placed in the ear
• Chemical dot thermometers – safe and acceptable plastic strips whose coloured dots change with heat, giving accurate readings to 0.1 of a degree when used orally or in the axilla.
    Use of the correct technique (especially for tympanic thermometry), and leaving the thermometer in place for the correct amount of time, are both vital steps – always check and follow manufacturers' guidelines. Correctly monitored, average oral temperature is around 0.4 to 0.7°C higher than axillary temperature (McGee 2007). Studies of tympanic thermometer differences are less consistent, with differences both above and below oral temperature being recorded in different studies. Poor technique can be a particular risk in tympanic temperature recording.

Finding fever

McGee (2007) defines fever (sometimes called pyrexia) as an oral temperature reading of 37.7°C or above, although you will find some other authors' definitions vary slightly. Fever is of serious concern in infants. NICE (2007a) place infants under 3 months old with a temperature of 38°C or higher, or 3 to 6 months old with a temperature of 39°C or higher, in the high-risk group for serious illness. They also give further helpful advice regarding a wide range of associated signs and symptoms of concern in the 0 to 5 age group, and on how their fever should be managed.

In from the cold

Hypothermia is defined by Bevan and Gawkrodger (2005) as a core temperature lower than 35°C, although other authors quote slightly higher figures.

Pulse

The patient's pulse reflects the amount of blood ejected with each heartbeat. Although learning to take a pulse is one of the first skills most healthcare practitioners learn, it is often not done as well as it could be, thereby missing vital information.

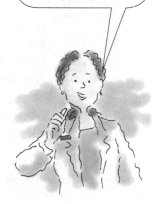

If the patient has an irregular heartbeat, a fast heartbeat or a pacemaker, be sure to count the pulse for a full minute.

Feeling the beat

To assess the pulse, palpate one of the patient's arterial pulse points (most usually the radial) with the pads of your index and middle fingers, and when you feel pulsations, note the rate, rhythm and volume (amplitude) of the pulse. If the rhythm is regular, count the beats for 30 seconds and then multiply by 2 to get the number of beats per minute (bpm). If the rhythm is irregular, fast or your patient has a pacemaker, count the beats for 1 minute. Counting for 15 seconds and multiplying by four yields too great a risk of inaccuracy.

Identifying normality

McGee (2007) suggests that 50 to 95 bpm should be regarded as the normal pulse rate for adults. However, the Resuscitation Council UK (2006) classify adult bradycardia at below 60 bpm, but recognise that lower pulse rates can be normal in some individuals (athletes commonly fall into this category). They also set under 40 bpm (excessive bradycardia) or over 140 bpm (excessive tachycardia) as the levels for emergency intervention in adults. Rates for children vary, with younger children normally having faster pulses. (See *Paediatric observations*, page 44.)

In any situation, it is also important to take account of other vital signs, other clinical factors and a normal baseline pulse where this is available. For example, a postoperative pulse of 85 to 90 bpm in a patient whose pre-operative pulse was 55 bpm and whose blood pressure is falling would be a cause for concern.

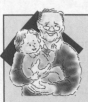

Ages and stages

Paediatric observations

In childhood the vital signs of heart rate, respiratory rate and blood pressure vary according to age – with the heart and respiratory rates decreasing with age, and the systolic and diastolic blood pressures increasing with age. The following table shows the average rates at different ages.

Age (years)	Heart rate (bpm)	Respiratory rate (breaths per minute)	Systolic blood pressure (range) (mmHg)	Diastolic blood pressure (mean average) (mmHg)
Under 1	110 to 160	30 to 40	70 to 90	53 (age 6/12 months)
1 to 2	100 to 150	25 to 35	80 to 95	56 (age 1 year)
2 to 5	95 to 140	25 to 30	80 to 100	55 (age 3 years)
5 to 12	80 to 120	20 to 25	90 to 110	61 (age 9 years)
>12	60 to 100	15 to 20	100 to 120	64 (age 12 years)

Heart rate, respiratory rate and systolic blood pressure: Mackway-Jones *et al.* (2005). Diastolic blood pressure; Second Task Force on BP in Children (1987) cited in Neil and Knowles *et al.* (2004).

Closer to your heart

The closer a pulse is to the heart, the more accurate the reflection of the heart's activity. Therefore, the carotid pulse or the apex beat itself are the most reliable sources of information in cardiovascular emergencies.

Paediatric pulse points

In babies and toddlers the radial pulse is often difficult or impossible to feel. Routine observation of infants' and toddlers' pulse rate is probably best achieved by listening to the apex beat of the heart (on the left side of the chest) via a stethoscope. Children's normal pulse rates decrease with age. (See *Paediatric observations*, above.)

Palpation pointers

Traditional advice has advocated avoiding using your thumb to count a patient's pulse because the thumb has a subtle pulse of its own. The radial pulse is certainly more easily palpated with the fingers. However, when assessing pulse shape (waveform) via the brachial pulse (see Chapter 9) or the carotid pulse, some experts now advocate using the thumb (Northridge *et al.* 2005) which is more able to feel subtle differences in pressure. When palpating the brachial pulse remember it sits in towards the medial aspect of the inner elbow. When palpating the carotids be sure not to place your fingers or thumb too laterally; the pulse is best felt in the groove either side of the Adam's apple. Avoid exerting a lot of pressure, which can stimulate the vagus nerve and cause reflex bradycardia, and *never* palpate both carotid pulses at the same time. Putting pressure on both sides of the patient's neck can impair cerebral blood flow and function.

Off beat

If you note an irregular pulse:
• Evaluate whether the irregularity follows a pattern. For example, it might slow down or speed up with inspiration/expiration. (For more on variation in pulse pattern/shape, see Chapter 9.)
• Auscultate the apical pulse to be sure of an accurate pulse rate. Also note whether the rate is higher than the radial pulse – if so, it is likely not all beats are being transmitted to the periphery.

Leaps and bounds

You also need to assess the pulse amplitude (sometimes called volume). This judgement tends to be somewhat subjective, but you will become more confident in your judgement with experience, especially if you ask others to check your findings whilst you are learning. Amplitude can be classified into different types:
• absent pulse – no pulse is palpable
• weak or thready pulse –hard to feel, easily obliterated by slight finger pressure
• normal pulse – easily palpable, obliterated by strong finger pressure
• bounding pulse – readily palpable, forceful, not easily obliterated by pressure from the fingers.
    If a peripheral pulse is not palpable, firstly consider ABC. If all is well, and a pulse closer to the heart is present, report/refer the patient urgently – they may require assessment by Doppler (an electronic blood flow measuring device), or emergency intervention such as splitting of a plaster of Paris.

Trust your fingers

Pulse oximeters, electronic blood pressure machines and cardiac monitors all electronically monitor pulse rate. But this can be inaccurate so be sure not to rely on these alone. Always regularly check the pulse manually, both to ensure accuracy and to detect rhythm and volume.

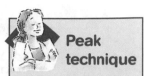

Peak technique

Pinpointing pulse sites

You can assess your patient's pulse rate at several sites, including those shown in the illustration below.

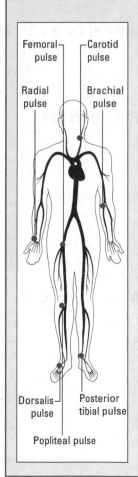

Femoral pulse

Carotid pulse

Radial pulse

Brachial pulse

Dorsalis pulse

Posterior tibial pulse

Popliteal pulse

Respirations

As you count respirations, be aware of the depth and rhythm of each breath. To determine the respiratory rate, count the number of respirations for 60 seconds. The Resuscitation Council UK (2006) cites the normal adult range as 12 to 20 breaths per minute. A faster rate is known as tachypnoea (above 20 breaths per minute) and a slower rate is known as bradypnoea (10 breaths per minute or less); both are of potential concern. A rate below 5 or above 36 breaths per minute requires emergency intervention (Resuscitation Council UK 2006). Be particularly alert to bradypnoea if your patient is receiving opiate analgesia. As with the pulse rate, normal respiratory rates in children are higher – see *Paediatric observations*, page 44.

Secret rate check

If the patient knows you're counting how often they breathe in and out, they may subconsciously alter the rate. To avoid this, count the respirations while you appear to be taking the pulse.

Rise and fall

Pay attention as well to the depth of the patient's respirations by watching the chest rise and fall. Is breathing shallow, moderate or deep? Observe the rhythm of the chest wall as it expands during inspiration and relaxes during expiration. Breathing should be regular and rhythmic in all but infants, for whom an irregular breathing pattern with pauses of 5 to 10 seconds is normal (Rennie 2005). Also observe symmetry of the expansion; be aware that skeletal deformity, fractured ribs and collapsed lung tissue can cause unequal chest expansion.

Accessory to the act . . . of breathing

Use of accessory muscles can enhance lung expansion when oxygenation drops. Patients may use neck muscles and abdominal muscles for breathing. Patient position during normal breathing may also suggest pathology; for example, a patient leaning forward on their hands to get more air into their lungs (sometimes called the 'tripod' position) may well have a respiratory problem such as chronic obstructive pulmonary disease. Normal respirations are quiet, so note any abnormal sounds such as wheezing and stridor. More information on this can be found in Chapter 8.

The big picture

As you assess the respiratory rate remember to look at the whole patient. Observe their colour carefully, both peripherally and centrally. Pallor or cyanosis should increase your concern. Record their oxygen saturation, noting the presence of any oxygen therapy; a saturation below 95% is a cause for concern (Hastings 2008). Is the patient distressed by difficulty in breathing, or are they relaxed in their breathing? All these factors should be considered alongside the rate, rhythm, depth and accessory muscle use as you interpret your findings.

Blood pressure

Blood pressure measurements are helpful in evaluating cardia output, fluid and circulatory status and arterial resistance. Blood pressure measurements consist of systolic and diastolic readings. The higher systolic reading reflects the maximum pressure exerted on the arterial wall at the peak of left ventricular contraction. In an adult a normal systolic pressure ranges from 100 to 140 mmHg, with a higher reading regarded as hypertensive (McGee 2007). An adult reading below 90 mmHg requires emergency intervention (Resuscitation Council UK 2006).

Aah – rest and relaxation!

The lower diastolic reading reflects the minimum pressure exerted on the arterial wall during left ventricular relaxation. This reading measures arterial pressure when the heart is at rest. Normal adult diastolic pressure ranges from 60 to 90 mmHg, with a pressure higher than 90 mmHg in the context of a normal or raised systolic blood pressure regarded as hypertensive (McGee 2007).

Little people, little pressure

Pressures in infants and children are much lower and gradually increase with age – see *Paediatric observations*, page 44.

Unpronounceable and indispensable

The sphygmomanometer, used to manually measure blood pressure, is a piece of equipment routinely used in healthcare practice but often used poorly. (See *Accurately taking the blood pressure*, page 49.)

As the cuff deflates, the sounds that the practitioner listens to with a stethoscope are known as Korotkoff sounds, and indicate the systolic pressure when the sound commences, and the diastolic

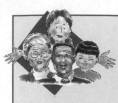

Bridging the gap

Blood pressure variations

Normal blood pressure may vary depending on a variety of factors.

Ethnicity

In particular, people of Afro–Caribbean origin tend to have higher blood pressure than Caucasian patients of the same age and gender. Although there may be some socioeconomic factors affecting this difference in some studies, it is also believed there is a genetic component possibly related to the activity of renin in the kidneys, and the retention of sodium (Seidel *et al.* 2003).

Gender

Gender is another factor that influences blood pressure readings. Premenopausal women have a lower blood pressure than men of the same age, whilst postmenopausal women have a higher blood pressure than men of the same age (Jarvis 2008).

Age

Age also influences blood pressure, with average readings steadily increasing with age. (See table in *Paediatric observations*, page 44.)

pressure when the last sound is heard. Blood pressure can be measured from most extremity pulse points. The brachial artery is used for most patients because of its accessibility.

Electric or manual?

Note that increasingly in healthcare, electronic devices are used to measure blood pressure. Like the sphygmomanometer, these machines are often poorly used and thus give inaccurate readings. Also, the patient staying still is key to a successful reading. Consequently, in some situations, notably paediatric settings, it is sometimes suggested that manual blood pressure recording with a sphygmomanometer is the only truly reliable reading. However, electronic devices are essential for blood pressure monitoring in infants, where it is extremely difficult to reliably hear the brachial pulse with a stethoscope.

Pain

Although assessment of pain is largely derived from the history, it is important as you physically examine the patient to be alert for signs of pain. In adults, take care to look at the patient's face, especially as they move in the bed or when you palpate. Notice if the patient

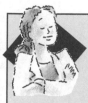

Peak technique

Accurately taking the blood pressure

- For accuracy and consistency, position your patient with their upper arm at heart level and palm turned up. The sphygmomanometer should also be positioned at the same height.
- Apply the cuff snugly on to the upper arm, 2.5 centimetres (cm) above the brachial pulse, as shown in the left hand photograph. It should ideally cover about 80% of the upper arm.
- If you have no idea what the systolic pressure might be, palpate the brachial or radial pulse with your fingertips while inflating the cuff so as not to over-inflate or under-inflate it.
- Inflate the cuff to 30 mmHg above the point where the pulse disappears (or the last systolic blood pressure if you are recording these regularly).
- Place the stethoscope over the brachial artery.
- Release the valve slowly and note the point at which the sounds reappear. The start of the pulse sound indicates the systolic pressure.
- The sounds will become muffled and then disappear. The last sound you hear is the diastolic pressure.

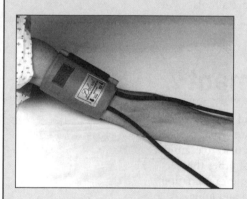 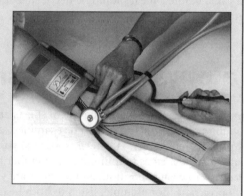

is holding themselves in an awkward position, or has an abnormal gait or shallow breathing; all may indicate pain. Pain is sometimes described as the fifth vital sign.

Taking the FLACC

In infants and younger children, observe behavioural cues; not only crying, but also cues such as drawing up the knees, adopting a rigid position, facial expression and being inconsolable. The revised

FLACC scale (Malviya *et al.* 2006) is a widely adopted behavioural scale used in infants and young children which considers these aspects.

Blood glucose monitoring

Blood glucose levels are a key component of your initial assessment of many patients. Consider this in any diabetic patient, any patient whose history is indicative of possible diabetes (for example, frequency of passing urine, frequent thirst), any patient with a reduced level of consciousness or any patient whose condition means that their intake or retention of diet and fluids has been compromised (for example, severe diarrhoea, vomiting or severe nausea).

A drop of blood

Local practice will dictate the monitoring device used for blood glucose, and practitioners should ensure that they receive expert guidance on how to use the device in their practice setting. Common to all monitoring is taking a drop of blood from the patient (usually from the fingertip, or the heel in an infant) and using this for instant analysis of the blood glucose level. The normal value before a meal should be between 4 and 7 mmols (Diabetes UK 2008).

Performing a physical assessment

During the physical assessment, the use of sheets and a gown will help to minimally expose the area to be examined, and to maximise patient privacy and dignity. Whatever system(s) you plan to examine, try to organise your steps to minimise the number of times the patient needs to change position, and to integrate your examination where appropriate. For example, listen to both heart and lung sounds at the same time whilst the patient is exposed. By using a systematic approach, you'll also be less likely to forget an area.

Hands first

Although approaches vary according to the systems being examined, it is often very helpful and reassuring for the patient if you start with the hands. Not only can a great deal be learned from examining the hands, but starting by touching the hands offers patients a 'safer' initial point of contact than immediately touching a more intimate area such as the chest or abdomen. From the hands the examiner then typically proceeds to the arms, head, neck, torso and legs in that order.

From the right

An interesting tradition is, where possible, standing at the right of the patient. Explanations for this vary – one being that it is the side you need to stand to view the jugular venous pressure in the neck. It is seldom essential clinically, and some room layouts may make it impossible, but standing on the right does achieve some sense of credibility with medical colleagues! Also, consistently approaching from the same side can help you develop more complex skills which require particular hand positions more easily.

General survey

The 'general survey' is the term used to describe a collection of assessment skills which are relevant to most clinical examinations, and often used as the starting point. The exact assessment varies between texts, but typically includes a careful initial overview of the appearance of the patient, assessment of the hands, the vital signs and inspection of the eyes, mouth, ears and neck. Many practitioners then add the thyroid gland, the cervical and axillary lymph nodes and the skin and hair. More details on these will be given in subsequent chapters.

Four key skills

When you perform your physical assessment, you'll use four key techniques: inspection, palpation, percussion and auscultation. These techniques are used in sequence in some examinations (for example, the respiratory examination), or in an adapted sequence (as often seen in the abdominal examination) or selectively (as in the musculoskeletal examination where you might just use inspection and palpation skills). It will be helpful to look at each step in the sequence, one at a time.

Inspection

Inspect the patient visually, also using your senses of smell and hearing, to observe normal condition and deviations. Performed correctly, thorough inspection can yield invaluable data. Inspection begins when you first meet the patient and continues throughout the health history and physical examination. As you assess the patient, you will inspect characteristics such as colour, size, location, movement, symmetry, odours and sounds. Note that use of the opthalmoscope and auroscope are also aspects of inspection.

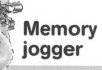

Memory jogger

To remember the order in which you should perform assessment of most systems, just think 'I'll Properly Perform Assessment.'

Inspection

Palpation

Percussion

Auscultation.

Palpation

Palpation requires you to touch the patient with different parts of your hands, using varying degrees of pressure. To do this, you need short fingernails and warm hands. Taking a radial pulse is an example of palpation, as is feeling the chest or abdomen for 'lumps and bumps', warmth, moisture, tenderness or pain. Always palpate tender areas last as that way patients will be more relaxed during the rest of the examination.

Fingers and palms

Note that feeing for 'lumps and bumps' is best done with the sensitive fingertips, whereas feeling for vibrations (such as cardiac 'thrills') is best done with a bony part of the hand such as the upper palm or the edge of your hand that runs down from your little finger (the ulnar edge). Tell your patient the purpose of your touch and what you're feeling with your hands. (See *Types of palpation*, page 53.) Don't forget to wear gloves when palpating areas such as mucous membranes or other areas where you might come in contact with body fluids.

Check out these features

As you palpate each body system, evaluate any abnormality according to the following features:
- texture – rough/craggy or smooth?
- temperature – warm, hot or cold?
- moisture – dry, wet or moist?
- mobility – tethered or mobile?
- consistency of structures – solid or fluid-filled?
- patient response – any pain or tenderness?

Percussion

Percussion involves tapping your fingers or hands quickly and sharply against parts of the patient's body, usually the chest or abdomen. The technique helps you locate organ borders, identify organ shape and position and determine whether an organ is solid or filled with fluid or gas. (See *Types of percussion*, page 54.)

Subtle sounds

Percussion requires a skilled touch and lots of practise to detect slight variations in sound. Organs and tissues, depending on their density, produce sounds of varying loudness, pitch and duration. For example, the resonance of the air-filled lungs is a notably different sound to the dullness of the liver. (See *Sounds and their sources*, page 55.)

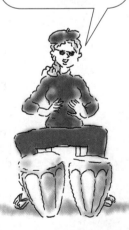

Percussion requires a skilled touch and a trained ear.

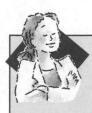

Peak technique

Types of palpation

The two types of palpation, light and deep, provide different types of assessment information, and are particularly useful when assessing the abdomen. For other areas such as the chest or a limb, the same techniques apply as for light palpation, but note that bony structures will usually prevent deep palpation in most other areas.

Light palpation

Perform light palpation to feel for surface abnormalities, including the underlying subcutaneous layers and musculature. On the abdomen, depress the skin around 1 to 2 cm with your finger pads, and palpate using light touch. Use a circling motion of your fingertips (or a snake-like motion) whilst keeping your hand fairly flat. Assess for texture, tenderness, temperature, moisture, elasticity, pulsations, superficial organs and masses.

Deep palpation

Deep palpation is used mostly to examine the abdomen, and allows you to feel internal organs and masses for size, shape, tenderness, symmetry and mobility. Position the hands as shown below, and then depress the skin 4 to 5 cm with firm, deep pressure. Sink the hand into the patient's skin, keeping it fairly flat. Again use the fingertips/upper fingers in a circling or snake-like motion to feel the underlying structures. Some examiners find using the second hand on top of the first helps them to exert firmer, more even pressure.

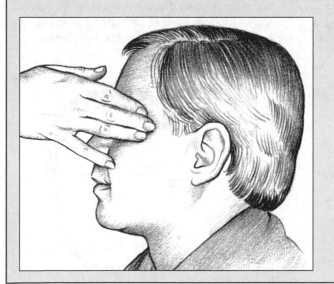

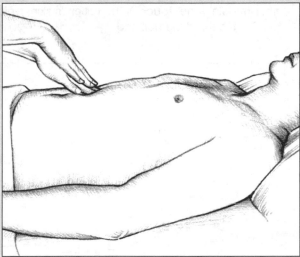

Peak technique

Types of percussion

You can perform percussion using the direct or indirect method.

Indirect percussion

Indirect percussion elicits sounds that give clues to the make-up of the underlying tissue. The sound penetrates below the skin surface and tells you whether underlying tissue is air filled or fluid filled/solid. To percuss:

- Press the distal part of the middle finger of your non-dominant hand firmly on the body part.
- Keep the rest of your hand off the body surface by lifting your palm and other fingers slightly away from the skin.
- Flex the wrist of your dominant hand, but keep your hand and finger firmly in an arched shape, and try to keep movement of the rest of the arm to a minimum.
- Then, moving from your wrist and using the tip of the middle finger of your dominant hand, tap quickly and directly two or three times (with intervals of about 0.5 seconds between each hit) over the point where your other middle finger touches the patient's skin; typically 1 to 2 cm behind the nail bed.

- Note that to do this successfully the nail of your percussing finger must be short, or your other finger will get sore very quickly!
- Listen to the sounds produced.

Direct percussion

Direct percussion reveals tenderness, such as when you tap on the inside of the wrist to assess the carpal tunnel, or the bones of the face to assess the sinuses. Using one or two fingers, tap directly on the body part. Ask the patient to tell you which areas are painful or tingling, and watch the face for signs of discomfort. Direct percussion is also sometimes used if you need to percuss on top of a bone, such as directly percussing the clavicle which lies over the lung apices.

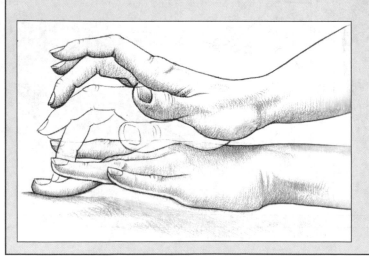

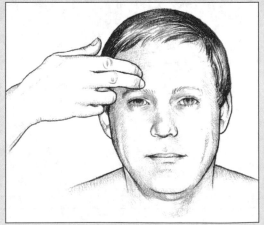

Sounds and their sources

As you practice percussion, you'll recognise different sounds. Each sound is related to the structure underneath. This chart offers a quick guide to percussion sounds and their sources.

Sound	Quality of sound	Where it's heard	Source
Tympany	Drum-like, musical	Over enclosed air	Air in bowel
Resonance	Hollow, clear	Over air-filled areas that are partially solid	Normal lung
Hyper-resonance	Booming, very hollow	Over large quantities of air	Lung with emphysema; normal infant lung
Dullness	Thud-like, muffled	Over solid tissue (sometimes with air-filled tissue underneath)	Liver, spleen, heart
Flatness	Flat, quiet, very dull	Over dense tissue	Muscle, bone

As you percuss, move gradually from areas of resonance to those of dullness and then compare sounds. Also, compare sounds on one side of the body with those on the other side.

Auscultation

Auscultation involves listening for various breath, heart, vascular and bowel sounds with a stethoscope. From this you can detect the presence or absence of sound, and also sound quality. To prevent the spread of infection among patients, clean the heads and end-pieces of the stethoscope with alcohol or a disinfectant before each use. Stethoscopes could well be a major source of hospital-acquired infection. (See *Using a stethoscope*, page 56.)

Recording your findings

Documenting findings clearly and concisely is an essential component of your assessment. As with history taking, some practitioners prefer to document their findings as they go along, whilst others prefer to make brief notes and write up their findings at the end.

Practice makes perfect

Note that documentation takes lots of practise, but is vital for effective communication between healthcare practitioners. It is difficult to give detailed guidance regarding how to document in a text such as this, because your clinical role and your local policy/practice for documentation (for example, written proformas, computerised documentation or freehand recording) will dictate

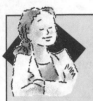

Peak technique

Using a stethoscope

Even if using a stethoscope is second nature to you, it might still be a good idea to brush up on your technique. First, your stethoscope should have these features:

- Snug-fitting ear plugs, which you'll position in your ears so that the ear pieces are angled toward your nose (Note: most good stethoscopes are clearly shaped to enable you to do this – put it back to front and you will wonder why you can't hear very much!)
- Tubing no longer than about 38 cm with an internal diameter no greater than 0.3 cm
- Diaphragm and bell (or an integrated diaphragm/ bell function).

How to auscultate

Hold the diaphragm *firmly* against the patient's skin, enough to leave a slight ring afterwards.

Hold the bell *lightly* against the patient's skin, just enough to form a seal. Holding the bell too firmly causes the skin to act as a diaphragm, obliterating low-pitched sounds.

A few more tips

Also keep these points in mind:

- Provide a quiet environment.
- Make sure the area to be auscultated is exposed. Don't try to auscultate over a gown or underwear because they can interfere with sounds or mimic crackles
- Warm the stethoscope head in your hand if it seems cold.
- If you find it hard to concentrate, try closing your eyes to help focus your attention.
- Listen to, and try to identify, the characteristics of one sound at a time.
- Hair on the patient's chest may mimic crackles. You can minimize this problem by lightly wetting the hair before auscultating.

your approach. But it is really important to familiarise yourself with local policy and documents, and then practise writing up the accounts of patients you have examined using it. Ask senior colleagues to give you feedback to help you develop this skill.

Order, order!

Whatever documents you use, begin your documentation with biographic information, including the patient's age/date of birth, gender and next of kin. This is likely to be followed by their weight, vital signs and comment regarding their general appearance. Next, precisely record all information you obtained from the history and the physical assessment. Just as you should follow an organised sequence in your examination, you should also follow an organised pattern for recording your findings. Document all information about one body system, for example, before proceeding to another. (See *Documenting your findings*, page 57.)

Documenting your findings

If you don't have a paper or computerised proforma to complete in your practice setting, and need to lay out your documentation of your history and examination from scratch, the following order may be helpful. Abbreviations in brackets are *not* recommended for use in the notes themselves despite being widely used, but they can be helpful as you make a quick list to jog your memory during or after the assessment.

History

- Biographical data
- Presenting complaint (PC) and history (detail) of presenting complaint (HPC)
- Past medical history (PMH) including allergies and medication
- Exposure to hazards (smoking, alcohol, recreational drugs, occupational)
- Family history (FH)
- Social history (SH)
- Lifestyle issues (diet, exercise, work, leisure, sleep, recent travel)
- Review of systems (ROS).

On examination

- Initial overview
- Skin
- Head, eyes, ears, nose, throat (HEENT)
- Respiratory system (RS)
- Cardiovascular system (CVS)
- Abdomen (gastrointestinal (GI), genitourinary (GU))
- Nervous system (central nervous system (CNS) and PNS)
- Musculoskeletal system (MSS).

Impression

Plan

Pt has VSD otherwise NAD . . .

You will find when you read others' notes it is commonplace to abbreviate, especially physical examination findings – for example, NAD meaning 'no abnormalities detected'. But be cautious about this and be mindful of the policy of your registering professional body and your employer on using abbreviations – many see them as detrimental to safe, effective practice. For example, the Nursing and Midwifery Council guidelines on record keeping (NMC 2007) state that abbreviations should not be used.

Locate landmarks

Learning and using anatomical landmarks to help you in your descriptions of findings can be really helpful. For instance, you might describe a heart sound as 'at the fifth intercostal space in the mid clavicular line'. In addition to using body structures as landmarks (for example, ribs), the anatomical reference lines (imaginary vertical lines down the chest and abdomen) help you to clearly communicate the location of findings – together they can work a bit like a grid reference on a map. (See *Respiratory assessment landmarks*, page 185 and *Identifying cardiovascular landmarks*, page 230.) You may also find a surface anatomy text (for example, Lumley 2008) really helpful.

Light reflection at 5 o'clock

With some structures, such as the tympanic membrane of the ear, you can pinpoint a finding by its position on a clock face. Breasts and abdomens tend to be referred to in quadrants; left upper quadrant, right lower quadrant and so on. Remember the purpose of documentation is effective written communication between yourself and others.

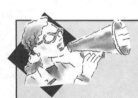

That's a wrap!

Physical assessment review

Performing a physical assessment

- Introduce yourself and try to alleviate the patient's anxiety.
- Explain the entire procedure, including expected duration.
- Briefly document essential information.

Initial impression

- ABC
- Level of consciousness – AVPU
- 'Track and trigger' score (for example, EWS) as indicated.

Initial overview

- Behaviour
- Demeanour
- Appearance.

Weight and height

- Obtain weight wherever possible, and height if indicated.

Body temperature

- Remember that normal body temperature ranges from 35.8 to 37.3°C.
- Select the most appropriate measuring route – oral, axilla or tympanic.

Pulse

- Remember that a normal adult pulse range is typically between 60 and 95 bpm but a pulse below 60 bpm is normal in some fit individuals, notably athletes.

(continued)

Physical assessment review *(continued)*

- To palpate a pulse, press the area over the artery using the pads of your index and middle fingers until you feel pulsations.
- Never palpate both carotid arteries at the same time.

Respirations

- Assess respiratory rate while taking the pulse to disguise what you are doing. Normal adult respiratory rate is 12 to 20 breaths per minute.
- Observe the number, depth and rhythm of the breaths and the symmetry of the chest.
- Watch for the use of accessory muscles, wheezing and stridor.

Blood pressure

- Remember that normal adult systolic pressure ranges from 100 to 140 mmHg; normal diastolic pressure is 60 to 90 mmHg.
- Use the brachial artery under normal circumstances.

Pain

- Assess pain using a validated scoring system appropriate to the age and condition of the patient.

Blood glucose

- Assess blood glucose if indicated. Normal value is 4 to 7 millimoles.

Physical assessment techniques

- Use drapes, exposing only the area being examined.
- Organise your approach: Start with the general survey. Then examine the required systems as appropriate.

Inspection

- Use your vision, smell and hearing to inspect the patient.
- Observe for colour, size, location, movement, texture, symmetry, odours and sounds.

Palpation

- Always tell the patient when and why you're going to touch him/her.
- Use different parts of your hand to touch the patient depending on purpose. Always palpate tender areas last.
- Use light palpation to assess for surface abnormalities, texture, tenderness, temperature, moisture, pulsations and masses.
- Use deep palpation to feel internal organs and masses.

Percussion

- Indirectly percuss quickly and sharply against parts of the patient's body to locate organ borders, identify organ shape and position, and determine consistency.
- Listen to the sounds produced; observe their loudness, pitch and duration.
- Use direct percussion to reveal tenderness.
- Use two or three sharp strokes with short intervals between them to maximise sound quality.

Auscultation

- Use a stethoscope to listen for breath, heart, vascular and bowel sounds.
- Hold the diaphragm of the stethoscope firmly against the patient's skin to listen for high-pitched sounds.
- Hold the bell of the stethoscope lightly against the patient's skin to listen for low-pitched sounds.
- Don't auscultate over a gown. Wet excess hair on the patient's chest if necessary to eliminate interference.

Documenting findings

- Begin by documenting general information.
- Next, document information you obtained from your assessment. Record your findings by body system to organise the information.
- Use anatomic landmarks in your descriptions.

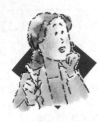

Quick quiz

1. The first technique in your physical assessment sequence is normally:

    A.   palpation.
    B.   auscultation.
    C.   inspection.
    D.   percussion.

2. The normal systolic blood pressure of an adult should be between:

    A.   80 and 120 mmHg.
    B.   100 and 140 mmHg.
    C.   120 and 160 mmHg.
    D.   140 and 180 mmHg.

3. The finding when percussing air-filled lung tissue is:

    A.   resonant.
    B.   tympanic.
    C.   dull.
    D.   flat.

4. The diaphragm of the stethoscope is:

    A.   best at eliciting low-pitched sounds.
    B.   best at eliciting high-pitched sounds.
    C.   is able to elicits both high-pitched and low-pitched sounds equally well.
    D.   is designed for accessing smaller areas of the body.

5. Which of the following is *not* part of the 'general survey'?

    A.   Examination of the hands
    B.   Examination of colour
    C.   Vital signs
    D.   Examination of the chest

For answers see page 398.

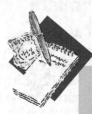

Just the facts

In this chapter, you'll learn:

♦ ways in which nutrition affects health

♦ questions to ask your patient during a nutritional health history

♦ methods for assessing body systems as part of a nutritional assessment

♦ the proper way to take anthropometric measurements

♦ specific laboratory tests to help diagnose nutritional problems

♦ abnormal findings that you may discover during a nutritional assessment.

A look at nutritional assessment

A patient's nutritional health can influence the body's response to illness and treatment, and its ability to heal. The poor nutritional status of many sick or hospitalised patients can lead to reduced resistance to infection, delayed wound healing and longer hospital stays. Yet it is an area of holistic care that is all too readily overlooked, especially in an acute care environment, leading to 'Benchmarks for Food and Nutrition' being a key component of *Essence of Care* (DH 2003). In contrast, obesity is increasingly being recognised as a major health risk in developed countries, linked with a range of conditions including coronary artery disease, diabetes, hypertension and some cancers. An evaluation of nutritional health and requirements should thus be a critical part of your total assessment. A better understanding of your patient's nutritional status can help you plan care more effectively. (See *Parts of a nutritional assessment*, right.)

Parts of a nutritional assessment

Remember the four parts of a nutritional assessment, shown here.

HEALTH HISTORY

LABORATORY TESTS

BODY SYSTEMS ASSESSMENT

ANTHROPOMETRIC MEASUREMENTS

Normal nutrition

Nutrition refers to the sum of the processes by which a living organism ingests, digests, absorbs, transports, uses and excretes nutrients. For nutrition to be adequate, a person must receive the five essential nutrients: proteins, fats, carbohydrates, vitamins and minerals. Also, the digestive system must function properly for the body to make use of these nutrients.

Break it down

The body breaks down the complex chemical compounds that make up most nutrients, either mechanically or chemically, to form simpler compounds for absorption from the gastrointestinal (GI) tract. The process is known as digestion. The mechanical breakdown of food begins in the mouth with chewing, and continues in the stomach and intestine as the food is churned. The chemical processes of digestion start with the salivary enzymes in the mouth and continue with acid and enzyme action throughout the rest of the GI tract.

Now . . . or later

Nutrients can be used for the body's immediate needs, or they can be stored for later use. For example, glucose – a carbohydrate – is stored in the muscles and the liver. It can be converted quickly when the body needs energy fast. If glucose is unavailable, the body breaks down stored fat, which acts as a source of energy during periods of starvation. (See *Anabolism and catabolism*, right.)

Famous five

The five main nutrient groups are all essential for optimal nutritional status, so it is helpful to explore a little more about each of them. Carbohydrate, protein and fats are sometimes called the macronutrients because they are required in large amounts, whereas vitamins and minerals tend to be known as micronutrients because only very small quantities are required by the body.

Count the carbs

Carbohydrate is the body's main source of energy. It is mainly stored in the liver and in muscle tissues. The body therefore needs carbohydrate frequently to maintain optimum energy levels. In the absence of carbohydrate, the body will use stored fat and protein for energy. Excessive intake of carbohydrate is stored in the body in the form of fatty tissue.

Anabolism and catabolism

Anabolism is a building-up process that occurs when simple substances such as nutrients are converted into more complex compounds to be used for tissue growth, maintenance and repair.

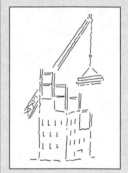

Catabolism is a breaking down process that occurs when complex substances are converted into simple compounds and stored or used for energy.

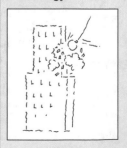

Protein power

The body needs protein to ensure normal growth and function, and to maintain body tissues. Protein is stored in muscle, bone, blood, skin, cartilage and lymph. Because the body preserves protein to maintain body functions, it breaks down protein as a source of energy only when the supply of carbohydrates and fat – the primary sources of energy for the body – is inadequate. Twenty different amino acids combine in different ways to form proteins, of which eight are deemed essential because they cannot be manufactured and have to be consumed.

Lipids on the loose

Lipids and other fats are also essential for the body's normal functioning, growth and development. They are also involved in the regulation of certain hormones, nerve impulse transmission and memory storage. Excessive fat is stored in fatty tissues around the body, and whilst excessive fat storage is problematic, some fat is needed to protect organs and provide insulation against heat loss.

Vital vitamins

Vitamins are essential for growth and development, and a wide variety of metabolic processes. They are divided into two groups, the water-soluble vitamins A, D, E and K, and the fat-soluble vitamins B and C. Note that vitamin B is further divided into various subtypes including thiamin (B_1), riboflavin (B_2), B_6 and B_{12}. The effects of vitamin deficiency vary depending on the vitamins involved; for example, bony deformity (vitamin D deficiency), prolonged clotting (vitamin K deficiency) and poor wound healing (vitamin C deficiency).

Magnificent minerals

Like vitamins, minerals are essential for growth and development. They are also essential for several different metabolic processes, including many processes related to cellular functioning. Examples include sodium, potassium, magnesium, iron, iodine and zinc. The role of sodium and potassium, for example, is crucial in maintaining the intracellular/extracellular fluid balance. Iron is essential in the creation of the haemoglobin needed to transport oxygen to the tissues.

Obtaining a nutritional health history

Screening nutritional status is a key component of any holistic patient assessment. Some patients will have a presenting complaint that has an obvious nutritional focus, but many patients will have more indirect nutritional risk factors in their history which need to be recognised and addressed.

A patient may present with one or more primary nutrition-related issues, such as:

- weight gain or loss
- changes in energy level, appetite or taste
- dysphagia (difficulty swallowing)
- GI tract problems, such as nausea, vomiting and diarrhoea
- other body system changes, such as skin and nail abnormalities.

Whilst some symptoms will be self-limiting or readily treatable, others will be indicators of more severe underlying disease. For example, unexplained/unplanned weight loss or difficulty swallowing are both symptoms that should be viewed seriously and investigated promptly. Also remember that any patient who is about to have major surgery or who is acutely unwell is automatically at increased risk of malnutrition compared with normal. Confusion and depression are also important risk factors for poor dietary intake.

After establishing the patient's presenting complaint/circumstances, ensure that their history includes a careful evaluation of their past and current nutritional status, and dietary habits.

Blast from the past

As you follow the guidelines covered in Chapter 1 for taking a comprehensive history, remember that many aspects of your questioning will allow you to explore issues regarding nutritional status and dietary habits. For example:

- The medication history may offer clues about certain medicines the patient takes, which could affect their nutritional status; for example, steroids are known to be associated with weight gain.
- The family history may reveal information about diabetes, metabolic disorders (for example, high cholesterol) or disorders of the GI tract. If the patient suffers from obesity, explore whether this has been a problem for other members of the family.
- The social history may suggest financial or housing concerns that limit the patient's ability to buy and/or prepare nutritious meals.

A day in the life

If you have concerns about the patient's dietary intake, ask them to describe their food intake over a typical day. Ask the patient firstly to recount what he/she ate yesterday (or in a typical day if for some reason the previous day was atypical) from breakfast through to supper. Use probes to try and explore portion sizes; for example, how many sausages? Were they large sausages or chipolatas? Also explore how the food was cooked; for example, were the sausages grilled or

The patient's description of a typical day can reveal important information about activity level and eating habits.

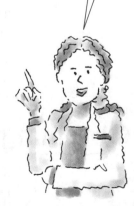

fried? This information not only tells you about the patient's usual intake but also gives clues about food preferences, eating patterns and even the patient's memory and mental status. (See *Understanding differences in food intake*, below.) You may then want to build on this information by asking the patient to make a food diary over the forthcoming week which they bring to their next appointment.

Remember though, patients may try to create a 'positive impression', and thus they may under-report the amount of puddings, sweets or chocolate eaten, and exaggerate the amount of vegetables and fruit. A 'self report' food history may only be a rough indicator of reality.

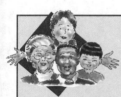

Bridging the gap
Understanding differences in food intake

What your patient eats depends on various cultural and economic influences. Understanding these influences can give you more insight into the patient's nutritional status:

- *Socioeconomic* status may affect a patient's ability to afford healthy foods in the quantities needed to maintain proper health. Low socioeconomic status can also lead to nutritional problems, especially for small children. Pregnant women who are malnourished may give birth to infants with low birth weights and/or may experience complications during labour.
- *Work schedule* can affect the amount and type of food a patient eats, especially if the patient works at night, works very long hours or doesn't have time to stop for regular breaks.
- *Religion* can restrict food choices, leading to avoidance of certain foodstuffs, particularly meat. Those eating a vegetarian diet may suffer with anaemia or excess bloating, for example, but are also likely to have lower cholesterol levels than those who consume meat.
- *Ethnic background* also influences food choices – for example, choosing spicy foods, foods rich in olive oil or foods rich in monosodium glutamate. Health conditions that restrict intake of these foodstuffs can have a profound effect on the patient and their family. Evidence is growing that diets prevalent in certain cultures may be healthier than others – for example the potential health benefits of consuming olive oil as opposed to other types of fat, or consuming red wine (in moderation) as opposed to other types of alcohol.

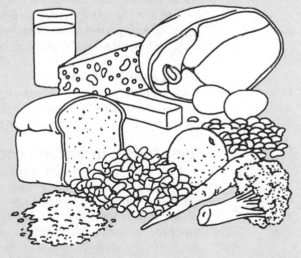

Performing the assessment

After completing the health history, there are various components of the physical assessment that can offer further information about nutritional status. You may also need to request or evaluate data from investigations such as blood tests. Remember that nutritional problems may be associated with various disorders or factors. (See *Tips for detecting nutritional problems*, page 67.)

Take a good look

All physical examinations should begin with a general overview of the patient. Rather than 'diving in' to look at the hands or whatever starting point you have chosen, take time to stand back and consider the patient's general appearance. From a nutritional perspective, consider whether height and weight appear to be in proportion? Are the clothes well fitting, or is there a suggestion that the clothes look too tight or too loose? Are clothes appropriate for the time of year? If not, the patient may be feeling unusually hot or cold. Does the patient seem particularly tired or lethargic? Is there pallor (paleness) of the skin, suggesting possible anaemia?

Assessing each body system

Further chapters will take you through the detailed examination of each body system. All systems relate in some way to nutritional status, and the following list will give you a number of pointers to keep in mind as you assess your patient. Considering these aspects could offer important information in relation to nutritional status, even if a nutritional problem is not the primary presenting complaint.

Ah, mucous membranes are pink and moist.

Skin, hair and nails
Is the patient's hair shiny and well kept, or dull and lifeless looking? Are there any skin blemishes and rashes? Is the skin a normal colour for that particular patient? Are there any nail abnormalities?

Eyes, nose, throat and neck
Is there any pallor of the conjunctiva of the eyes, indicating possible anaemia? Are there any signs of corneal arcus (white rings around the irises) suggesting possible raised cholesterol? Is there any discolouration of the tongue, or other tongue abnormalities such as cracking or leisons? Are there any ulcers or lesions in the mouth, which could suggest poor nutritional status or ill-fitting dentures? Does the patient have any difficulty in swallowing?

Tips for detecting nutritional problems

Nutritional problems may stem from physical conditions, medication, diet or lifestyle factors. Listed below are factors that might indicate your patient is particularly susceptible to nutritional problems and/or has particular nutritional requirements. Remember that children, some elderly people and some people with disabilities are reliant on their parents/carers for their dietary intake. So be sure, where appropriate, to assess lifestyle factors in relation to the parent/carer as well as the patient.

Physical conditions

- Chronic illnesses such as diabetes, neurological, cardiac or thyroid problems
- Family history of diabetes or heart disease
- Draining wounds or fistulas
- Obesity
- Planned or unplanned weight loss
- Cystic fibrosis
- History of GI disturbances
- Anorexia nervosa or bulimia
- Depression or anxiety
- Severe trauma

- Recent chemotherapy, radiation therapy or bone marrow transplantation
- Physical limitations, such as paralysis
- Recent major surgery
- Pregnancy
- Burns
- Mouth, tooth or denture problems
- Mobility problems.

Medication and diet

- Weight-reducing diets that fail to offer a balanced nutritional intake
- Steroid, diuretic or antacid use
- Strict vegan diet
- Nil by mouth prior to or post surgery, or unable to take solid food.

Lifestyle factors

- Living alone, especially those who have recently been widowed or separated from a partner
- Financial problems or poor housing
- Rural location and/or lack of access to transport
- Excessive working hours or other factors that lead to an over-reliance on processed foodstuffs, 'ready meals' or snacking
- Excessive alcohol intake
- Recreational drug use.

Cardiovascular system

Are heart rate, rhythm and volume normal? Is blood pressure normal for the patient's age? Are extremities free from swelling?

Respiratory system

Are the patient's lungs clear or is there a possibility that they are aspirating (taking fluid or food particles into the lungs due to swallowing difficulties)?

Body mass index

To calculate the BMI, divide the patient's weight in kilograms (Kg) by their height in m, and then divide the answer by height in m again (you will probably need a calculator!). So, for example:

If weight is 70 Kg and height is 1.67 m, then:

> 70 divided by 1.67 = 41.9

> 41.9 divided by 1.67 = BMI 25

Or use the helpful tool given on the body mass index calculator website (see page 420).

GI system

Is the patient an appropriate weight for their height? What is their body mass index (BMI)? (See *Body mass index*, above.) Does the patient need help with eating and drinking? Are there any problems with poor appetite, indigestion, nausea, diarrhoea, constipation or vomiting? Are there striae (stretch marks) on the abdomen resulting from current or previous weight gain?

Note that this is just a brief overview; the GI assessment will be central to any comprehensive nutritional assessment. Full detail is offered in Chapter 11.

Neurological system

Is there any evidence of muscle wasting? Is there any leg pain (especially when walking) or numbness that might indicate vascular disease?

Musculoskeletal system

Does the patient have any evidence of osteoporosis, for example, frequent fractures or fractures that have occurred with minimal impact? Are there mobility issues that might affect the patient's ability to shop for or prepare food?

Anthropometric measurements

Anthropometric measurement is the rather grand term sometimes used for measuring nutritional status more precisely, using a variety of instruments. These measurements can help identify nutritional problems, especially in patients who are seriously overweight or underweight. Weight and height are two key components in most nutritional assessments. Like many routine aspects of patient assessment, these are not always conducted as accurately as they could be.

Measuring height and weight

Despite advances in technology making digital/electronic weighing scales increasingly commonplace, many clinical settings still advocate the use of a manual calibrated balance beam scale to maximise accuracy. Whatever scale is used, it should be calibrated regularly, and if the same patient is being measured on a number of occasions, the same set of scales should be used. Guidance regarding how to safely and accurately weigh patients and measure their height is given in Chapter 2. (See *Measuring height and weight*, page 40 and *Obtaining paediatric measurements*, page 41.)

> Discussing a patient's weight may seem like a heavy topic, but don't be shy. Being significantly overweight or underweight can have serious health consequences.

Mass-ive formula

Historically, a variety of charts have been used by practitioners to calculate whether patients are underweight or overweight. However, their accuracy is limited by cultural and socioeconomic variations. Increasingly, the most widely accepted way of evaluating a patient's weight is by using BMI. The BMI is a measure of body fat based on height and weight. For guidance on calculating BMI, see *Body mass index*, page 68.

The following scale (NHS Direct 2008a) classifies the BMI as follows:

- underweight for height – BMI less than 18.5
- normal weight for height – BMI between 18.5 and 24.9
- overweight for height – BMI between 25 and 29.9
- obese – BMI between 30 and 39.9
- very obese – BMI of 40 or greater.

B . . . MI cautious

The standard BMI formula is only valid for use in adults. It does not work reliably with children unless it is adapted to take account of age and gender. Adapted charts are increasingly felt to be reliable measures for use with children (SIGN 2003), although there is still some debate on the issue, and they are not suitable for infants and toddlers. The alternative is validated centile charts, which allow you to plot a child's weight and height against national normal values. See NICE (2006: 213) for further guidance. Also see *Overweight children*, page 75.

BMI should not be used with pregnant or breastfeeding women. It can also be inaccurate for athletes with a very high muscle mass. Accuracy has recently been questioned in relation to its use with older people, although NICE (2006) feels it is still a useful tool in this age group. There is also concern regarding accuracy for Asian people, with suggestions that lower values for obesity and overweight may be more applicable in some high-risk Asian groups. A level of 27.5 for obesity and 23.00 for overweight has been suggested (NICE 2006).

Waist width

In patients with a BMI of less than 35, waist circumference may give more accurate information than BMI about their abdominal fat, with a high abdominal fat content being linked to increased risk of certain diseases, including cardiovascular disease and type 2 diabetes. Using a tape measure, measure midway between the top of the hip bone and the lowest rib (usually this is the narrowest point), with the tape level and pulled snugly against the skin without compressing it. The patient should have just breathed out.

Men with a waist circumference of 94 cm or more and women with a waist circumference of 80 cm or more are judged to be at increased risk (NICE 2006). Again there are cultural variations in normal values, with the 'at risk' waist measurement values for Asian men set at a lower 90 cm (Diabetes UK 2006).

Apples or pears?

The ratio of hip to waist measurement has recently been suggested as an accurate way of distinguishing the higher risk 'apple shape' from the lower risk 'pear shape'; with 'apples' at greater risk of cardiovascular disease and type 2 diabetes. To calculate the hip to waist ratio, measure the waist measurement as described above. Then measure around the hips/bottom at the widest point. The ratio is the waist measurement divided by the hip measurement. For example, for waist 85 cm and hip 100 cm:

85 (waist) divided by 100 (hip) = 0.85

In men the ratio should be no more than 1.0 and in women no more than 0.85 (McGee 2007). Higher values suggest an 'apple shape' rather than a 'pear shape' and carry greater risk.

McGee (2007) cites evidence that the waist to hip ratio may be a better predictor of health outcomes than waist circumference or BMI in relation to a number of conditions, including diabetes, hypertension and heart attack. It may also be a more appropriate tool for assessing older people (Price *et al.* 2006). Importantly though, NICE (2006) notes the need for more good quality research in this area; it is therefore important not to overlook the value of other measures.

MUST consider malnutrition

Detecting malnutrition or risk of malnutrition is also a very important part of nutritional care. A BMI below 18.5 is one factor that might alert you, but assessment of malnutrition is more complex. The Malnutrition Universal Screening Tool (BAPEN 2003, revised 2008) offers very helpful guidance here, considering BMI alongside unplanned weight loss and the effect of acute disease as a predictor of malnutrition or risk of malnutrition. Using such tools to calculate risk will help you recognise the need for close monitoring of weight and dietary intake, and also to determine when intervention such as prompt referral to a dietician or enhanced nutritional intake is required.

Anthropometric alternatives

Other specialised anthropometric measurements, usually undertaken by dieticians, include mid-arm circumference, mid-arm muscle circumference and skin-fold thickness. These measurements are used to evaluate muscle mass and subcutaneous fat, both of which relate to nutritional status. There are also formulae to help you estimate height by measuring the ulnar length, knee height or arm span in patients who cannot stand. All of these measurements need specialist training in order to perform them accurately. If you have any concerns about your patient's nutritional status, an early referral to a dietician for further assessment can be a really important part of their plan of care.

Laboratory studies

Laboratory studies are used to evaluate the levels of various substances in the patient's blood. Below are some common biochemical investigations that may be performed as part of a nutritional assessment, as well as possible outcomes and interpretations. Note that other tests, such as thyroid function tests, serum electrolytes and vitamin levels, may also be ordered.

All about albumin

The serum albumin level is used to assess protein levels in the body. Albumin makes up more than 50% of total proteins in the blood serum. It affects the cardiovascular system because it helps maintain plasma osmotic pressure, which is needed to balance the amount of fluid in the tissues and the amount in the circulatory system. It also functions as a carrier protein for various substances which are important for nutritional health, such as iron. The serum albumin level is decreased with serious protein deficiency and loss of blood protein, and may also result from conditions such as burns, malnutrition, liver or renal disease, heart failure, major surgery, infections, dehydration or cancer. A low serum albumin level can also result in peripheral oedema. However, albumin can be stored in the body for several weeks, so serum albumin measurement may not be a reliable early indicator of protein malnutrition

Carry on with transferrin

Transferrin is a carrier protein that transports iron. The molecule is synthesised mainly in the liver. A serum transferrin level reflects the patient's protein status more accurately than the serum albumin level. The level decreases along with protein levels and indicates depletion of protein stores. Decreased values may also indicate inadequate protein production resulting from liver damage, protein loss from renal disease, acute or chronic infection' or cancer. Elevated levels may indicate severe iron deficiency.

Here's to haemoglobin!

Haemoglobin is the main component of red blood cells, which transport oxygen. Its formation requires an adequate supply of protein in the form of amino acids. Haemoglobin values help to assess the blood's oxygen-carrying capacity and are useful in diagnosing anaemia, protein deficiency and hydration status. A decreased haemoglobin level suggests iron-deficiency anaemia, protein deficiency, excessive blood loss or overhydration. An increased haemoglobin level suggests dehydration or polycythaemia.

Don't omit haematocrit

Haematocrit reflects the proportion of red blood cells (that is, red cell volume) in a whole blood sample. This test helps diagnose anaemia and dehydration. Decreased values suggest insufficient haemoglobin formation, indicative of iron-deficiency anaemia, excessive fluid intake or excessive blood loss. Increased values suggest severe dehydration or polycythaemia. Haemoglobin and haematocrit findings should therefore be interpreted together, and alongside other serum blood results.

Next comes nitrogen

A nitrogen balance test involves collecting all urine passed during a 24-hour period to determine the adequacy of a patient's protein intake. Proteins contain nitrogen, and when they are broken down into amino acids, nitrogen is excreted in the urine as urea. Nitrogen excretion should therefore be equal to protein intake. Results may vary in patients with such conditions as burns and infection or who are recovering from serious illness.

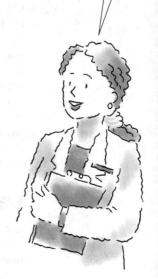

Serum transferrin is the most accurate predictor of a patient's protein status. A low serum transferrin level indicates a low protein level.

Trust in triglycerides

Triglycerides are the main storage form of lipids. Measuring triglyceride levels can help with early identification of hyperlipidaemia and thus the risk of cardiovascular disease. However, increased levels alone aren't diagnostic; further studies such as cholesterol measurements are required. Patients who consume large amounts of sugar, sugary fizzy drinks or refined carbohydrates commonly have elevated triglyceride levels. Decreased triglyceride levels commonly occur in those who are malnourished.

Count the cholesterol

A diet which is high in saturated fats raises cholesterol levels by stimulating lipid absorption. Two types of cholesterol are commonly described. Low-density lipoproteins are sometimes called 'bad' cholesterol as high levels are linked with cardiovascular disease. In contrast, high-density lipoproteins are 'good cholesterol' and have a protective effect against atherosclerosis.

Blood tests to measure cholesterol should be taken after the patient has fasted for 8 hours. This is usually done after an overnight fast, but if done during the day the patient should be encouraged to drink plenty of water during the fast. Increased levels of low-density lipoproteins indicate a higher risk of coronary artery disease, myocardial infarction, stroke and peripheral vascular disease. Decreased cholesterol levels may indicate malnutrition.

Abnormal findings

Patients with nutritional problems may experience such signs and symptoms as excessive weight loss or gain, loss of appetite or muscle wasting. Remember that clinical signs of nutritional deficiencies can often appear late.

I was fine when I came in . . .

Also, be aware that previously healthy hospitalised patients are at risk of developing a nutritional disorder. A variety of factors contribute to this risk, such as being nil by mouth for a period of time, being restricted to clear or intravenous fluids for a period of time, having a reduced appetite relating to illness or surgery or simply not liking the food provided by the hospital. These risk factors are easily overlooked. If you work in a hospital ward setting, consider who clears up the meal trays. Do you know how much lunch the patients you are caring for have eaten? Also be aware that many patients are malnourished on admission, with hospitalisation increasing their risk, hence the importance of the screening processes discussed earlier.

Excessive weight loss

Patients with nutritional deficiencies often experience weight loss. Weight loss may result from decreased food intake, decreased food absorption, increased metabolic requirements or a combination of the three. Other possible causes include endocrine disorders (for example, diabetes), cancer and GI disorders. Also consider chronic disease, infection and neurological lesions that cause paralysis and dysphagia (difficulty swallowing). Other important considerations are psychiatric disorders including anorexia nervosa and bulimia.

Dental deterrent

Excessive weight loss may also occur if the patient has a condition that prevents them from consuming a sufficient amount of food, such as painful oral lesions, ill-fitting dentures or a loss of teeth. In addition, poverty, 'faddy' diets, excessive exercise or certain drugs may contribute to excessive weight loss.

Excessive weight gain

When a person consumes more calories than the body requires for energy, the body stores excess adipose tissue, resulting in weight gain. Emotional factors (such as anxiety, guilt and depression) as well as social factors can trigger overeating, resulting in excessive weight gain. Excessive weight gain is also a primary sign of many endocrine disorders. In addition, patients with conditions that limit activity, such as cardiovascular or respiratory disorders, may also experience excessive weight gain, as might patients taking certain medication.

A huge concern

The risks of obesity to future health in Western countries cannot be overestimated, and is likely to be the cause of a growing number of health problems and premature deaths if the trend is not reversed. Increasingly, healthcare practitioners are looking to address the trend in children and young people, with the aim of creating a healthier next generation. (*See Overweight children*, page 75.)

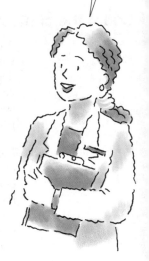

Excessive weight loss or weight gain may be a sign of an endocrine disorder.

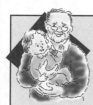

Ages and stages

Overweight children

Like adults, the number of children considered overweight has dramatically increased in recent years. Most overweight children become overweight or obese adults. This has led to a government campaign in England, 'Healthy Weight, Healthy Lives' (DH 2008) with similar initiatives in other UK countries.
Initiatives include:

- early indication of at-risk families
- promotion of breastfeeding
- marketing to promote healthy eating and increased physical activity
- ensuring all schools are 'healthy schools', including cooking being part of the national curriculum
- lobbying for greater advertising restrictions on unhealthy food.

All healthcare practitioners have a role in promoting healthy diet and lifestyle to children, young people and their parents.

More weight, more risks

Children who are overweight are more likely to develop high cholesterol and high blood pressure (risk factors for heart disease) as well as type 2 diabetes. They also tend to suffer from poor self-esteem and depression because of their weight.

Counting causes

During your nutritional assessment, look for these common causes of excessive weight gain in children:

- lack of exercise
- sedentary lifestyle (involving an excessive amount of watching television, using computers or playing video games)
- unhealthy eating habits, including excessive consumption of sugary drinks, fast foods and sweets.

Remember to use age and gender adapted BMI charts or validated centile charts rather than standard BMI charts to assess obesity in children.

Healthy habits

Children who are overweight need a carefully and individually planned weight and lifestyle management programme which involves the whole family. Professional opinions still vary about the optimum approaches to managing obesity in childhood, so any plan needs to be carefully thought through by those involved.

(continued)

Overweight children *(continued)*

For younger overweight children a weight loss programme may not be appropriate. Instead, a weight maintenance programme that enables them to 'grow into their weight' may be safer and more realistic. Finding healthy foodstuffs that they enjoy, and a type of exercise that particularly appeals to them, can often be helpful motivators, as can rewards for reaching certain goals.

Wanting to change

Enabling the child or young person to recognise the problem, accept the risks and want to change is key. Identifying short-term benefits, such as a reduction in teasing/bullying, may be a more powerful motivator than talking about long-term risks such as heart disease in middle age.

It is important to ensure that children don't feel labelled. For this reason and others, long-term follow up of children after the problem appears to have been resolved is important. This will ensure that weight is being managed and that excessive weight gain, or even excessive weight loss, in later childhood/ adolescence is not a problem.

For more information on obesity in children, see NICE (2006) or SIGN (2003).

Anorexia

In medical terms, anorexia is simply defined as a lack of appetite despite a physiologic need for food, and commonly occurs with GI and endocrine disorders. It can also result from anxiety, chronic pain, poor oral hygiene and changes in taste or smell that normally accompany ageing. Short-term anorexia rarely jeopardises health, but chronic anorexia can lead to life-threatening malnutrition.

Girls at risk – and boys too . . .

Anorexia nervosa (sometimes referred to simply as anorexia, hence the potential for confusion), is a psychological condition in which the patient severely restricts their food intake, usually as a result of an unfounded belief that they are overweight. This results in excessive weight loss which, if left untreated, can have major physiological consequences and at its worst be a cause of death. If you suspect a patient might be suffering from anorexia nervosa (for example, a thin patient may tell you they feel fat or that their periods have stopped) then a prompt referral to an expert is important. Note that whilst the condition mostly affects teenage girls and young women, other groups including children, older women and adolescent boys/men can also suffer from the condition.

Muscle wasting

Usually a result of chronic protein deficiency, muscle wasting or atrophy, results when muscle fibres lose bulk and length. The muscles involved shrink and lose their normal contour, appearing emaciated or even deformed. Associated symptoms include chronic fatigue, apathy, anorexia, dry skin, peripheral oedema, and dull, sparse, dry hair.

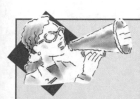

That's a wrap!

Nutritional assessment review

Evaluating nutritional status

- Nutrition is the sum of the processes by which a living organism ingests, digests, absorbs, transports, uses and excretes nutrients.
- Nutrition includes the adequate intake of the five key nutritional groups – proteins, fats, carbohydrates, vitamins and minerals, as well as adequate intake of water.
- Nutrients can be used for the body's immediate needs, or they may be stored for later use.

Obtaining a nutritional health history

- Determine the patient's presenting complaint and/or risk of nutritional concern.
- Obtain the patient's relevant previous medical history, family history, social history and a list of current medications (including vitamins, supplements and herbal preparations).

- Ask the patient about routine activity levels and eating habits.
- Ask the patient about what they ate yesterday or eat in a typical day.

Performing a nutritional physical assessment

- Perform a general inspection.
- Assess key body systems in relation to nutritional status: skin, hair and nails; eyes, nose, throat and neck; cardiovascular system; respiratory system; GI system; neurological system and musculoskeletal system.
- Obtain anthropometric measurements: height, weight and BMI. Consider value of waist measurement and/or hip to waist ratio. Refer for further assessment by a dietician where indicated.
- Assess for risk of malnutrition.

Evaluating laboratory tests

- Albumin – decreased levels indicate protein deficiency, liver or renal disease, heart failure, infection or cancer.

(continued)

Nutritional assessment review *(continued)*

- Transferrin – levels reflect protein stores.
- Haemoglobin – decreased levels indicate iron-deficiency anaemia, overhydration or excessive blood loss.
- Haematocrit – decreased values indicate anaemia; increased values indicate dehydration.
- Nitrogen – output should be equal to intake.
- Triglycerides – levels reflect lipid stores.
- Cholesterol – high levels indicate an increased risk of coronary artery disease and other heart/vascular diseases.

Abnormal nutritional findings

- Weight loss reflects decreased food intake, decreased food absorption, increased metabolic requirements or a combination of the three.
- Weight gain occurs when ingested calories exceed body requirements for energy, causing increased adipose tissue storage.
- Anorexia refers to a lack of appetite despite the physiologic need for food.
- Muscle wasting occurs when muscle fibres lose bulk and length, causing a visible loss of muscle size and contour.

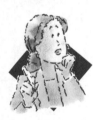

Quick quiz

1. The six main vitamins are:
   A. ABCDEF.
   B. ABDEGK.
   C. ABCDFK.
   D. ABCDEK.

2. A serum albumin test assesses:
   A. protein levels in the body.
   B. the ratio of protein to albumin.
   C. how well the liver metabolises proteins.
   D. protein anabolism.

3. A BMI of 27 would be classified as:
   A. normal.
   B. overweight.
   C. underweight.
   D. obese.

4. Haematocrit refers to:
   A. the proportion of red blood cells to white blood cells.
   B. the amount of haemoglobin in the blood.
   C. the proportion of red blood cells in the full blood sample.
   D. the amount of oxygen in the blood.

For answers see page 398.

4 Mental health assessment

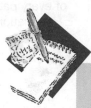

Just the facts

In this chapter, you'll learn:

♦ methods for establishing a therapeutic relationship with a patient

♦ ways to obtain important information during the patient interview

♦ techniques for assessing mental health status

♦ abnormal findings that may be revealed by a mental health assessment

♦ ways to identify mental health disorders.

A look at mental health assessment

Effective holistic patient assessment requires consideration of the psychological as well as the physiological aspects of health. Snadden *et al.* (2005) suggest that mental health and behavioural disorders may affect as many as 20% of the UK population, and account for as many as 40% of the consultations in primary care. Although the comprehensive assessment of patients with a primary presenting mental health problem requires expertise beyond the scope of this book, it is important to recognise that any patient who seeks medical help for a problem with their physical health may also have a mental health concern. The patient presenting with headaches, for example, may also need to be assessed for anxiety and depression. The patient presenting with a cut may have self-harmed. It is, therefore, essential that all who carry out health assessments have a sound understanding regarding how to assess patients for potential mental health concerns, and how to refer them appropriately. In addition to the material in this chapter, knowing the brain's basic function and structures will help you to perform a comprehensive mental health assessment and recognise abnormalities. (See Chapter 14 for a quick review.)

Safety first

You should think of your own safety and that of the patient during *any* consultation, and although it's important not to stigmatise people with mental health concerns, safety may be particularly pertinent in such situations. So consider the following points:
• Does the patient seem agitated, excited or aggressive?
• Are they under the influence of recreational drugs or alcohol?
• What does their body language tell you?
• Is the environment safe for you to assess and care for the patient?
• Is there a means of escape and are there other people around, or is the room isolated and without call buttons?

Suspending judgement

As in any assessment, it is important when undertaking a mental health assessment not to jump to premature conclusions. Patients may make statements that seem offensive or shocking, but these statements may also convey the patient's inner turmoil and distress. It is important to remain as objective as possible within the assessment process.

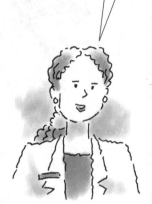

Any illness can affect a patient's mental outlook. Be sure to include a psychological assessment as part of every patient evaluation.

Obtaining a health history

An effective assessment of a mental health problem begins with a detailed health history. For this assessment to be effective, you need to establish a therapeutic relationship with the patient that's built on trust. You must communicate to the patient that his/her thoughts and behaviours are important. Effective communication involves not only speech but also non-verbal communication, such as eye contact, posture, facial expressions, gestures, clothing and even silence. All convey a powerful message. (See *Therapeutic communication techniques*, page 81.)

Patient interview

A patient interview establishes a baseline and provides clues to the underlying or precipitating cause of their current problem.

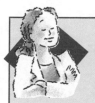

Peak technique

Therapeutic communication

Therapeutic communication is the foundation of any good practitioner – patient relationship. Here are some effective techniques for developing that relationship. They will be useful in any patient encounter, but are particularly useful to consider in relation to a mental health assessment.

Listening

Listening intently to the patient enables you to hear and analyse everything they are saying, and alerts you to the patient's communication patterns.

Rephrasing

Succinct rephrasing of key patient statements helps ensure that you understand, and emphasises important points in the patient's message. For example, you might say 'You're feeling angry and you think it's because of the way your friend treated you yesterday?'

Broad openings and general statements

Using broad openings and general statements to initiate conversation encourages the patient to talk about any subject that comes to mind. These openings allow the patient to focus the conversation and also demonstrate your willingness to interact. An example of this technique is: 'Is there something you would like to talk about?'

Clarification

Asking the patient to clarify a confusing or vague message demonstrates your desire to understand what they are saying. It can also elicit precise information crucial to their recovery. An example of clarification is: 'I'm not sure I understood what you said.'

Focusing

In the technique called focusing, you can help the patient redirect attention toward something specific. It fosters their self-control and helps avoid vague generalisations, so they can accept responsibility for facing problems. 'Let's go back to what we were just talking about,' would be one example of this technique.

Silence

Silence has several benefits. It gives the patient time to talk, think and gain insight into problems. It may also allow you to gather more information. Use this technique judiciously, however, to avoid giving the impression of disinterest or judgement.

Suggesting collaboration

When used correctly, the technique of suggesting collaboration gives the patient the opportunity to explore the 'pros and cons' of a suggested approach. It must be used carefully to avoid directing the patient. An example

(continued)

Therapeutic communication *(continued)*

of this technique is: 'Would it be possible to meet with your parents to discuss the matter?'

Sharing impressions

In the technique called sharing impressions, you attempt to describe the patient's feelings and then seek corrective feedback from the patient. Doing so allows the patient to clarify any misperceptions. For example, you might say 'Tell me if my understanding of what you're saying is right. I think you are telling me that . . .'

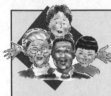

Bridging the gap

Transcultural communication

Communication styles vary among cultures. Qualities viewed as desirable in one culture (such as maintaining eye contact, having a certain degree of openness, offering insight and portraying emotional expression) may not be considered appropriate in another culture. For example:

- Direct eye contact is considered inappropriate and disrespectful in some cultures.
- Some cultures and religions focus primarily on the present; viewing the future as something to be accepted as it occurs, rather than planned.
- In many cultures there can be a tendency for the patient to want to please the healthcare practitioner and/or maximise harmony. As a result, they may nod, smile and provide answers they feel are expected to maintain harmony or gain approval, rather than expressing their true feelings and concerns.
- Gender roles in some cultures may make it difficult to assess a patient's history first hand; a partner may be present in the interview and give most of the answers. Try to address questions to the patient as much as you can and sensitively encourage their own response.

Remember, the patient may not be a reliable source of information, particularly if they have impaired cognition, reasoning, perception or are under the influence of substances such as alcohol. If possible (taking account of confidentiality but also patient 'best interest'), verify responses with family members, friends or healthcare personnel. Also, where you can, check hospital records of previous admissions and compare the patient's past behaviour, symptoms and circumstances with your current findings.

Presenting complaint

During your health interview, you or others may note that the patient seems to be having difficulty coping, is making poor eye contact, lacks emotional response (sometimes called 'flattened affect') or is exhibiting unusual behaviour. Often, mental health problems reveal themselves as physical symptoms, such as difficulty sleeping or headaches. If you note any such concerns, try to explore more deeply using a mnemonic such as OLD CART or PQRSTU. (See Chapter 1, *What's the story?*, page 16.) This will help you assess factors such as the onset and severity of current symptoms, as well as the patient's insight into the problem. This will then inform your plan of care or an appropriate referral. When documenting the patient's response, write it word for word if you can and enclose it in quotation marks.

History of mental illnesses

Discuss any past mental health concerns – such as episodes of anxiety, delusions, depression or drug/alcohol abuse and any previous psychiatric treatment, including the prescription of medication such as antidepressants. Also ask about any family history of psychiatric illness or substance abuse.

Socioeconomic data

Patients living in poor socioeconomic situations are more vulnerable to some types of mental health problem. Sensitively gathered information about the patient's educational level, family, social networks, housing conditions, income and employment status may provide clues to the current situation/problem. Note that social isolation is an important risk factor to consider in depression and risk of suicide.

Medication history

Certain prescribed medication can cause symptoms of mental illness. Review any medications that the patient is taking, including over-the-counter and herbal preparations such as St John's Wort, and check for interactions. If the patient has been prescribed medication to address a mental health concern, ask if the medication is being taken as prescribed, whether the symptoms have improved and if there have been any adverse reactions. Remember that several prescribed drugs used to treat mental health problems, such as many antidepressants, can take 2 weeks or longer to have a noticeable effect.

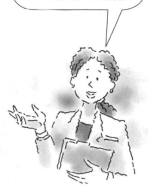

Always review the patient's medication history, keeping in mind that certain medications can cause symptoms of mental illness.

Drugs and alcohol

Assessing the patient's use of alcohol and recreational drugs may reveal important clues regarding their mental health. There are well-established links between dependence on such substances and mental health problems; with the term 'psychoactive' substances sometimes being applied to alcohol and recreational drugs, and indeed also to tobacco and caffeine.

Physical illnesses

Find out if the patient has a history of physical illnesses that may cause distorted thought processes, disorientation, depression or other symptoms of mental illness. For example, is there a history of renal or hepatic failure, severe infection, thyroid disease, raised intracranial pressure or a metabolic disorder? Other life events, such as menopause, have also been linked to some mental health concerns, for example depression.

Assessing mental health status

Most of a mental health status assessment can be done during an interview. Jarvis (2008) suggests there are four main components to assessing mental health status:
• appearance – including dress, grooming, hygiene and posture/body movement
• behaviour – including level of consciousness, mood and speech
• cognition – including orientation to time, place and person, as well as attention span and memory
• thought processes – including logical thought, perceptions and self-destructive behaviour or intent.

Appearance

Much about a patient's mental state can be determined by observing appearance and how the patient handles themselves in your presence. Appearance helps to indicate his/her emotional and mental health status. Is the patient adequately groomed or obviously struggling to maintain hygiene? Is clothing appropriate to the season and situation? Unkempt or inappropriate dress/appearance may alert your concern. Is the patient's posture erect or slouched? Is their head lowered? Note facial expression. Do they look alert, or stare blankly? Do they appear sad or angry? Do they maintain eye contact, and is it appropriate?

Behaviour

Note the patient's demeanour and overall attitude as well as any extraordinary behaviour, such as speaking to a person who isn't present. Also record any mannerisms such as nail biting or fidgeting. Do they display any tics or tremors? How do they respond to you? Is the patient cooperative, friendly, hostile or indifferent?

Mood

Does the patient appear anxious or depressed? Any crying, sweating, breathing heavily or trembling? Ask the patient to describe current feelings in concrete terms and to suggest possible reasons for these feelings. Note inconsistencies between body language and mood (such as smiling when discussing an anger-provoking situation). Asking patients whether they feel they have anything to look forward to can be a good way of assessing mood; a negative answer should alert your concern. Also note feelings of self-worth, as a patient who feels worthless may be more vulnerable in respect of mental illness.

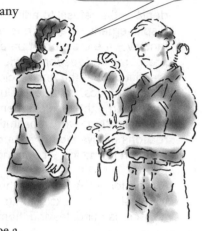

You seem distracted. Would you like to talk about it?

Defence mechanisms

The patient who's faced with a stressful situation may adopt mechanisms to help them cope with it – behaviours that operate on an unconscious level to protect the ego. Examples include denial, displacement, fantasy, identification, projection and repression. Listen for an excessive reliance on these mechanisms. (See *Exploring coping mechanisms*, page 86.)

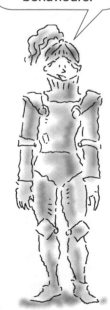

Patients faced with stressful situations may adopt defensive behaviours.

Cognitive function

Evaluate the patient's orientation to time, place and person, noting any confusion or disorientation. For example, you might ask them the date, day of the week or month, their demographic details and where they are right now.

Listen for any indication that the patient might be having delusions, hallucinations, obsessions, compulsions, fantasies or daydreams (more detail regarding these is given later in the chapter).

Exploring coping mechanisms

The use of coping, or defence, mechanisms helps to relieve anxiety. Common coping strategies include:

- denial – the refusal to admit truth or reality
- displacement – transferring an emotion from its original object to a substitute
- fantasy – the creation of unrealistic or improbable images to escape from daily pressures and responsibilities
- identification – the unconscious adoption of another person's personality characteristics, attitudes, values or behaviours
- projection – the displacement of negative feelings onto another person
- rationalisation – the substitution of alternative reasons for the real or actual reasons motivating behaviour
- reaction formation – behaving in a manner opposite from the way the person feels
- regression – the return to the behaviour of an earlier, more comfortable time
- repression – the exclusion of unacceptable thoughts and feelings from the conscious mind, leaving them to operate in the subconscious.

Attention please

Evaluation of short-term memory can be helpful. Tell the patient a short fictitious address or a list of four or five objects, and ask them to repeat it back to you. Then ask them to remember it and check again in 10 to 15 minutes to see if they can still recall it. Also consider assessing remote or long-term memory. To some extent the history so far will already have given you clues about this, but consider asking about key life events such as weddings, significant birthdays or holidays. A partner or other family member may be able to verify the accuracy of what the patient describes.

Intellectual function can be assessed by numerical skills, such as counting backwards from 20. Sensory perception and coordination can be assessed by asking the patient to make or copy a simple drawing (for example, draw a square or circle, or copy a pentagon).

For a systematic assessment of these cognitive functions consider using a validated tool such as the Mini Mental State Examination, which combines tests of orientation, learning, short-term memory, language and calculation. For example, see the tool described by Patient UK (2007b).

Thought processes

Assessment of thought processes enables you to consider what the patient is thinking about and the ways in which they are thinking.

Are their thoughts logical or illogical? Are there any suggestions of harmful intent to themselves or others?

Spee-eech

Note any speech characteristics that may indicate altered thought processes, including monosyllabic responses, irrelevant or illogical replies to questions, convoluted or excessively detailed speech, slurred speech, repetitive speech patterns, a 'flight of ideas' (when the patient moves illogically from one idea to another) or sudden silence without obvious reason.

Insight

Assess the patient's insight by asking if he/she understands the significance of their illness, the plan of treatment and the effect the illness is having/will have on their life.

Potential for self-destructive and suicidal behaviour

In any patient with a mental health concern, the practitioner needs to be alert to the risks of suicidal or self-destructive behaviour.

Feelin' alive

Not all self-destructive behaviour is suicidal in intent. Some patients engage in self-destructive behaviour because it makes them feel alive. A patient may cut or mutilate body parts to focus on physical pain, which may be less overwhelming than emotional distress. Be aware in particular of looking at the patient's wrists and forearms, as this is a common place where such cutting may take place. Look for signs of both new scars and well healed scars from past events, which may present as fine white lines only visible in a good light.

Higher risk when they're low

Assess the patient for suicidal tendencies, particularly if he/she reports symptoms of depression. Not all such patients want to die; indeed, suicide attempts are sometimes described as a 'cry for help'. However, the incidence of suicide attempts, including death as a result of these, is higher in patients with certain mental illnesses such as depression.

Practitioners are often worried about how to assess suicidal intentions. Importantly though, do not assume the best thing to do is 'not to mention it', for fear of 'putting the idea into the patient's head'. Experts advise that whenever the practitioner thinks the patient may be at risk of harm to themselves (or indeed others) then this must be explored further (Snadden *et al.* 2005). Try if possible to wait until later in the interview when a rapport has been established, as this may help to facilitate an honest answer.

Careful questioning

Questions may be difficult to phrase. A good starting point to determine whether the patient may be depressed can be the two-question test designed by Whooley *et al.* (1997).

> 'During the last month, have you often been bothered by feeling down, depressed or hopeless?'

> 'During the last month, have you often been bothered by little interest or pleasure in doing things?'

This may then lead to a more direct question about whether the patient has any plans to harm themselves, and any expressed intent can then be explored more precisely to help assess the degree of risk. If you are in any doubt regarding the patient's response and the risk it indicates, check out your findings with a senior colleague before allowing the patient to go home. An urgent mental health referral may be required to ensure the patient's immediate safety.

Note that, inevitably, some patients will choose not to tell you the truth in answer to these questions. However, others will feel relieved at the opportunity to share their feelings and thus give open and honest answers.

Psychological and mental status testing

Although much can be learned about mental health during an interview, you may need to evaluate particular aspects of your patient's mental status in more detail. These aspects can be assessed using psychological and mental status tests. Other than the Mini Mental State Examination, a variety of other tests exist; for example, the Beck Depression Inventory II (Beck *et al.* 1996) or the Hospital Anxiety and Depression Scale (Zigmond and Snaith 1983). However use of these tests requires experience in mental health assessment, and some may only be used by licensed or registered test users who have purchased them for use in their clinical setting, so seek guidance from senior colleagues. Also check the age range for which the test is validated – for example, the Beck Depression Inventory II is designed for use with those aged 13 to 80. It is also very important to

I've never been good at taking tests.

Don't worry. This isn't the type of test on which you'll receive a grade.

remember that although tests are carefully validated, no such test is 100% accurate. Findings suggestive of low risk should not cloud your clinical judgement; if you have any doubts refer the patient urgently for further assessment.

Abnormal findings

During your assessment, you may detect abnormalities in thought processes, thought content and perception.

Abnormal thought processes

During the interview, you may identify some of these abnormalities in your patient's thought processes:
- flight of ideas – the patient jumps abruptly from topic to topic in a continuous flow of speech
- neologisms – words are distorted or invented
- confabulation – the patient fabricates facts or events to fill gaps in their memory
- clanging – the patient chooses a word based on the sound rather than the meaning
- echolalia – the patient repeats words or phrases that others say
- incoherence – the patient's speech is incomprehensible.

Abnormal thought content

With careful questioning, you may also detect abnormalities in thought content during the interview. Be sure to follow the patient's lead. For example, 'You told me a few minutes ago that your mother was responsible for your illness; can you tell me a bit more about that?' With this type of questioning, you can find abnormalities in thought content, which may include:
- obsessions – recurrent, uncontrollable thoughts about a particular issue, topic or situation
- compulsions – repetitive behaviours that result from attempts to alleviate an obsession
- phobia – an irrational and disproportionate fear of objects or situations
- depersonalisation – the feeling that one has become detached from one's mind or body or has lost one's identity
- delusions – false, fixed beliefs that aren't shared by others
- paranoia – unfounded suspicion that someone or something is trying to cause one harm
- poverty of content – thoughts that give little information because of vagueness, empty repetition or obscure phrases.

Perception abnormalities

You can assess a patient's perception abnormalities in the same way that you assess his/her thought content. Ask direct questions about perceptions, such as 'What did the voice say to you when you heard it speaking? How did you feel?' If the patient doesn't talk about abnormal perceptions, you can ask if he/she ever hears peculiar voices or frightening sounds. Perception abnormalities include:

*   illusions – misinterpretations of external stimuli
*   hallucinations – auditory, visual, tactile (touch), somatic (feeling) or gustatory (taste) sensory perceptions when no external stimuli are present.

> To detect mental health abnormalities, follow your patient's lead and ask direct questions about his/her perceptions.

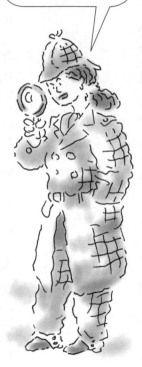

Understanding more about mental health

There are many conditions which can affect a patient's mental health. For further information regarding such conditions, see O'Carrol and Park (2007) or Callaghan and Waldock (2006).

Child and Adolescent Mental Health Services (CAMHS)

It is sometimes easy to think that mental health problems predominantly affect adults. In recent years though, there has been growing recognition of the importance of child and adolescent mental healthcare. CAMHS seeks to promote the mental health and psychological wellbeing of children and young people, and to ensure effective assessment, treatment and support for them and their families (Department of Children, Schools and Families 2008).

Specialist input from those with training and experience in CAMHS is essential for the care of many children and young people with mental health problems. However, initial recognition of children who may need further assessment or treatment is the responsibility of the wider healthcare team, as well as others such as schoolteachers and social services. If you have any concerns about the mental health or psychological well-being of a child or young person in your care, discuss this with a more senior colleague or refer them to a specialist CAMHS practitioner.

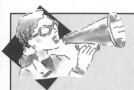

That's a wrap!

Mental health assessment review

Obtaining a mental health history

- Establish a trusting, therapeutic relationship.
- Choose a quiet, private setting.
- Maintain a calm, non-threatening tone of voice to encourage open communication.
- Determine the patient's presenting complaint, and any associated problems or concerns, using the patient's own words to document it.
- Discuss past mental health problems and previous psychiatric or psychological treatment, if any, and also family history of mental health problems.
- Obtain the patient's demographic and socioeconomic data.
- Discuss cultural and religious beliefs as appropriate.
- Obtain a medication history.
- Ask about a history of medical disorders; some conditions may adversely affect the patient's mental health.

Mental status checklist

- Appearance
- Behaviour

- Mood – including inconsistencies between body language and mood
- Defence mechanisms
- Cognitive function – including orientation to time, place and person, as well as and any confusion or disorientation
- Short-term memory
- Ability to recall events
- Intellectual function
- Speech characteristics that indicate altered thought processes
- Insight
- Potential for self-destructive or suicidal behaviour
- Psychological and mental status test results.

Abnormal mental health findings

- Abnormal thought processes – flight of ideas, neologisms, confabulation, clanging, echolalia, incoherence
- Abnormal thought content – obsessions, compulsions, phobia, depersonalisation, delusions, phobias, poverty of content
- Abnormal perceptions – illusions, hallucinations.

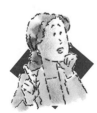

Quick quiz

1. Which psychological and mental status test helps assess the patient's cognitive functioning?

    A. The Mini Mental State Examination

    B. The Sad Person's Scale

    C. The Beck Depression Inventory

    D. The CAGE scoring system

2. You notice that your patient jumps from topic to topic in a continuous flow of speech. You identify this abnormal thought process as:
   A. flight of ideas.
   B. echolalia.
   C. confabulation.
   D. clanging.

3. A good way to evaluate short-term memory is to:
   A. ask the patient to tell you when their wedding anniversary is.
   B. ask the patient what they ate for lunch yesterday.
   C. give the patient a short list of objects and ask them to repeat it back to you 10 minutes later.
   D. give the patient a piece of paper and ask them to draw a square.

4. An irrational and disproportionate fear of objects or situations is:
   A. obsession.
   B. delusion.
   C. compulsion.
   D. phobia.

For answers see page 399.

Part II

Assessing body systems

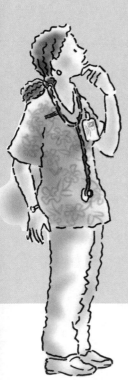

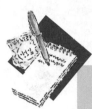

(5) Skin, hair and nails

Just the facts

In this chapter, you'll learn:

♦ components of skin, hair and nails

♦ changes in skin, hair and nails that occur normally with age, as well as those that signal a health problem

♦ questions to ask about skin, hair and nails during the health history

♦ techniques for assessing skin, hair and nails

♦ abnormalities of skin, hair and nails and their causes.

A look at skin, hair and nails

The skin covers the internal structures of the body and protects them from the external world. It's sometimes described as the largest organ in the body, comprising about 16% of body weight (Bevan and Gawkrodger 2005). Along with hair and nails, the skin provides a window for viewing changes taking place inside the body. Careful examination of the skin is therefore a very important part of patient assessment.

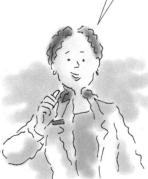

The skin, hair and nails are like windows into a patient's health.

Anatomy and physiology of skin, hair and nails

To perform an accurate physical assessment, you'll need to understand the anatomy and physiology of the skin, hair and nails. Let's review them one by one.

Skin

Also called the integumentary system, the skin is the body's largest organ and has several important functions, including:
• protecting the tissues from trauma and bacteria
• preventing the loss of water and electrolytes from the body
• sensing temperature, pain, touch and pressure
• regulating body temperature through sweat production and evaporation
• synthesising vitamin D
• promoting wound repair by allowing cell replacement of surface wounds.

Layers of the skin

The skin consists of two distinct layers: the epidermis and the dermis. Subcutaneous tissue lies beneath these layers. (See *What's in your skin*, below.)

What's in your skin

This cross-section of the skin illustrates major skin structures.

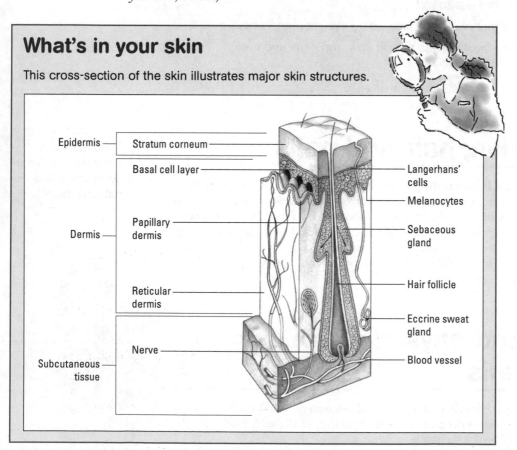

Epidermis
— Stratum corneum
— Basal cell layer

Dermis
— Papillary dermis
— Reticular dermis

Subcutaneous tissue
— Nerve

Langerhans' cells
Melanocytes
Sebaceous gland
Hair follicle
Eccrine sweat gland
Blood vessel

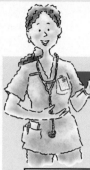

Identifying primary lesions

Are you having trouble identifying your patient's lesion? Here are a number of common lesions that your patient may have. Remember to keep a centimetre ruler handy to accurately measure the size of the lesion.

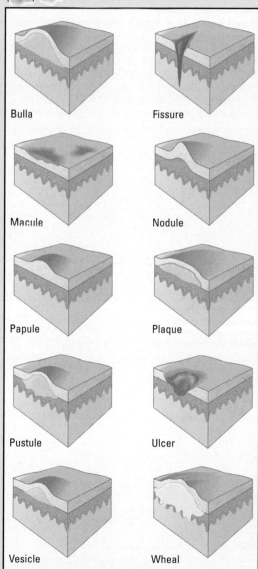

Bulla
Elevated, serous fluid-filled lesion, larger than 1 cm in diameter. Thin walled, ruptures easily. Example: blister.

Fissure
Usually painful, crack-like lesion of the skin that extends into at least the dermis. Example: athlete's foot, cracked heels.

Macule
Flat, circumscribed area of altered skin colour, less than 1 cm. Examples: freckle, flat mole, some viral rashes.

Patch
Macule larger than 1 cm. Examples: café-au-lait spot, Mongolian spot.

Nodule
Raised solid lesion. Extends up into the epidermis but also down deeper into the dermis than a papule. Usually more than 1 cm in diameter. Example: fibroma.

Papule
Raised, circumscribed, solid area; generally less than 1 cm. Examples: elevated mole, wart, some viral rashes.

Plaque
Papule or merged group of papules larger than 1 cm. Example: psoriasis.

Pustule
Elevated pus-filled lesion. May contain a hair. Example: acne.

Ulcer
A crater-like lesion of the skin that extends to the dermis. Examples: venous ulcer, pressure sore.

Vesicle
Circumscribed, elevated lesion; contains serous fluid; less than 1 cm. Example: early chickenpox.

Wheal
Superficial, raised, reddish area. Transient (may appear and disappear quickly). Likely to be itchy. Example: allergic reaction.

Urticaria
Wheals that merge into each other (coalesce) to form a larger rash. Very itchy. Example: allergic reaction.

Text adapted from *Health Assessment Made Incredibly Visual* (2007) and Jarvis (2008).

ABCDE of malignant melanoma

To remember what to assess when evaluating a lesion, think of the letters ABCDE.

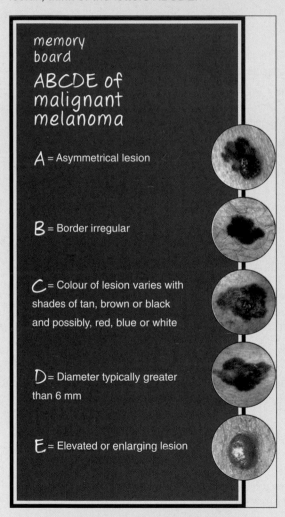

memory
board

ABCDE of
malignant
melanoma

A = Asymmetrical lesion

B = Border irregular

C = Colour of lesion varies with shades of tan, brown or black and possibly, red, blue or white

D = Diameter typically greater than 6 mm

E = Elevated or enlarging lesion

Adapted from Health Assessment Made Incredibly Visual, p. 19, Philadelphia: Lippincott Williams & Wilkins (2007).

Images from Anatomical Chart Co. (A to D) and from Nettina, S.M. (2001) The Lippincott Manual of Nursing Practice, 7th edn. Philadelphia: Lippincott Williams & Wilkins (E).

Recognising common skin disorders

On this page and the pages that follow, you'll find photos of common skin disorders along with brief descriptions of each. Use the photos to guide your assessment of abnormal skin findings.

Basal cell carcinoma

The most common type of skin cancer, basal cell carcinoma results from sun exposure. It usually appears as a small waxy-looking nodule that ulcerates and forms a central depression. Basal cell carcinoma usually starts as a skin-coloured papule (may be deeply pigmented) with a translucent top and overlying telangiectases. It rarely metastasises and commonly appears on the head and neck.

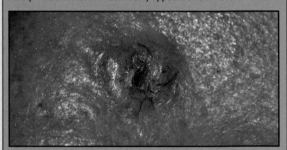

From Goodheart, H.P. (2003) Goodheart's Photoguide of Common Skin Diseases, 2nd edn. Philadelphia: Lippincott Williams & Wilkins.

Squamous cell carcinoma

Squamous cell carcinoma results from sun exposure and can metastasise. It appears as a raised border with a central ulcer and may be rough, thickened or scaly. It most commonly appears on the face and neck as an erythematous scaly patch with sharp edges.

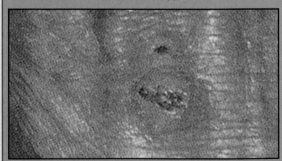

Reprinted with permission from Bickley, L.S. (2003) Bate's Guide to Physical Examination and History Taking, 8th edn. Philadelphia: Lippincott Wilkins & Wilkins.

Recognising common skin disorders *(continued)*

Lupus erythematosus (discoid or systemic)

The typical sign of lupus erythematosus appears as a red, scaly, sharply demarcated, butterfly-shaped rash over the cheeks and nose. The rash may extend to other areas of the face or to other exposed areas, such as the ears and neck.

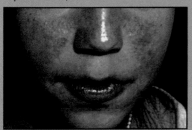

From Goodheart, H.P. (2003) *Goodheart's Photoguide of Common Skin Diseases,* 2nd edn. Philadelphia: Lippincott Williams & Wilkins.

Spider naevi

Spider naevi (sometimes called spider angiomas) are small dilated blood vessels, typically looking like a spider. They usually occur on the face, arms and trunk. They can be normal in isolation, but are abnormal if more than five or six are present, and may indicate liver disease. They also occur in pregnancy.

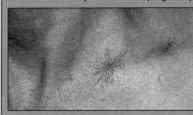

From Goodheart, H.P. (2003) *Goodheart's Photoguide of Common Skin Disorders,* 2nd edn. Philadelphia: Lippincott Williams & Wilkins.

Vitiligo

Vitiligo is a slowly progressive disease of hypopigmentation that causes irregular areas of pigmented skin around milk-coloured patches. These areas commonly appear on the face, hands and feet.

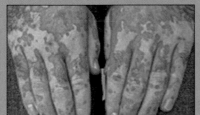

Stedman's Medical Dictionary, 27th edn. (2000). Philadelphia: Lippincott Williams & Wilkins.

Psoriasis

Psoriasis is a chronic disease of marked epidermal thickening. Plaques are symmetrical and generally appear as red bases topped with silvery scales. The lesions, which may connect with one another, occur most commonly on the scalp, elbows and knees.

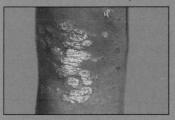

Reprinted with permission from Bickley, L.S. (2003) *Bate's Guide to Physical Examination and History Taking,* 8th edn. Philadelphia: Lippincott Williams & Wilkins.

Contact dermatitis

Contact dermatitis is an inflammatory disorder that results from contact with an irritant. Primary lesions include vesicles, large oozing bullae and red macules that appear at localised areas of redness. These lesions may itch and burn.

From Goodheart, H.P. (2003) *Goodheart's Photoguide of Common Skin Diseases,* 2nd edn. Philadelphia: Lippincott Williams & Wilkins.

Urticaria (hives)

Occurring as an allergic reaction, urticaria appears suddenly as pink, oedematous papules or wheals (round elevations of the skin). Itching is intense. The lesions may become large and contain vesicles.

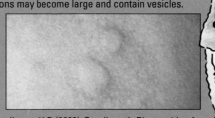

From Goodheart, H.P. (2003) *Goodheart's Photoguide of Common Skin Diseases,* 2nd edn. Philadelphia: Lippincott Williams & Wilkins.

(continued)

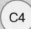

Recognising common skin disorders *(continued)*

Eczema

Eczema may be acute or chronic and may be accompanied by severe itching. Mostly affecting the antecubital and popliteal areas, these lesions may be red and papular, vesicular or pustular. Lesions cause blisters, oozing and crusting. Thickening, excoriation and extreme dryness of the skin can also occur.

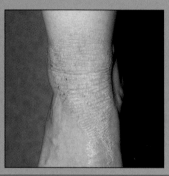

Impetigo

Impetigo is a rash that usually appears on the face. It's caused by a bacterial infection. When ruptured, fragile vesicles in the rash ooze a honey-coloured fluid and crusts may form. It is important to distinguish this rash from herpes simplex (cold sore) as they are similar in appearance, but impetigo is bacterial wheras herpes simpex is viral. Swabbing may be required.

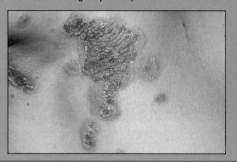

Candidiasis

Candidiasis is a fungal infection that produces erythema and a scaly, papular rash. Because the fungus thrives in moist environments, it most commonly occurs under the breasts and in the axillae, in the genital area and orally and in the nappy area in infants

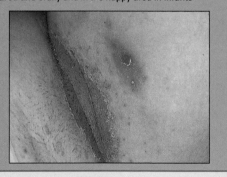

Herpes zoster

Herpes zoster appears as a group of vesicles or crusted lesions along a nerve root. The vesicles are usually unilateral and appear mostly on the face, hands and neck. These lesions cause severe pain.

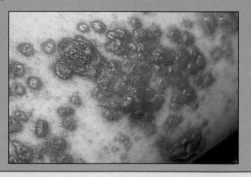

All images on this page are from Goodheart, H.P. (2003) *Goodheart's Photoguide of Common Skin Diseases,* 2nd edn. Philadelphia: Lippincott Williams & Wilkins.

Skimming the surface

The epidermis – the outer layer – is made of squamous epithelial tissue. It's thin but also tough, and contains no blood vessels. The two major layers of the epidermis are the stratum corneum – the most superficial layer – and the deeper basal cell layer, or stratum germinativum.

The superficial stratum corneum is made up of cells that form in the basal cell layer, then migrate to the skin's outer surface, dying as they reach it. However, because epidermal regeneration is continuous, new cells are constantly being produced.

The basal cell layer contains melanocytes, which produce melanin and are responsible for skin colour. Hormones, the environment and hereditary factors influence melanocyte production. Because melanocyte production is greater in some people than in others, skin colour varies considerably.

Laying it on thick

The dermis – the thick, deeper, supportive layer of the skin – consists of connective tissue called collagen and an elastic, extracellular material called matrix, which contributes to the skin's strength and pliability. Blood vessels, lymphatic vessels, nerves and hair follicles are located in the dermis, as are sweat and sebaceous glands. Because it's well supplied with blood, the dermis delivers nutrition to the epidermis. In addition, wound healing and infection control take place in the dermis.

Give the glands a hand!

Sebaceous glands, found primarily in the skin of the scalp, face, upper body and genital region, are part of the same structure that contains the hair follicles. Their main function is to produce sebum, which is secreted onto the skin or into the hair follicle to make the hair shiny and pliant.

There are two types of sweat glands:
•   The eccrine glands are located over most of the body and produce a watery fluid that helps regulate body temperature. They are mature from 2 months old.
•   Apocrine glands secrete a milky substance and open into the hair follicle. They're located mainly in the axillae and the genital areas. They become active during puberty and secretion is stimulated by emotion or sexual arousal.

Affects of ageing on skin

As people age, skin thins and loses its elasticity. A loss of collagen increases the risk of tearing-type injuries, and a reduction in sweat and sebaceous glands means that skin becomes dry. Vascularity of the skin diminishes and blood vessels become more fragile, leading

Ages and stages

How skin ages

This table lists skin changes that normally occur with ageing.

Change	Findings in older people
Pigmentation	Increased likelihood of: • cherry angiomas – small, flat 'cherry red' lesions, usually on the trunk • 'liver spots' (lentigo) – small pale brown patches particularly on the hands • seborrhoeic keratoses – raised pale to dark brown wart-like lesions that feel waxy, sometimes with a craggy surface; they have a 'stuck on' appearance • local patches of red/purple discoloration in response to trauma
Thickness	Wrinkling, especially on the face, arms and legs Parchment-like appearance, especially over bony prominences and on the dorsal surfaces of the hands, feet, arms and legs
Moisture	Dry, flaky and rough
Turgor	'Tents' and stands alone, especially if the patient is dehydrated
Texture	Numerous creases and lines

to dark-red discoloured patches occurring as a result of trauma. (See *How skin ages*, above.)

Affects of sunlight on the skin

Exposure to sunlight, especially of lighter coloured (less pigmented) skin, causes important changes, including reduction in elasticity, uneven colouring and changes in texture. In addition, the increased incidence of skin cancer, particularly basal cell carcinoma and melanoma, is a growing health problem. This is due to increased exposure to the sun caused by a variety of factors including environmental damage, greater access to foreign travel and widespread acceptance of sunbathing as a 'normal' part of a summer holiday. (See *ABCDE of malignant melanoma*, colour plate C2.)

Hair

Hair is formed from keratin and produced by matrix cells in the dermal layer. Each hair lies in a hair follicle and receives nourishment from a papilla, a loop of capillaries at the base of the

A close look at hair

The illustration below shows a hair shaft and its associated glands.

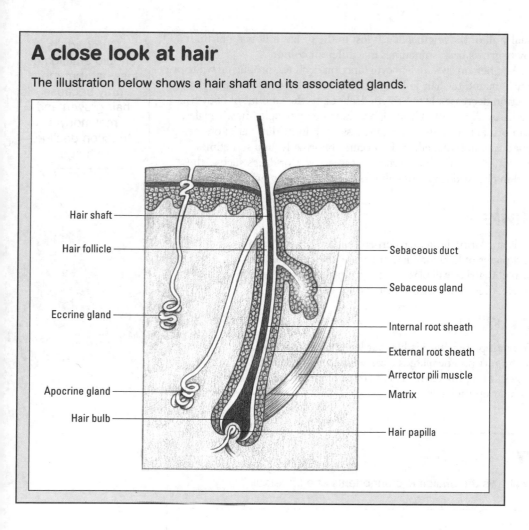

Hair shaft

Hair follicle

Eccrine gland

Apocrine gland

Hair bulb

Sebaceous duct

Sebaceous gland

Internal root sheath

External root sheath

Arrector pili muscle

Matrix

Hair papilla

follicle. At the lower end of the hair shaft is the hair bulb. This contains melanocytes, which determine hair colour. (See *A close look at hair*, above.)

Each hair is attached at the base to a smooth muscle called the arrector pili. This muscle contracts during emotional stress or exposure to cold and elevates the hair, causing goose bumps.

Hair today, gone tomorrow

A newborn baby's skin is covered with lanugo, which is a fine, downy growth of hair. Lanugo can be located over the entire body but occurs mostly on the shoulders and back. Most of the lanugo is shed within 2 weeks of birth. The amount of hair on a newborn's head varies, and usually all of the original hair is lost in the weeks following birth. It slowly grows back, sometimes in a different colour.

As a person ages melanocyte function declines, producing white or grey hair, and the hair follicle itself becomes drier as sebaceous gland function decreases. Hair growth declines, so the amount of body hair decreases. Age-related balding occurs in many people, mostly males, as a normal part of the ageing process, with individual variations being genetically determined. It also occurs abnormally (and sometimes reversibly), as a result of certain diseases, stress or drugs such as those used in chemotherapy; this abnormal hair loss is known as alopecia.

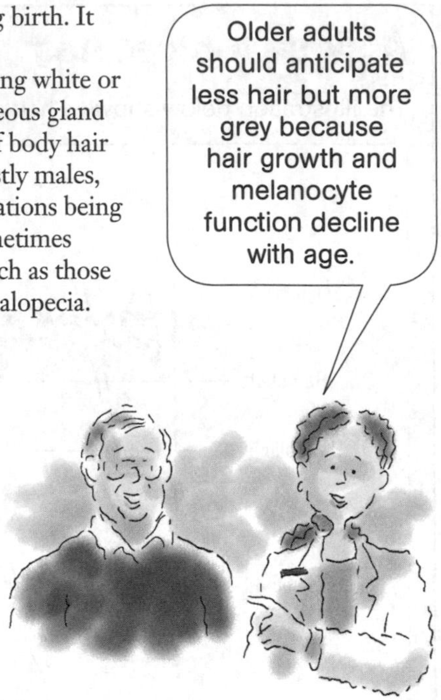

> Older adults should anticipate less hair but more grey because hair growth and melanocyte function decline with age.

Nails

Nails are formed when epidermal cells are converted into hard plates of keratin. They are made up of the nail root (or nail matrix), nail plate, nail bed, lunula, nail folds and cuticle. (See *Nail anatomy*, below.)

What's on your plate?

The nail plate is the visible, hardened layer that covers the fingertip. The plate is clear with fine longitudinal ridges. The pink colour results from blood vessels underlying vascular epithelial cells.

Nail anatomy

The illustration below shows the anatomic components of a fingernail.

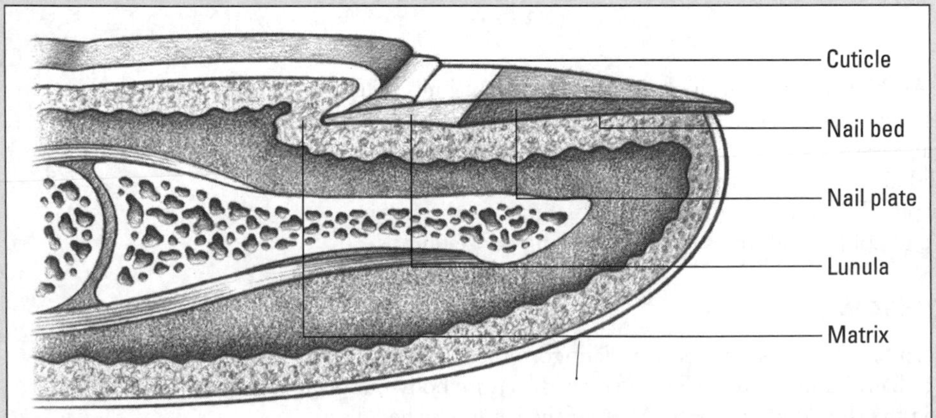

- Cuticle
- Nail bed
- Nail plate
- Lunula
- Matrix

What is the matrix?

The nail matrix is the site of nail growth. It's protected by the cuticle. At the end of the matrix is the white, crescent-shaped area, known as the lunula, which extends beyond the cuticle.

Not hard as nails anymore

With age, nail growth slows and the nails lose their lustre, becoming brittle and thin. Longitudinal ridges in the nail plate become much more pronounced, making the nails prone to splitting.

Obtaining a health history

When assessing a problem related to skin, hair or nails, keep in mind that these abnormalities may result from a medical problem related to the patient's presenting complaint, but the patient may not realise their significance.

Asking about the skin

Many skin disorders involve itching, rashes, lesions, pigmentation abnormalities or changes in existing lesions. Use the PQRSTU or OLD CART mnemonic (page 16) to help you frame the questions needed to explore the condition fully.

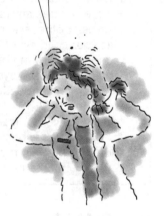

Itching is one of the most common skin complaints.

Rash judgements

If the patient has a skin rash or lesion there are number of particular questions you will want to consider.
• How has the rash or lesion changed between when the patient first noticed it and today?
• Is there any bleeding, itching or fluid leakage?
• Has the patient noticed similar skin changes in any other areas of the body?
• Does the patient have any sense of what might have caused the problem initially, such as an insect bite, new washing powder or new toiletries?
• Does the patient have any other symptoms such as vomiting, a fever, joint pain or recent weight loss?

Other important factors to explore include family history of any skin diseases; conditions such as psoriasis, for example, may be inherited. It is also important to remember that there are particular considerations in relation to children. (See *Additional history questions for infants and children*, page 102.)

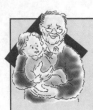

Ages and stages

Additional history questions for infants and children

Remember to consider asking parents these questions when obtaining a history for infants and children:

- Does the child have any birthmarks that are still present, or did they have any that have now faded?
- Have you noted any rashes, abnormal bruises or other skin changes?
- Has your child ever had any jaundice (yellowing of the skin or white areas of the eyes) either at birth, or subsequently? If so, how was it treated?
- Have you ever noticed your child looking 'blue', especially around the mouth or on their face? If so, what tends to cause this?

- Has the child ever had, or been recently exposed to, any contagious conditions – such as scabies, lice or impetigo, or any contagious illnesses such as chickenpox?
- Have you noticed any mottling of the skin? (Note that mottled skin in a sick child can be a sign that he/she is seriously unwell.)
- Has the child had all the relevant immunisations against infectious childhood illnesses? (If you are unsure of the current schedule see the regularly updated NHS Immunisation website, page 420.

Skin SMART

From a health-promotion perspective it is valuable to consider the amount of time the patient spends in the sun, either due to work or leisure, and whether they are using adequate skin protection. It is important to remember that children's skin and fair skin is especially vulnerable, but also to remember that darker skinned people are also at risk.

The Australian 'slip–slap–slop' slogan (that is, **slip** on a T-shirt, **slap** on a hat, **slop** on some sun cream) can be a useful 'easy to remember' piece of advice. More comprehensively, Cancer Research UK (2006a) developed the 'SunSmart' guideline:

- **S**pend time in the shade between 11 a.m. and 3 p.m.
- **M**ake sure you never burn
- **A**im to cover up with a T-shirt, hat and sunglasses
- **R**emember to take extra care with children
- **T**hen use factor 15+ sun cream (sunscreen).

Health practitioners all have a part to play in reinforcing these messages, as well as in the early detection of possible malignancy. (See *ABCDE of malignant melanoma*, page C2.)

Asking about the hair

Most concerns about the hair refer either to hair loss or hirsutism – an increased growth and distribution of body hair.

Getting to the root of the problem

Again systematically use a mnemonic to explore the patient's presenting problem. Note that common causes of hair loss or hirsutism include skin infections, ovarian or adrenal tumours, increased stress, prescribed medication such as steroids, or systemic diseases such as hypothyroidism and malignancies. So be sure to cover these points in your systematic history taking.

Asking about the nails

Most complaints about the nails concern changes in growth, shape, colour or structure. Each of these problems may result from infection, nutritional deficiencies, systemic illnesses or stress.

Nailing down the details

In addition to using a mnemonic to systematically explore the problem, remember that nails can offer important clues to a wide variety of systemic illnesses/conditions, such as cardiovascular disease, respiratory disease, liver disease and psoriasis. So ensure that your questioning is broad enough to consider these possibilities. If you observe damage to the nails, consider causes such as recent application of 'artificial nails' or excessive recent use of nail varnish. Patients may also mistake normal age-related changes (for example, increases in the ridges on the nails) as an indication of an underlying problem.

Assessing skin, hair and nails

To assess skin, hair and nails, you'll use the techniques of inspection and palpation. Before beginning the examination, make sure the room is well lit and comfortably warm. Wear gloves during your examination if appropriate, particularly if examining open skin lesions.

Skin

Start by observing the skin's overall appearance. Such observation can help you to identify areas that need further assessment, and to make comparison between normal skin for that patient and the area of concern. Inspect and palpate the area of the skin where the problem exists, and if possible a comparable area of normal skin (for example, the other leg) to facilitate a comparison. Focus on factors such as colour, texture, turgor (that is, elasticity), moisture and temperature.

Colour

Look for localised areas of bruising, cyanosis (blue-tinged skin), pallor (white or pale skin), jaundice (yellow or orange hue) and erythema (redness). Acute central or peripheral cyanosis requires urgent intervention. Unexplained jaundice should always be investigated. Also check the skin for uniformity of colour and hypopigmented or hyperpigmented areas. Also be aware of the particular areas of the body where colour changes can best be detected in people with darker skin. (See *Detecting colour variations in dark-skinned people*, below.)

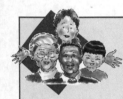

Bridging the gap

Detecting colour variations in dark-skinned people

Cyanosis

Examine the lower conjunctivae (inside the lower eyelids), palms, soles, buccal mucosa (lining of the mouth) and tongue. Look for dull, dark or bluish colour.

Erythaema

Palpate the area for warmth.

Jaundice

Examine the sclerae (white area of the eyes) and hard palate in natural, not fluorescent, light if possible. Look for a yellow colour.

Pallor

Examine the lower conjunctivae, especially the outer edge nearest the eyelashes (outer rim) for pallor. Also note pallor in the buccal mucosa, tongue, lips, nail beds, palms and soles. Look for a pale ashen colour. Pallor can also sometimes be seen in the skin depending on how dark the skin tone is.

Petechiae

Examine areas of lighter pigmentation such as the abdomen. Look for tiny, purplish red dots.

Rashes

Palpate the area for skin texture changes. Use a good light source and shine it across the skin to detect raised areas/changes more clearly.

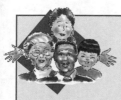

Bridging the gap

Mongolian spots

Mongolian spots, sometimes called Mongolian blue spots, are irregularly shaped areas of deep blue pigmentation. They most commonly occur over the sacral and gluteal areas but may also appear on the shoulders, arms, abdomen or thighs. These bluish discoloured areas are normal variations of the skin, much more prevalent in darker-skinned children. They are most frequently seen in Afro–Caribbean children, with 90% having Mongolian spots. They are rarest, but do sometimes occur, in Caucasian children (Jarvis 2008).

Mongolian spots are present at birth and usually remain visible into adulthood, although they often fade over time. They result from deposits of embryonic pigment in the epidermal layer left behind from foetal development.

Mongolian spots are completely benign and require no treatment. However, when assessing children, be careful not to confuse these spots with bruises, which may cause an erroneous safeguarding concern.

Skin exposed to the sun may have a darker pigmentation than other areas. Be aware that some local skin colour changes are normal variations that appear in certain cultures. (For example, see *Mongolian spots*, above.)

Texture and turgor

Inspect and palpate the skin's texture, noting its thickness and mobility. It should look smooth and be intact. Rough, dry skin is common in patients with hypothyroidism, psoriasis and excessive keratinisation.

Turgor-nomics

Palpation also helps you evaluate the patient's hydration status. Dehydration causes poor skin turgor. Note however, that because poor skin turgor may also be caused by ageing, it may not be a reliable indicator of an older patient's hydration status. (See *Evaluating skin turgor*, page 106.)

Observing oedema

Oedema, on the other hand, causes skin to appear swollen and spongy, and when pressed, the indentation of the finger may take some time to flatten out; this is known as pitting oedema. Oedema may be

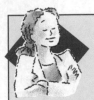

Peak technique

Evaluating skin turgor

To assess skin turgor in an adult, gently squeeze the skin on the forearm, back of the hand or abdomen between your thumb and forefinger, as shown in the upper picture. In an infant, roll a fold of loosely adherent abdominal skin between your thumb and forefinger.

Then release the skin. If the skin quickly returns to its original shape, the patient has normal turgor. If it returns to its original shape slowly over 30 seconds, or maintains a tented position as shown in the lower picture, the skin has poor turgor. Note that this may indicate moderate to severe dehydration, but also remember that reduction in turgor may well be a normal finding in elderly people.

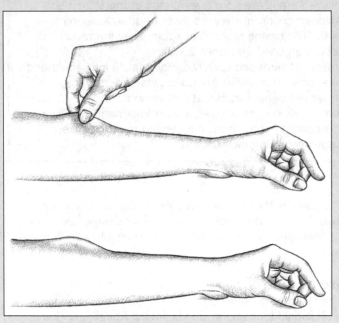

systemic or localised. Unexplained oedema should be investigated further as it can be indicative of a wide variety of conditions of varying severity. For example, oedema of the ankles and/or sacrum may indicate cardiovascular disease.

Moisture

The skin should be relatively dry, with a minimal amount of perspiration. Skin-fold areas should also be fairly dry. Overly dry skin appears red and flaky.

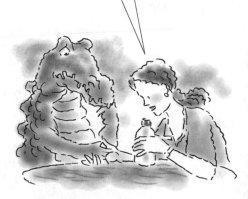

All in a sweat

Overly moist skin is normal as a result of strenuous activity or an environment that's too warm. It may also be triggered by anxiety or obesity, or an illness that increases metabolic rate. Heavy sweating, or diaphoresis, usually accompanies fever. Other systemic causes include cardiac and pulmonary diseases, such as tuberculosis for example.

Temperature

Palpate the skin bilaterally for temperature, which can range from cool to warm. The dorsal surface (back) of the hands tends to be the most sensitive for detecting temperature changes. Hot or cool skin may just relate to the external environment, or may signify an underlying disorder. Distinguish between generalised and localised coolness and warmth.

That's cool

Localised temperature variations may be observed; for example, finding one limb cooler than the other may be a result of vasoconstriction associated with impaired arterial circulation to a limb. General coolness or coolness of all four limbs can result from such conditions as shock or hypothyroidism. In either situation be sure to check the peripheral circulation as described later in the chapter. (See also *Assessing skin temperature*, right.)

Hot and bothered

Localised warmth occurs in areas that are infected, inflamed or burned. Generalised warmth occurs with fever or systemic diseases such as hyperthyroidism. Be sure to check skin temperature bilaterally.

Lesions and rashes

During your inspection, you may notice variations in the skin's texture and pigmentation. Remember to familiarise yourself with the different types of rashes and skin lesions that exist, and the different ways they may be distributed. (See *Identifying primary lesions*, page C1, and *Recognising common lesion configurations*, page 109.)

Denoting disease

Red lesions caused by vascular changes include haemangiomas, telangiectases, petechiae, purpura and ecchymoses, and may indicate disease. These are described later in the chapter.

Stamp of approval

Normal variations include birthmarks, freckles or moles. Birthmarks are generally flat and range in colour from tan to red or brown.

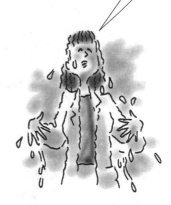

Fever, strenuous activity, disease or factors that elevate the metabolic rate can cause heavy sweating.

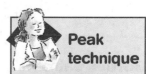

Peak technique

Assessing skin temperature

When you're trying to compare subtle temperature differences in one area of the body with another, use the dorsal surface (that is, back) of your hands and fingers. They're the most sensitive to changes in temperature.

They can be found on all areas of the body. Freckles are small, flat macules located primarily on the face, arms and back. They're usually red brown to brown. Moles are either flat or raised and may be pink, tan or dark brown. Like birthmarks, they can be found on all areas of the body.

New or not?

When investigating a lesion, start by classifying it as primary or secondary. A primary lesion is new. Changes in a primary lesion constitute a secondary lesion. Examples of secondary lesions include fissures, scales, crusts, scars and excoriations.

It's what's inside that counts

Determine whether the lesion is solid or fluid-filled. Macules, papules, nodules, wheals and hives are solid lesions. Vesicles, bullae, pustules and cysts are fluid-filled lesions. (See *Illuminating lesions*, page 109.)

Lesion low-down

After you've identified the type of lesion, you'll need to describe its characteristics, pattern, location and distribution. A detailed description can help you or others determine whether the lesion is a normal or pathological skin change.

Border patrol

Examine the lesion to see if it looks symmetrical. Also, check the borders to see if they're regular or irregular. An asymmetrical lesion with an irregular border may indicate malignancy. Itching or inflammation may also suggest malignancy. (See *ABCDE of malignant melanoma*, page C2.)

Colour changer

Lesions occur in various colours and can change colour over time. Therefore, watch for such changes in your patient. For example, if a lesion such as a mole has changed from a single colour to more than one colour (which can vary from dark brown to fawn or red) the lesion might be malignant.

Follow the pattern

Pay close attention as well to the configuration and distribution of the lesions. Many skin diseases have typical configuration patterns. Identifying those patterns can help to determine the cause of the problem. (See *Recognising common lesion configurations*, page 109.)

Change in a lesion's colour may indicate malignancy.

Recognising common lesion configurations

You may be able to identify the configuration of your patient's skin lesion by matching it to one of these diagrams.

Discrete

Individual lesions are separate and distinct.

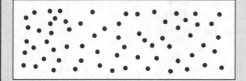

Annular

Lesions are arranged in a single ring or circle.

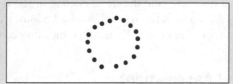

Grouped

Lesions are clustered together in one or more groups.

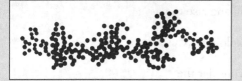

Polycyclic

A number of annular lesions are arranged in multiple circles.

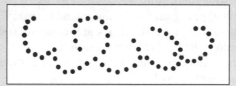

Confluent

Lesions merge so that individual lesions aren't visible or palpable.

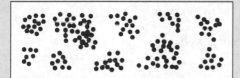

Arciform

Lesions form arcs, curves or twists.

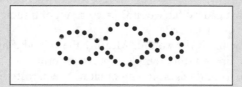

Reticular

Lesions form a mesh-like network.

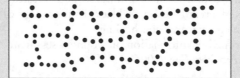

Linear

Lesions form a line. Note: a linear rash along a nerve root distribution is known as Zosterform, as in Herpes Zoster (Shingles).

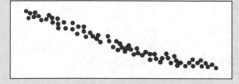

Peak technique

Illuminating lesions

Illuminating a lesion can help you see it better and learn more about its characteristics. Here are two techniques worth considering.

Macule or papule?

To determine whether a lesion is flat or raised (for example, a macule or a papule), use this technique. Reduce the direct lighting and shine a pen torch at a right angle to the lesion. If the light casts a shadow, the lesion is a papule. Macules are flat and don't produce shadows.

Solid or fluid-filled?

To determine whether a lesion is solid or fluid-filled, place the tip of pen torch against the side of the lesion. Solid lesions don't transmit light. Fluid-filled lesions transilluminate with a red glow.

Sizing up the situation

Measure the diameter of the lesion using a millimetre–centimetre (mm–cm) ruler. If you estimate the diameter, you may not be able to determine subtle changes in size. Although an increase in the size or elevation of a mole over many years may be normal. It is important that any moles which are getting bigger, or becoming elevated, are investigated for possible malignancy. Moles that are 6 mm or larger are linked with a greater risk.

If you note any fluid drainage, document the type, colour and amount. Also note if the lesion has a foul odour, which can indicate a superimposed infection. Remember, bleeding can also be a sign of melanoma.

Wound Assessment

When assessing a wound, it is important to pay attention to the following factors adapted from Enoch (2006).

Wound wisdom

- What caused the wound? Is it a result of trauma, burns, pressure sore or other factor?
- How big is the wound? Measure the wound if healing problems are anticipated (for example, a pressure sore).
- Are wound edges sloping or clearly demarcated?
- Where is the wound on the body?
- Is the wound superficial or deep?
- Is the surrounding skin healthy looking, or is it oedematous, red or otherwise abnormal?
- Are there indications that the wound is oozing? If so, what does the exudate look like? Look at the wound itself, and also the surrounding skin and removed dressing.
- Is the patient experiencing wound pain? If so, explore fully using a pain assessment tool.

If the wound has been present for a while, also consider the following.
- Is it healing as expected, or is healing delayed?
- What colour is the bed of the wound? Healthy, healing tissue is pink. Red, cream, yellow or black tissue is a sign of possible infection or problems with wound healing.

For further information on wound assessment see *Wound Care Made Incredibly Easy* (2006).

Hair

Depending on the presenting complaint, it may be appropriate to inspect hair over the patient's entire body, not just on his/her head. Note the distribution, quantity, texture and colour. The quantity and distribution of head and body hair varies between patients, particularly on the male body where huge individual variations are seen. Note, however, it is usual for hair distribution to be symmetrical.

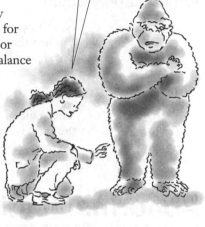

Hmm. The hair is definitely evenly distributed.

Too much or too little?

Check for patterns of hair loss and growth. If you notice patchy hair loss, look for regrowth. Also, if relevant, examine the scalp for erythema, scaling or encrustation. Also, note areas of excessive or inappropriate hair growth, which may indicate a hormone imbalance or be a sign of a systemic disorder such as Cushing's syndrome.

Having a bad hair day?

The texture of scalp hair also varies between patients, and whilst healthy hair is often described as being shiny and soft, hair products (especially colouring products) and ageing often lead to hair being dry, coarse or brittle. This means that although hair changes can be indicative of systemic illness or nutritional deficiency, as an isolated finding such changes are often difficult to interpret in terms of their significance.

Extension errors

There is a growing trend towards using hair extensions to add length and/or decoration to existing hair. These are often so realistic that it can be very difficult to distinguish the patient's hair from the artificial hair. Patients also occasionally have hair transplants. So be sure to check whether the hair you are assessing is actually the patient's own.

Nails

Assessing the nails is vital for two reasons. Firstly, the appearance of the nails can be a critical indicator of systemic illness, and secondly, their overall condition tells you a lot about the patient's grooming habits and ability to care for himself/herself. As part of the general survey, or as part of your respiratory, cardiovascular or gastrointestinal examination, it is vital to examine the nails for colour, shape, thickness, consistency and contour.

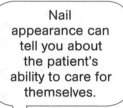

Nail appearance can tell you about the patient's ability to care for themselves.

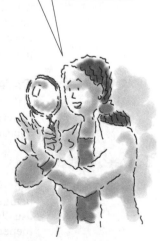

Nail that colour

First, look at the colour of the nails. Light-skinned people generally have pinkish nails. Dark-skinned people generally have pinkish or brown nails. Brown-pigmented bands in the nail beds are normal in dark-skinned people and abnormal in light-skinned people. Yellow nails may occur in smokers as a result of nicotine stains.

Circulation check

Nail beds can be used to assess a patient's capillary refill. (See Chapter 8.)

What shapely nails!

Next, inspect the shape and contour of the nails. The surface of the nail bed should be either slightly curved or flat. The edges of the nail should be smooth, rounded and clean.

What's the angle?

The angle of the nail base (where the base of the nail runs under the skin) is normally less than 180 degrees. An increase in the angle suggests clubbing, indicative of cardiovascular, respiratory or gastrointestinal disease. (See *Evaluating clubbed fingers*, page 117.)

> Are you feeling self-conscious about your nails?

Abnormal findings

Various abnormalities may be found when assessing the skin, hair and nails. Because these abnormalities may be visible to others, the patient may experience some degree of emotional stress. Carefully document all abnormal findings, pertinent health history and as much information as possible from the physical examination.

Skin abnormalities

The signs and symptoms you detect during your assessment may be caused by a wide variety of disorders. This section describes the most common skin abnormalities. (You can also refer to the chart *Skin colour variations*, page 113, and the colour photographs on pages C2–C4 for more on skin abnormalities.)

Café-au-lait spots

Café-au-lait spots appear as flat, light brown, uniformly hyperpigmented macules or patches on the skin surface. They usually appear during the first 3 years of life but may develop at any age.

Coffee, anyone?

Café-au-lait spots can be differentiated from freckles and other benign birthmarks by their larger size and irregular shape. They usually have no significance; however six or more café-au-lait spots (depending on their size) are one of the criteria for diagnosing the neurological disorder neurofibromatosis.

Interpretation station

Skin colour variations

To consider the possible causes of skin colour variations, this chart may be helpful.

Colour	Distribution	Possible cause
Absent pigmentation	• Small, circumscribed areas • Generalised	• Vitiligo • Albinism
Blue/grey	• Around lips, buccal mucosa or generalised	• Cyanosis. Note: in some dark-skinned people, blue/grey gums are normal
Tan to brown	• Facial patches	• Chloasma of pregnancy
Tan to brown–bronze	• Generalised (not related to sun exposure)	• Addison's disease
Yellow to yellowish brown	• Sclera or generalised	• Jaundice from liver dysfunction. Note: in dark-skinned people and the elderly, a slight yellowing of the periphery of the sclera can be normal
Yellowish orange	• Palms, soles and face; not sclera	• Carotenemia (carotene in the blood). Note: unlike jaundice, the sclera will not be affected

Cherry angiomas

Cherry angiomas are tiny, bright red, round macules or papules that may become brown over time. These clinically insignificant lesions occur extremely commonly in individuals older than 30 and increase in number with age. They occur mostly on the trunk.

Macules and papules

Macules are small (less than 1 cm in diameter), flat lesions that are often red to purple in colour, and tend to appear collectively as a macular rash. In contrast, papules are small (less than 1 cm in diameter), raised, sometimes discoloured (red to purple) lesions that again tend to occur collectively. Either rash may erupt anywhere on the body in various configurations, and may be acute or chronic. Macules and papules characterise a wide variety of skin disorders; they may also result from allergies, and from infectious, neoplastic or systemic disorders. Often a rash is made up of a combination of macules and papules known as 'macular-papular' (for example, measles).

Patches and plaques

A large macule (bigger than 1 cm in diameter) is known as a patch; for example, a café-au-lait spot or a Mongolian blue spot. A papule larger than 1 cm in diameter is known as a plaque; for example, the skin change in psoriasis.

Port-wine stain

Port-wine stains are vascular malformations that usually present at birth and commonly appear on the face and upper body as flat purple marks.

Pruritus

Pruritis is an unpleasant itching sensation is the most common symptom of skin disorders. Patients commonly scratch the area to obtain relief.

I've got you under my skin

Pruritus may also result from a local or systemic disorder, drug use, emotional upset or contact with skin irritants. It may be exacerbated by increased skin temperature, poor skin turgor, local vasodilation and stress. Persistent pruritis should be investigated as it may be an indicator of underlying disease; for example liver disease or some cancers.

Purpuric lesions

Purpuric lesions are important as they are different to most other rashes. Normally, the blood causing the skin discoloration remains in the blood vessels. In contrast, a purpuric lesion is caused by red blood cells and blood pigments which sit under the skin. Consequently, whereas the blood still in the vessels will 'blanch' (disappear revealing the normal skin tone) when pressed, a purpuric lesion doesn't blanch under pressure.

On the spot

The three types of purpuric lesions are:
- petechiae – red or brown pinpoint lesions generally caused by capillary fragility in diseases such as bacterial endocarditis, meningitis and thrombocytopenia
- ecchymoses – bluish or purplish discolorations resulting from blood accumulation in the skin after injury to the vessel walls
- haematomas – masses of blood that accumulate in a tissue, organ or body space after a break in a blood vessel.

Cruisin' for a bruisin'

Purpuric lesions may also produce deep red or reddish/purple bruising that may be caused by bleeding disorders such as disseminated intravascular coagulation or meningococcal septicaemia.

Looking in the glass

An easy way to work out whether a rash is purpuric or not is to press it firmly with the side of a clear drinking glass. If the rash disappears (blanches) it is unlikely to be purpuric. This test is an important part of the advice parents are given in the detection of meningococcal septicaemia; any unexplained non-blanching rash, especially in a febrile child, should be viewed as a medical emergency. (See *Meningitis Trust* (2007) for further details.) But also remember, in the early stages the rash may blanch, so don't rule out septicaemia with the glass test alone.

Telangiectases

Telangiectases are permanently dilated, small superficial blood vessels that typically form a web-like pattern, although they can be so close together that they appear as a uniform redness.

Spider naevi

Spider naevi, a type of telangiectasis, are small, red lesions that appear as a red central dot with 'legs'. They usually appear on the face, neck, arms, chest or back, and in isolation may be normal. Alternatively they may be associated with pregnancy or liver disease. As a general rule, any patient with more than five or six spider naevi should have further assessment for possible liver disease.

Urticaria

Urticaria is a vascular skin reaction characterised by the eruption of transient itchy wheals – smooth, slightly elevated patches of various shapes and sizes with well-defined red margins and pale centres.

Allergy alert

Urticaria lesions, also called hives, are produced by the local release of histamine or other vasoactive substances as part of a hypersensitivity reaction. Common causes include certain drugs, foods, insect bites, inhalants or contact with certain substances. Urticaria may also result from emotional stress or environmental factors. Any patient with an acute onset of urticaria needs to be closely observed for signs of swelling of the subcutaneous tissue and respiratory distress.

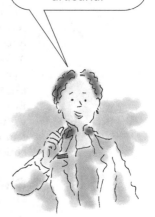

Remember: in addition to allergies, stress and environmental factors can cause urticaria.

Vesicular rash

A vesicular rash is a scattered or linear distribution of blister-like lesions – sharply circumscribed and filled with clear fluid. The lesions, which are less than 1 cm in diameter, may occur singly or in groups. They sometimes occur with bullae – fluid-filled lesions larger than 1 cm in diameter. A vesicular rash may be mild or severe, and temporary or permanent. It can result from infection, inflammation or allergic reactions. It is perhaps most commonly seen in chickenpox.

Hair abnormalities

Typically stemming from other problems, hair abnormalities can cause patients emotional distress. Among the most common hair abnormalities are alopecia and hirsutism.

Alopecia

Alopecia occurs more commonly and more extensively in men than in women. Diffuse hair loss, although commonly a normal part of ageing, may occur as a result of infections, chemical trauma, ingestion of certain drugs and endocrine or other disorders. Tinea capitis, trauma, chemotherapy and third-degree burns can cause patchy or total hair loss, as can stress.

Hirsutism

Excessive hairiness in women, or hirsutism, can develop on the body and face, affecting the patient's self-image. Localised hirsutism may occur on pigmented naevi. Generalised hirsutism can result from certain drug therapy or from such endocrine problems as Cushing's syndrome and acromegaly.

Nail abnormalities

Although many nail abnormalities are harmless, some point to serious underlying problems. Common nail problems include Beau's lines, clubbing, koilonychia, onycholysis, paronychia and Terry's nails.

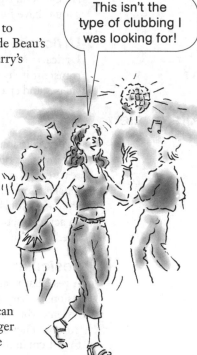

This isn't the type of clubbing I was looking for!

Beau's lines

Beau's lines are transverse depressions in the nail. They occur with acute illness, malnutrition, anaemia and trauma which temporarily impairs nail function. A dent appears first at the cuticle and then moves forward as the nail grows.

Clubbing

With clubbed fingers, the proximal edge of the nail (where it goes under the skin at its base) elevates so the angle when you look across it appears curved or convex, greater than 180 degrees. The nail is also thickened and curved at the end, and the distal phalanx looks rounder and wider than normal. Whilst advanced clubbing is distinctive, giving the fingers a 'drumstick appearance', early clubbing can be harder to spot. To check for clubbing, view the index finger in profile and note the angle of the nail base, or perform the 'diamond test'. (See *Evaluating clubbed fingers*, page 117.)

Koilonychia

Koilonychia refers to thin, spoon-shaped nails with lateral edges that tilt upwards, forming a concave profile. The nails tend to be white and opaque. This condition is associated with some types of anaemia, chronic infections, Raynaud's disease and malnutrition.

Peak technique

Evaluating clubbed fingers

When you see a patient whose fingers are clubbed there are many possible cardiac or respiratory diseases associated with it, including cystic fibrosis, lung cancer, tuberculosis and congenital heart failure. It is also linked with some gastrointestinal problems such as ulcerative colitis and Chron's disease. Many but not all of the changes relate to chronic hypoxia; hence the reasons clubbing occurs are not fully understood. For a full list of associated conditions and further information on clubbing, see Knott (2007).

To examine a patient's fingers for clubbing, hold the nail at eye level and look across it. The normal angle is about 160 degrees. In clubbing, the angle is greater than 180 degrees, as shown. Also gently palpate the bases of the patient's nails. Normally they'll feel firm, but in early clubbing they'll feel spongy.

Another helpful test is the diamond test (or Schamroth's window test). Ask the patient to place the nails of their index, middle or ring fingers together. Normal nail bases are concave and so they create a small, diamond shape as shown above. In early clubbing the diamond of light may vanish, and in later clubbing the now convex nail bases can touch easily but the nails themselves may not meet, as shown.

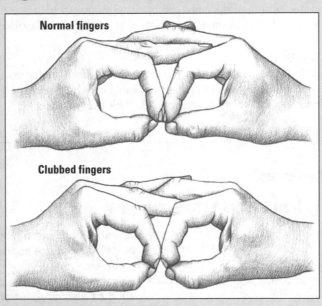

Normal fingers

Clubbed fingers

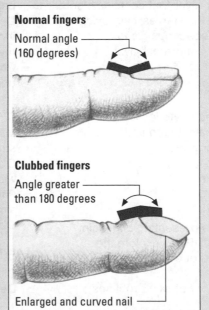

Normal fingers

Normal angle (160 degrees)

Clubbed fingers

Angle greater than 180 degrees

Enlarged and curved nail

Onycholysis

Onycholysis is the loosening of the nail plate with separation from the nail bed. It's associated with minor trauma to long fingernails, and such disease processes as psoriasis, contact dermatitis, hyperthyroidism and pseudomonas infections. Note that psoriasis can also cause pitting of the nails, giving an appearance which is similar to the effect of pushing a toothbrush into a piece of plasticine.

Terry's nails

Terry's nails are characterised by transverse bands of white that cover the nail, except for a narrow band at the distal end which remains pink. They are most commonly associated with liver disease.

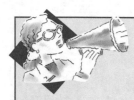

That's a wrap!

Skin, hair and nails review

Skin

Skin structures

- Epidermis – thin outer layer composed of epithelial tissue
- Dermis – thick, deeper layer that contains blood vessels, lymphatic vessels, nerves, hair follicles as well as sweat and sebaceous glands
- Subcutaneous tissue – innermost layer.

Functions

- Protects tissues
- Prevents water and electrolyte losses
- Senses temperature, pain, touch and pressure
- Regulates body temperature
- Synthesises vitamin D
- Promotes wound repair.

Health history

- Determine the patient's presenting complaint.
- Use PQRSTU or OLD CART to explore the symptoms. Ask detailed questions about any skin lesion or rash.
- Ask about a family history of skin problems including skin cancer.

- Ask about any other skin problems, hair loss or gain and about sudden or gradual nail changes.
- Ask about associated signs and symptoms, such as discharge, fever, weight loss and joint pain.
- Determine which medications the patient takes, including over-the-counter and alternative medicines.
- Check patients' experience of sun exposure and understanding of the risks.

Assessment

- Inspect and palpate the texture – it should be smooth and intact.
- Observe for moisture content – it should be dry with a minimal amount of perspiration.
- Palpate the skin for temperature, checking each side for localised temperature changes.
- Observe for skin lesions.

Lesion assessment

- Classify the lesion as primary or secondary.
- Determine whether it's solid or fluid-filled.

(continued)

Skin, hair and nails review *(continued)*

- Check for symmetry, and check the borders to see if they're regular or irregular.
- Note the lesion's colour as well as its pattern, location and distribution.
- Measure the lesion's diameter using a millimetre–centimetre (mm–cm) ruler. Note any enlargement or elevation.
- Describe any drainage, noting the type, colour, amount and odour.

Abnormal findings

- Café-au-lait spots – flat, light brown, uniformly hyperpigmented macules or patches on the skin surface
- Cherry angiomas – tiny, bright red, round papules that may become brown over time
- Macular rash – small, flat red or purple lesions
- Papular rash – small, raised, circumscribed and perhaps discoloured (red to purple) lesions appearing in various configurations
- Port-wine haemangiomas – flat, purple marks usually present at birth that may appear on the face and upper body
- Pruritus – unpleasant itching sensation
- Purpuric lesions – petechiae (brown, pinpoint lesions), ecchymoses (bluish or purplish discolourations), haematomas (masses of accumulated blood)
- Telangiectases – permanently dilated, small blood vessels sometimes in a web-like or spider pattern
- Urticaria – vascular skin reaction of transient itchy wheals
- Vesicular rash – scattered or linear distribution of blister-like lesions filled with serous fluid.

Hair

Structures

- Formed from keratin
- Lies in a hair follicle, receiving nourishment from the papilla, and is attached at the base by the arrector pili.

Assessment

- Inspect and palpate the hair over the patient's entire body, noting distribution, quantity, texture and colour.
- Check for patterns of hair loss and growth.
- Inspect the scalp for erythema, scaling and encrustations.

Abnormal findings

- Alopecia – hair loss
- Hirsutism – excessive hairiness in women.

Nails

Structures

- Nail root (or nail matrix) – site of nail growth
- Nail plate – visible, hardened layer that covers the fingertip
- Lunula – white, crescent-shaped area that extends beyond the cuticle.

Assessment

- Examine the nails for colour, shape, thickness and consistency.

Abnormal findings

- Beau's lines – transverse depressions in the nail extending to the bed
- Clubbing – proximal end of the nail elevates so the angle is greater than 180 degrees
- Koilonychia – thin, spoon-shaped nails with lateral edges that tilt upward
- Onycholysis – nail-plate loosening with separation from the nail bed
- Terry's nails – transverse bands of white that cover the nail.

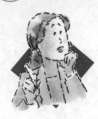

Quick quiz

1. Asymmetric borders on a lesion suggest a:
    A.   benign lesion.
    B.   malignant lesion.
    C.   normal variation.
    D.   vesicular lesion.

2. Skin temperature is best assessed with the:
    A.   fingertips.
    B.   fingers.
    C.   palm of the hand.
    D.   back of the hand.

3. Hirsutism refers to:
    A.   hair loss.
    B.   excessive hairiness, especially in women.
    C.   dry skin.
    D.   dark lines across the nails.

4. A small, blister-like, raised fluid-filled lesion, less than 1 cm in diameter, is known as a:
    A.   macule.
    B.   papule.
    C.   vesicle.
    D.   bullae.

5. As you assess your patient, you note clubbed fingers. This is a sign of:
    A.   malnutrition.
    B.   cardiovascular disease.
    C.   bacterial infection.
    D.   allergic reaction.

For answers see page 399.

6 Eyes

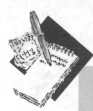

Just the facts

In this chapter, you'll learn:

♦ the importance of eye assessments

♦ eye structures and their functions

♦ questions to ask about the eyes during the health history

♦ techniques for assessing the eyes

♦ ways to recognise normal and abnormal variations in the eyes.

A look at the eyes

The eyes are a major source of sensory information. Disorders in vision can interfere with a patient's ability to function independently, perceive the world and enjoy beauty. A thorough assessment of your patient's eyes and vision can help you to identify problems that can affect their health and quality of life. In many cases, early detection can lead to successful, sight-saving treatment.

The eyes have it!

Many changes to the eye which cause visual problems occur as a result of the ageing process. Thus the overall incidence of severe sight problems is likely to rise as the population ages. Primary causes of severe sight problems or vision loss in older people include diabetic retinopathy, glaucoma, cataracts and macular degeneration – conditions more common in older patients than in younger ones.

Other threats to sight include infections such as toxoplasmosis or cytomegalovirus retinitis, or infections associated with human immunodeficiency virus and acquired immunodeficiency syndrome.

Infants and children are at risk of particular sight problems. Infants can be born with congenital cataracts, congenital glaucoma or retinoblastomas. Children's sight can be affected by strabismus (squint). This needs correcting before the age of 7 or 8 years, or visual impairment may be permanent in the affected eye due to lack of use (Patient UK 2008). A similar problem can occur if a child is very short sighted or long sighted in one eye, causing the brain to rely on the other eye and not use the affected one.

Structures of the eye

In this section, we'll look at the external (extraocular) structures as well as the internal (intraocular) structures of the eye. (See *A close look at the eye*, below.)

A close look at the eye

This cross-section details important anatomic structures of the eye.

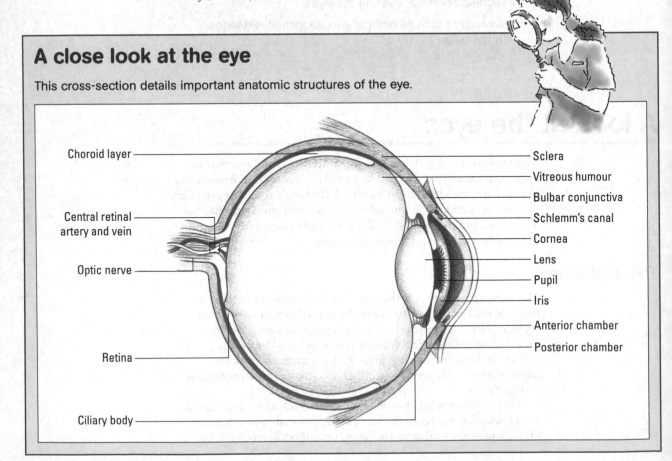

Choroid layer

Central retinal artery and vein

Optic nerve

Retina

Ciliary body

Sclera

Vitreous humour

Bulbar conjunctiva

Schlemm's canal

Cornea

Lens

Pupil

Iris

Anterior chamber

Posterior chamber

Extraocular structures

The eyes are delicate sensory organs equipped with many protective structures. On the outside, the bony orbits protect the eyes from trauma. Eyelids (or palpebrae), lashes and the lacrimal apparatus (tear ducts) protect the eyes from injury, dust and foreign bodies.

Conjunctiva

A thin, transparent membrane, the conjunctiva lines the eyelid (the palpebral conjunctiva). It also covers and protects the anterior portion of the white sclera (the bulbar conjunctiva).

Extraocular muscles

Also included as part of the extraocular structures are the six extraocular muscles. Innervated (stimulated) by the cranial nerves (III oculomotor, IV trochlear and VI abducens), these muscles control the movement of the eyes. The coordinated actions of these muscles allow the eyes to move in tandem, ensuring clear vision.

Intraocular structures

The eye contains multiple structures that function together to provide vision. Some structures are easily visible, whereas others can only be viewed with special instruments. Here's a brief review of these structures.

Sclera and choroid

The white coating on the outside of the eyeball, the sclera, maintains the eye's size and shape. The choroid, which forms the middle layer between the sclera and the inner retina, is darkly pigmented, and contains a network of arteries and veins that maintain blood supply to the back of the eye.

Cornea

The cornea is a smooth, avascular, transparent tissue that merges with the sclera at the limbus (the border between cornea and sclera) to cover the iris and pupil. It refracts, or bends, light rays entering the eye. The cornea is innervated by the sensory ophthalmic branch of cranial nerve V (the trigeminal nerve). Stimulation of this nerve triggers cranial nerve VII, the facial nerve, to initiate a protective blink, this is known as the corneal reflex.

Iris

The iris is a circular, contractile diaphragm that contains smooth and radial muscles, and is perforated in the centre by the pupil. Varying amounts of pigment granules within the smooth-muscle fibres give the iris its colour. Its posterior portion contains involuntary muscles that control pupil size and so regulate the amount of light entering the eye.

Pupil

The pupils are normally round and equal in size. The pupil permits light to enter the eyes. Depending on the patient's age, normal adult pupil diameter in daylight or a well-lit room ranges from 3 to 5 millimetres (Bickley and Szilagyi 2007). Small and unresponsive to light at birth, the pupil enlarges during childhood and then progressively decreases in size throughout adulthood.

Anterior and posterior chambers

The anterior chamber is the space between the cornea and the iris, whereas the posterior chamber is a ring-like space between the iris and the lens. Both chambers are filled with clear aqueous humour. The production and drainage of the fluid is controlled in order to maintain a constant pressure in the eye, circulating from the posterior chamber to the anterior chamber through the pupil, and then draining out through Schlemm's canal. Drainage problems lead to a build-up of pressure – acute or chronic glaucoma. The aqueous humour gives the front of the eye its shape and provides nourishment to the cornea and lens.

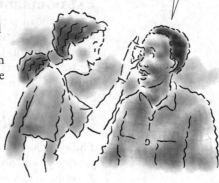

I can tell by the shape of your eyeball that you clearly have a great sense of aqueous humour.

Lens

Located directly behind the iris at the pupillary opening, the lens consists of avascular, transparent fibrils in an elastic membrane called the lens capsule. The lens refracts and focuses light onto the retina, and its shape varies to adjust for near or far vision.

Ciliary body

The ciliary body connects the iris and the choroid. Within it are the ciliary muscles, which control the shape of the lens. The ciliary body also produces the aqueous humour.

Vitreous chamber

The vitreous chamber, located behind the lens, occupies four-fifths of the eyeball. This chamber is filled with vitreous humour, a thick, gelatinous substance that fills the centre of the eye and maintains the placement of the retina and the shape of the eyeball.

Retina

The retina is the innermost layer of eyeball. It receives visual stimuli and converts the light into electrical impulses which are transmitted to the brain for processing.

Various vessels

There are four sets of retinal blood vessels, which are visible through an ophthalmoscope. Each set of vessels contains an artery and a vein. Arteries are lighter red, narrower and brighter, whereas veins are darker and wider. As the vessels leave the optic disc, they become progressively thinner, intertwining as they extend to the periphery of the retina.

Optic disc and physiologic cup

The optic disc is a well-defined, round or oval area within the retina's nasal portion. It is the opening through which the ganglion nerve axons (fibres) exit the retina to form the optic nerve (cranial nerve II). This area is known as the 'blind spot' because no light-sensitive cells (photoreceptors) are located there. Abnormal swelling of the optic disc will enlarge the blind spot.

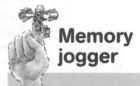

Memory jogger

To remember that cones are cells that respond to colour, think of a brightly coloured ice cream cone!

Cup and cover

The physiologic cup is a light-coloured depression within the temporal (outer) side of the optic disc where blood vessels enter the retina. It is not always visible, but if it is, it should be no larger than half the diameter of the disc.

Photoreceptor neurones

Photoreceptor neurones make up the retina's visual receptors. Not visible through the ophthalmoscope, these receptors – some shaped like rods and some like cones – are responsible for vision. Rods respond to low-intensity light, but they don't provide sharp images or colour vision. Cones respond to bright light and provide high-acuity colour vision.

Macula and fovea centralis

Located laterally from the optic disc, the macula is slightly darker than the rest of the retina and contains no visible retinal vessels. Because its borders are poorly defined, the macula is difficult to see on an ophthalmologic examination. It's best identified by asking the patient to look straight at the ophthalmoscope's light.

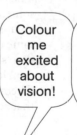

Colour me excited about vision!

What colour? I don't see any colours.

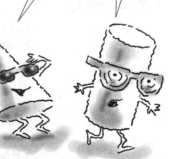

Cone container

The fovea centralis, a slight depression in the macula, appears as a bright reflection when examined with an ophthalmoscope. Because the fovea contains the heaviest concentration of cones, it acts as the eye's clearest, sharpest vision and colour receptor. Patients with macular degeneration lose their central vision, and thus the ability to read and to see small objects clearly.

Obtaining a health history

Now that you're familiar with the normal anatomy and physiology of the eyes, you're ready to obtain a health history of them. The most common eye-related complaints include double vision (diplopia), visual floaters (seeing small, dark shadowy spots or lines), photophobia (light sensitivity), vision loss, visual field loss (partial loss of sight in one or both eyes), eye pain, decreased visual acuity (clarity), defects in colour vision and difficulty seeing at night. Distinguishing between symptoms that have occurred gradually and symptoms that have come on suddenly is a key part of your assessment; typically, symptoms of sudden onset require more urgent intervention.

Eye emergencies

The extent of your interview, and the point at which you refer someone for specialist review, will vary. Certain presenting complaints which have occurred *suddenly* need to be referred the same day for specialist review. These include pain, multiple floaters or a 'shower' of floaters, flashing lights, blurred or distorted vision, double vision, halos, photophobia, loss of vision and visual field loss. Chemical or penetrating injury to the eye is a medical emergency that requires immediate intervention.

Ask anyway

Even if a patient's reason for seeking care isn't primarily eye-related, its often important to gather some information about his/ her eyes and vision. Keep in mind that poor vision can affect the patient's ability to comply with treatment. A patient complaining of a gradual recent change in close or distance vision requires non-urgent review by an optometrist (sometimes referred to as a prescribing optician).

Asking about eyes

If the patient's presenting complaint relates to an eye problem, use the PQRSTU or OLD CART mnemonic (page 16) to gain a

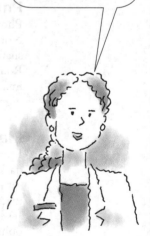

Even if the patient's presenting complaint isn't eye-related, you still need to ask questions about eyes and vision.

comprehensive picture of the signs and symptoms. In addition, it will be useful to explore the following points:
• Does the patient wear glasses or contact lenses for distance vision and/or for reading?
• Does the patient have any visual problems not currently corrected by glasses or lenses, including difficulty seeing at a distance or reading/seeing close objects?
• Do they have, or have they ever experienced, blurred vision, blind spots, floaters, double vision, discharge, a squint (strabismus), colour blindness or unusual sensitivity to light?
• Does the patient have trouble seeing at night? Is this a new or long-term problem?
• Has the patient ever had an eye injury or eye surgery?
• Is the patient experiencing eye pain or recurrent headaches?

Asking about general health

Now that you've asked the patient questions about their eyes, broaden your assessment to include questions about other diseases, medications, work issues and smoking habits.

Family matters

Ask the patient if there is a history of hypertension, diabetes, stroke, Grave's disease, multiple sclerosis, syphilis or human immunodeficiency virus. Find out if anyone in the family has glaucoma, cataracts, vision loss, diabetes, retinal detachment or retinitis pigmentosa. A family history may increase risk to the patient of these conditions, so frequent testing will be indicated. UK patients with diabetes or glaucoma, those over 40-years-old with a close relative who has glaucoma and all children and patients over 60-years-old, are entitled to free eye checks from the National Health Service.

Drug connection

Ask the patient about medication. Note that some drugs can affect vision. For example, digoxin (Lanoxin) overdose can cause a patient to see yellow halos around bright lights. Remember to ask about over-the-counter drugs, herbal preparations and eye drops/eyewashes too.

All in a day's work

Ask the patient about their work and leisure activities to assess potential risks to their eyes. Is he/she exposed to chemicals, fumes, flying debris or infectious agents? If so, do they wear eye protection? All patients should wear protective eyewear when working with substances that may injure the eye.

Igniting a problem

If your patient smokes, warn them that smoking increases the risk of vascular disease and macular degeneration, which can lead to blindness or damaged vision.

A view of the situation

If your patient has impaired vision, ask them how well they can manage activities of daily living. Assess whether they need assistance with adaptations in the home, or a referral to an agency that helps people with impaired vision. Occupational therapy referral may be appropriate in this instance, or offering the patient contact details of a charitable organisation that helps the visually impaired. Some optometry practices have a specialist who can recommend for those with impaired vision.

Kiddin' around

If your patient is a young child you may have to rely on the parents for some of the answers, but try to include the child as much as possible. For example, ask if he/she has difficulty at school seeing the whiteboard, the computer or their reading book. Do they have problems playing ball sports or with other sporting activities that require good vision? In contrast, parents may be better placed to tell you if they have noticed a squint (strabismus), where the child's eyes don't seem to move in parallel. Remind parents that eye examinations are free for children, and encourage them to attend for regular check ups. (See *Seeing things differently*, page 129.)

Assessing the eyes

An eye assessment includes inspecting the external eye and lids, testing visual acuity, assessing eye muscle function, palpating the nasolacrimal sac and examining intraocular structures with an ophthalmoscope.

Gather your gear

Before starting your examination, gather the necessary equipment. You are likely to need a good light source, a pen torch, two opaque 'cover cards', an ophthalmoscope, a Snellen chart (vision-test chart) and a pen with a bright coloured (ideally red) cap. Make sure that the patient is seated comfortably and that, where appropriate, you're seated facing the patient at eye level.

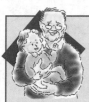

Ages and stages

Seeing things differently

You'll need to modify your health history for a child or an older adult.

Infants

- Find out whether the infant seems to see clearly. Does the infant respond to the parents' facial expressions and make eye contact? Do they reach out for toys and other objects? Do they follow an object moved in front of their eyes?
- If the patient is a neonate with an eye infection, ask if the infant was delivered vaginally, and if so whether the mother may have had an infection at the time? (Inform the parents that sexually transmitted infections such as chlamydia, gonorrhoea, genital herpes or candidiasis can be contracted at birth and cause eye problems in infants.)

Children

- Is the child reaching normal developmental milestones? If there are any delays, consider whether vision might be a problem.
- Does the child seem to have any problems at school? Note: inattention or bad behaviour sometimes turns out to be linked to the child being bored because they can't see the board or computer screen properly.

- Has the parent ever noticed that both eyes don't always seem to move in parallel, indicating strabismus?
- Does the child seem to screw their eyes up excessively when trying to look at things, suggesting difficulty in focusing?

Older people

- Check if your patient has any difficulty climbing stairs or driving. Offer urgent safety advice if appropriate.
- Does the patient tend to trip or fall frequently? This could be related to sight problems.
- Is the patient being tested regularly for glaucoma? They should be checked once every 2 years by an optometrist.
- Does the patient have diabetes? If so, are their eyes checked regularly for diabetic retinopathy?
- Have they noticed any changes or deterioration in their vision in recent months or years. Remember that cataracts and macular degeneration are also common problems in older people.

Inspecting the eyes

Start your assessment by observing the patient's face. With the scalp line as the starting point, check that the eyes are in a normal position. They should be level, about one-third of the way down the face and about one eye's width apart from each other. Note that dysmorphic features (unusual facial features) may be indicative of underlying congenital abnormalities.

Eye shape and eyelids

As you look at the eyes, check the shape of opening between the upper and lower lids (the palpebral fissures). This should be oval/almond shaped and symmetrical, although note there will be some cultural and individual variations. Each upper eyelid should cover only the top of the iris, and none of the pupil. Look for a 'drooping eyelid', known as a ptosis. If they have one, ask if it's longstanding or a recent change. It may be linked to a problem with cranial nerve III.

What big eyes you have

Also check for an excessive amount of visible sclera above (and possibly below) the iris – this is known as lid retraction and is often associated with thyroid disease. Visible sclera above the irises as the patient looks down is known as lid lag; again associated with thyroid disease. A fixed visible sclera above the eyes with partial coverage of the lower iris ('sunset' eyes) is linked with hydrocephalus in infants. Protrusion of the eyeballs, which is associated with thyroid disease, Grave's disease and orbital tumour, is known as exophthalmos.

Also assess the lids for redness, oedema, inflammation, lumps or lesions. For example, a 'stye' (a hordeolum) is a common eyelid lesion.

Crying or drying?

Inspect the eyes for excessive tearing or dryness. The eyelid margins should be pink, and the eyelashes should turn outward. Observe whether the lower eyelids turn inward toward the eyeball, called entropion (if seen, check for corneal abrasions), or excessively outward, called ectropion.

Pressing the point

If indicated by a history of excessive tears being produced from the eye, palpate the nasolacrimal sac (which drains tears from the eye). Ask the patient to look up, and with a gloved finger gently palpate the area just inside the lower orbital rim close to the medial (inner) canthus, noting tenderness, swelling or discharge through the lacrimal point. This indicates possible blockage of the nasolacrimal duct. Avoid doing this if the area is very inflamed and tender.

Conjunctiva

To inspect the conjunctiva (the delicate mucous membrane that covers the exposed surface of the sclera) ask your patient to look up. Gently pull the lower eyelid down or ask the patient to do this for you. The conjunctiva should be clear and shiny. Note excessive

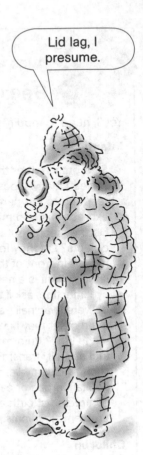

Lid lag, I presume.

redness or exudate, or excessive pallor especially on the outer edge next to the eyelashes, indicating possible anaemia. Also look for any other abnormal colour changes, foreign bodies or oedema.

It is also possible to inspect under the upper eyelids if indicated, but this is a specialised technique that should only be undertaken by a practiced examiner or under the supervision of one.

True colours

Also, observe the sclera's colour, which should be white or creamy white. In darker-skinned patients, you may see flecks of tan. A yellowy discoloration may be a relatively early sign of jaundice, which is not yet visible elsewhere. A bluish discoloration may indicate scleral thinning, or in children a condition called 'brittle bones' (ontogenesis imperfecta).

Anterior chamber, cornea and iris

The cornea should be clear and without lesions. The irises should be the same size, colour and shape. The iris should appear flat, and the cornea should appear convex. Excess pressure in the eye – such as that caused by glaucoma – may push the iris forward, but this is very difficult to recognise. Glaucoma is a major preventable cause of sight loss. All patients over 40-years-old should have an expert glaucoma check from an optometrist every 2 years, as initial onset of chronic glaucoma may be asymptomatic. For more information on glaucoma, see Royal National Institute for the Blind (2007).

Pupil

The pupils should be round and equal in size, about 3 to 5 millimetres (mm) in diameter in normal room light. Cranial nerves II (optic) and III (oculomotor) are responsible for maintaining pupil size and shape. Some people, about one in five, have minor (less than 0.5 mm) inequality in pupil size without disease – anisocoria (Bickley and Szilagyi 2007). Try to establish whether pupil inequality is new or 'has always been that way'. If it occurred recently, unequal pupils may indicate neurological damage, iritis, glaucoma or therapy with certain drugs. A fixed pupil that doesn't react to light can be an ominous neurological sign.

In perfect agreement

Test the pupils for direct and consensual response to light; this is controlled by cranial nerve III. In a darkened room, ask the patient to look into the distance to dilate the pupils. Bring a pen torch in from the side, about 10 cm from the patient, and shine it on the pupil (check it's not shining in the other eye at all). Note the speed and extent of constriction of the pupil you're testing (direct response) and the opposite pupil (consensual response). They should both react the same way due to their link via the optic chiasma. Note any sluggishness or inequality in the response. Repeat the test with the other pupil.

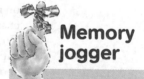

Memory jogger

To make sure that your pupil assessment is complete, think of the acronym **PERRLA**.

Pupils

Equal

Round

Reactive to

Light and

Accommodation

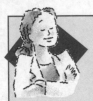

Peak technique

Tips for assessing corneal sensitivity

Corneal sensitivity testing is only undertaken when clinically indicated, as it is uncomfortable for the patient and not without risk. To test corneal sensitivity, touch a wisp of cotton from a cotton wool ball onto the cornea, approaching from the side.

The patient should blink. Not blinking suggests they may have suffered damage to the sensory fibres of cranial nerve V (trigeminal) or to the motor fibres controlled by cranial nerve VI (facial).

Keep in mind that people who wear contact lenses may have reduced sensitivity because they're accustomed to having objects in their eyes.

Just a wisp

Remember that a wisp of cotton wool is the only safe object to use for this test. Even though a gauze pad or tissue is soft, it can cause corneal abrasions and irritation.

Willing to accommodate

Accommodation is the ability of the eye to change in order to focus on near and far objects, involving cranial nerves III and IV. A key change is in the shape of the lens, but you cannot see this happening. What you can see is pupil convergence and constriction when the patient looks at a near object. To test this, place a pen or your finger about 10 cm from the bridge of the patient's nose. Ask the patient to look at a distant object directly in front of the pen, and then tell them to look at the pen/your finger. Their pupils should constrict and their eyes converge (move inwards) as they focus on the near object. To remind yourself what to look for, remember there are two c's in accommodation – one for convergence and one for constriction.

Testing visual acuity

To test your patient's central vision there are a range of eye testing charts. For distance vision, use a Snellen chart. Near vision can be tested with a near-vision chart. To test peripheral vision, use the confrontation test.

Before each test, consider if it is necessary to ask the patient to remove corrective lenses, if worn. Whilst an optometrist's eye test is typically done without correction, tests as part of a cranial nerve assessment (CN II), or to assess a sudden change in the eyes, are probably better performed with vision corrected. This allows you to assess changes compared with what is 'normal' for the patient. Remember when you document the results to note whether the vision was corrected or uncorrected.

Snellen chart

Ask the patient to sit or stand 6 m from the chart (or 3 m if a reversed chart is being reflected into a mirror) and then ask them to cover their left eye with an opaque cover card. (This is better than the hand as it makes the pupil dilate less, making testing the second side easier. It also prevents cheating!) Ask the patient to read the letter on the top line of the chart and then to move downwards to the increasingly smaller lines until it becomes apparent he/she can no longer discern all of the letters. Allow several seconds for refocusing of the previously covered eye, and then ask the patient to repeat the test covering the right eye. (For illustrations and guidance regarding documentation, see *Visual acuity charts*, page 134.)

Can't see it!

If the patient can't see any of the letters from 6 m, stand them 3 m away and record the findings accordingly. If that also fails, assess whether they can count the number of fingers you are holding up, and failing that whether they can differentiate light and dark.

The Big E

Use the Snellen E chart or the Snellen picture chart to test visual acuity in young children and other patients who can't read. The picture chart is a visual recognition test of common objects. (Although if the patient struggles, check they can recognise the object when shown to them close up!) The E test requires the patient to have a copy of the E shape on the chart, and to hold it in the correct orientation to indicate which way the letter faces. Or ask a child to pretend it's a table with three legs and point their fingers in the same direction as the legs. It is also possible to obtain charts with letters from other alphabets.

If your patient can't read, use the Snellen E!

Near-vision chart

If indicated, also test near vision. Ask the patient to cover one eye as before, and hold a near-vision testing card 35 cm from his/her eyes. Ask them to read the line with the smallest letters he/she can see. Repeat the test with the other eye. Scoring follows similar principles

Visual acuity charts

The most commonly used charts for testing vision are the Snellen alphabet chart (left) and the Snellen E chart (right), which is used for young children and adults who can't read. Both charts are used to test distance vision and measure visual acuity. The patient reads each chart at a distance of 6 m.

Documenting findings

Note just above or below each line there is a tiny number. This refers to the line that an average typical patient could see from that distance. For example, the top letter is often the 60 line – an average patient would see this from 60 m away. Towards the bottom will be the line marked with a 6. This is the line that an average patient can see from 6 m (your test distance); that is, normal vision.

20/20 vision

North America measures normal vision at 20 feet rather than 6 m, hence the phrase 20:20 vision. In the UK this is recorded in m; 6/6 vision. Any other finding is recorded with the first number a 6 (that is, the patient 6 m away) and the second number indicating the line the patient was able to read. For example, 6/6 left eye, 6/9 right eye.

Getting one letter wrong is typically recorded as −1, for example 6/6−1. More than two mistakes generally means the patient failed on that line, and the result is usually recorded as the line above.

Some charts have lines for 'better than average' vision – enabling a patient to score 6/4, for example (that is, they can see at 6 m what an average person could only see from 4 m).

Snellen alphabet chart

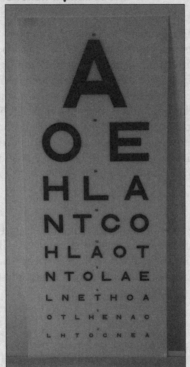

Snellen E chart

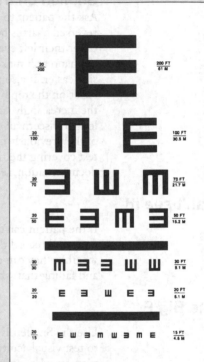

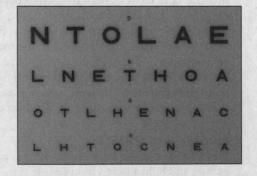

Visual acuity charts *(continued)*

Screening children

Children usually need to be aged between 3 and 4 years before they can cope with even an E chart or a picture chart test. Use of a 3 m chart is often recommended. Note that in children, 6/6 vision is not achieved until the age of around 6 to 7 years. Levels which require referral to an optician are 6/15 for 3-year-olds and 6/12 for 4 to 5-year-olds. A score of 6/9 in 4 to 5-year-olds should be rechecked in a year. A difference between eyes of two lines or more should also be referred.

to the Snellen chart, although a greater variety of near-vision testing cards exist. If you don't have an appropriate chart, use a magazine or newspaper with small print. Either way, ask the patient to tell you if they feel their vision has *suddenly* deteriorated compared with what is normal for them.

Peripheral vision

To assess peripheral vision, use a method known as visual fields by confrontation. This test can help to identify abnormalities in the visual field, which may include partial loss of the visual fields in one or both eyes. (See *Testing visual fields by confrontation*, page 136.)

Assessing eye muscle function

A thorough assessment of the eyes includes an evaluation of the extraocular muscles. To evaluate these muscles, you'll need to assess the corneal light reflection and the cardinal positions of gaze, and then, if indicated, perform the cover – uncover test (see below).

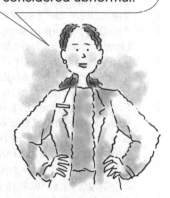

When you cover and then uncover the patient's eye, it should remain still. Any movement is considered abnormal.

Ages and stages

Strabismus in children

Strabismus is the most common abnormal eye movement in children. Although severe strabismus is readily apparent, mild strabismus must be confirmed by tests for misalignment, such as the corneal light reflex test and the cover–uncover test.

To perform a cover–uncover test, ask the child to stare at a wall on the other side of the room. Then cover one eye, and as you do so watch for movement in the uncovered eye. Movement is abnormal – a normal response is a steady fixed gaze. Remove the eye cover and watch for movement in the newly uncovered eye; again movement is abnormal. Repeat the test with the other eye.

Such testing is crucial because early corrective measures help to preserve vision, and also enhance cosmetic appearance. Be aware that mild strabismus is a rare but important sign of retinoblastoma.

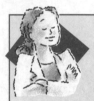

Peak technique

Testing visual fields by confrontation

There are several variations of the tests for assessing peripheral vision. However, this test (Jarvis 2008) is designed to give you a precise assessment of your patient's visual fields. Remember you can't do this test if you don't have normal peripheral vision yourself:

- Sit directly across from the patient and ask them to focus their gaze on your eyes.
- Ensure you are close enough to put your hand on the patient's shoulder.
- Get the patient to cover one eye with a cover card, and cover your own eye on the same side of the room (for example, the patient's left eye, your right eye).
- Place a brightly topped marker pen (top downwards) as high as you can, halfway between you and the patient, so that neither of you can see it. Check the patient can't see it.
- Ask the patient to keep their head and eyes still, looking directly ahead.
- Now move the pen *slowly* down, coloured end first, asking the patient to tell you when they see it. You and the patient should both see it at about the same time – the typical angle being about 50 degrees (assuming looking forward is 0 degrees and directly above is 90 degrees).
- Repeat this from below (normal angle 70 degrees) and then from the nasal (covered) side of the eye you are examining (normal angle 60 degrees).
- Now to examine the temporal side, uncover your own eye and place the pen behind the patient's ear. Bring it forward in an arc and ask them to tell you when they see it. Normal temporal peripheral vision is greater than 90 degrees (which is why the examiner can't just hold their hand out at arms length to check this as the full angle wouldn't be tested).

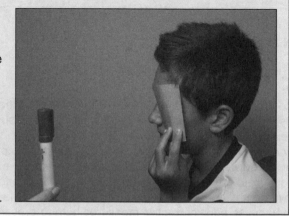

- If vision is normal, the patient should see the pen just before it gets level with their eye.
- Note: it is good practise, especially if you have any abnormal findings on any of the four fields, to also test the four diagonals in the same way as the first three fields. For an alternative, simple screening test, see Chapter 14.

Corneal light reflection

To assess the corneal light reflection (sometimes called the corneal light reflex), ask the patient to look straight ahead, then shine a pen torch on the bridge of the nose from about 40 cm away, and ask the patient to look at the light. The light should fall at the same spot on each cornea. If it doesn't, the eyes aren't being held in the same plane by the extraocular muscles. This commonly occurs in a patient who lacks muscle coordination (that is, strabismus). This is not an unusual finding, but if it is something that the patient was unaware of, it is best checked out by an optometrist. Acute onset strabismus is likely to result in double vision, and would require same-day referral.

Cardinal positions of gaze

Cardinal positions of gaze evaluate cranial nerves III (oculomotor), IV (trochlear) and VI (abducens) and the extraocular muscles they supply. There are six cardinal positions of gaze. Abducens is responsible for lateral eye movement (looking sideways), trochlear for downward–inward movement (such as when walking down stairs) and oculumotor is responsible for the rest (medial, upward–inward, downward–outward and upward–outward). (See *Cardinal positions of gaze*, below.)

Cardinal positions of gaze

The illustration below identifies the six cardinal positions of gaze in each eye.

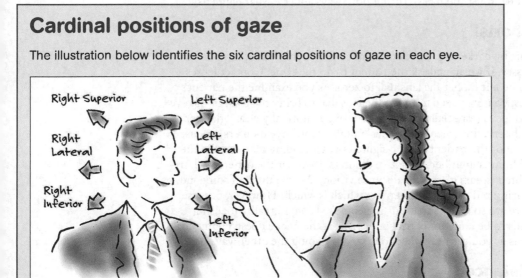

Right Superior   Left Superior

Right Lateral   Left Lateral

Right Inferior   Left Inferior

Eyeballs on the move

Techniques for this test vary; the H test (Bickley and Szilagyi 2007) is probably most comfortable for the patient. To perform this test, sit directly facing the patient. Hold a marker pen or other similar object at a distance of about 45 cm. Ask the patient to follow the object with their eyes, without moving their head. Taking your starting point at eye level, draw an imaginary H starting in the middle of the horizontal bar (this should be opposite the bridge of the nose). Then, without 'taking your pen off the page', move the object in a H-shaped pattern, making the H large enough to move the eyeballs fully through all six cardinal positions of gaze.

The patient's eyes should remain parallel as they move. Note abnormal findings such as any loss of parallel movement or any nystagmus (a sideways oscillation or flickering of the eyeballs, although a slight flicker on extreme lateral gaze is normal).

Examining intraocular structures

The ophthalmoscope allows you to directly observe the eye's internal structures. Take a few moments to familiarise yourself with the opthalmoscope and how it works. Get used to looking through it at your hand; focus on a ring, your nail or your watch perhaps. Practise holding it in both hands. Get used to putting your finger on the lens dial to adjust the focus. Turn it both ways and see what happens.

Green long, red shorts!

Start by darkening the room as much as possible. Remove your glasses, if worn, and ask the patient to do the same. Contact lenses can be left in. Set the lens dial to zero. As you examine the patient's eyes, you may need to adjust the lens dial to bring the back of the eye into focus (especially if one or both of you normally wears glasses). In theory, the green/black 'plus' numbers (positive diopters) are used if you or the patient is long-sighted (wears reading glasses), and the red 'minus' numbers (negative diopters) if you or the patient is short-sighted (wears glasses for distance vision). Maybe think of someone wearing red shorts to remember which is which! However, because there are so many variations in people's vision, in reality focusing tends to be a matter of trial and error! If the image doesn't come into focus as you turn the wheel one way, try going the other way.

Gazing into the distance

As you begin the examination, ask the patient to focus on a point behind you. Tell them that you'll be moving into their visual field and blocking their view, but to keep staring into the distance. Also,

Seeing eye to eye

This illustration shows the correct position for the examiner and the patient when an ophthalmoscope is used to examine the eye's internal structures.

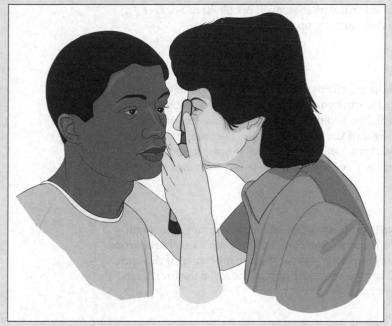

explain that you'll be shining a bright light into their eye, which may be uncomfortable but not harmful. Tell them to blink if they need to. (See *Seeing eye to eye*, above.)

Closing in on the cornea

With the lens dial at zero, hold the ophthalmoscope about 30 to 40 cm from the patient's eye, and position yourself at a 10 to 20 degree angle away from the 'face to face' position, so that you are turned slightly towards the patient's nose. Feel free to close one eye, if you can, as this will help you to concentrate; some texts advocate keeping both eyes open to enhance your binocular vision, but this takes lots of practise! Placing your other hand on the patient's forehead or shoulder can also help you to orientate yourself correctly.

Red eye

Then direct the light through the pupil to elicit the red reflex, a reflection of light off the choroid. This looks a bit like the 'red eye' reflection you see in some photographs taken with flash. Check the red reflex for depth of colour. Remember that it may be more orange than red, and that darker-skinned people have a darker choroid. Note if there are any opaque areas.

Zoom in

Now, keeping the pupil clearly in view, move the ophthalmoscope closer to the eye. Imagine you are aiming the light through the centre of the pupil. You should end almost touching the patient's eyelashes. If the light of the opthalmoscope reflects off the cornea, adjust your position fractionally. If the lens is opaque, indicating cataracts, you may not be able to complete the examination.

On the move

The first thing to remember is that as you look through the pupil with a standard ophthalmoscope you will only see a small proportion of the retina at any one time – about the circumference of the optic disc. So you will have to move the ophthalmoscope fractionally to see different structures.

Rotating to the retinal structures

To examine the retina, start with the dial turned to zero. If necessary, rotate the lens dial into the plus or minus numbers to adjust the focus. It is likely that the first retinal structures you'll see are the blood vessels, and it is often easiest to focus on these. The arteries will look thinner and brighter than the veins, and may have a narrow strip of light reflecting from them.

Pick a vessel and follow it

All the blood vessels you will see branch out from the optic disc. If you don't see the optic disc initially, follow one of the vessels along its path towards the nose until you reach it. The vessels get bigger as they get nearer the disc.

Diggin' the disc and depression

The optic disc is a creamy pink to yellow–orange structure with a clear border and a round-to-oval shape. With practise, you'll be able to identify the physiologic cup, a small depression that occupies up to a half of the disc's diameter. The nasal border of the disc may be somewhat blurred. Note any abnormalities of the disc such as abnormal colour (redness or pallor), blurring, swelling or a larger than expected physiologic cup.

Riveting on the retina

Completely scan the retina by following blood vessels from the optic disk to different peripheral areas (although remember in an undilated pupil you cannot see right to the peripheries). The retina should have a uniform colour and be free from scars and pigmentation. As you scan, look for lesions or haemorrhages. (See *A close look at the retina*, page 142.)

Movin' in on the macula

Finally, move the light laterally from the optic disc to locate the macula. It is about the same size as the optic disc and about two disc widths away from it. It is the part of the eye most sensitive to light, and appears as a darker structure, free from blood vessels. Your view may be fleeting because most patients can't tolerate having a beam of light fall on the macula. To have the best chance of locating it, ask the patient to shift their gaze into the light.

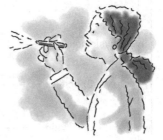

The macula is the part of the eye that's most sensitive to light.

Lastly the lens

Before completing the examination, adjust the dial into the positive numbers (about +6 if you saw the retina from 0) so you can focus on the anterior chamber and lens. Look for clouding, debris or other opacities. Many texts suggest doing this first. However, when you are first learning, it is easier to examine the retina first.

Abnormal findings

Common abnormalities which you may detect during an eye assessment include arteriolar narrowing, decreased visual acuity, diplopia, eye discharge, eye pain, periorbital oedema, ptosis, strabismus, vision loss, visual floaters and visual halos.

Arteriolar abnormalities

Typically, arterioles of the inner eye are between two-thirds and three-quarters of the width of veins and have a brighter appearance. When these minute arteries narrow, they appear to be about one-half as wide as veins, although spotting this difference

A close look at the retina

This illustration shows the complex anatomy of the retina and its structures.

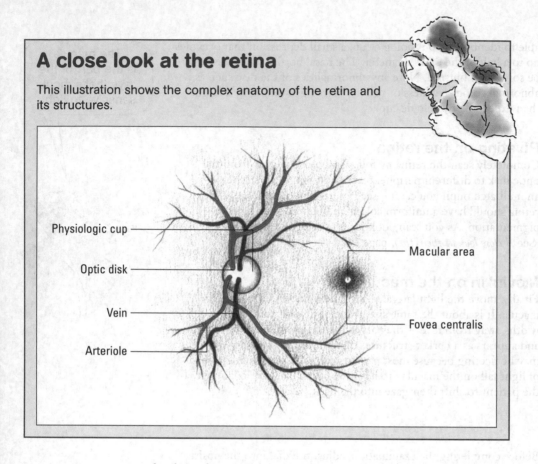

Physiologic cup

Optic disk

Vein

Arteriole

Macular area

Fovea centralis

takes lots of practise! Arteriolar narrowing commonly occurs in patients who have hypertension.

You're nicked

Examine any areas where arteries and veins cross for arteriovenous 'nicking'. This happens when an artery presses on a vein. The vein may look as if it stops abruptly either side of the artery, or look narrow directly under the crossing point and wider either side of it. This is seen in hypertension and arteriosclerosis.

Decreased visual acuity

Decreased visual acuity – problems with the ability to see clearly – commonly occurs with refractive errors. In short sightedness, or myopia, the eye focuses the visual image in front of the retina, causing objects in close view to be seen clearly while those at a distance appear blurry. In long-sightedness, or hyperopia, the eye focuses the visual image behind the retina, causing objects in close view to appear blurry while those at a distance seem clear. Both problems result from an abnormal shape of the eyeball and are likely to require correction with glasses or contact lenses.

> Is your patient seeing double? It must be diplopia.

Lost elastic

Presbyopia is a gradual age-related decline in the ability to focus on close objects due a loss of elasticity in the lens and ciliary muscles. This occurs increasingly commonly from the age of 40, accounting for the very high percentage of middle-aged and older people requiring reading glasses.

Diplopia

When the extraocular muscles are misaligned, the visual axes aren't directed at the object of sight at the same time. This results in double vision, or diplopia.

Discharge

The excretion of any substance from the eyes other than tears is known as a discharge. A common finding, discharge may occur in one or both eyes and may be scant or copious. The discharge may be purulent, frothy, mucoid, cheesy, serous, clear or have a stringy, white appearance. Eye discharge commonly results from inflammatory and infectious eye disorders, such as conjunctivitis, but it may also occur in certain systemic disorders.

Exudates and red dots

As you examine the retina with an ophthalmoscope, you may see tiny grey 'cloud-like' structures called 'exudates'; these occur with diabetes, hypertension, lupus and subacute bacterial endocarditis. Also look for red dots. Red dots with blurred irregular edges are intraretinal haemorrhages, and similar red dots with smooth edges are microaneurysms. Both are linked to hypertension and diabetes. Diabetic retinopathy, as indicated by these and other findings, is a leading cause of blindness in adults, making screening of huge importance. In England, the National Service Framework for Diabetes (DH 2001) mandates regular surveillance for diabetic retinopathy in adults with diabetes. Similar schemes are supported by the other UK countries, with some country-specific variations.

Lid retraction and lid lag

These two terms are often confused. Lid retraction refers to being able to see the sclera above (and sometimes below) the eyelids when the patient is looking directly ahead; that is, the lids are *retracted* (pulled or pushed back). Lid lag refers to the whites of the eyes becoming or remaining visible as the patient looks at an object when it is moved downwards; that is, the lids *lag* behind. Both conditions are linked to thyroid disease, notably hyperthyroidism.

Pain

Eye pain may signal an emergency and requires immediate attention. Diseases causing eye pain include acute glaucoma, iritis and keratitis. Trauma, or corneal damage caused by a foreign body or abrasion, can also cause eye pain. Conjunctivitis may cause significant eye pain, depending on the severity of the infection; milder infections may present with a gritty sensation.

Papilodema

Papilodema is a swelling of the optic disc associated with raised intracranial pressure. It makes the disc appear reddened, congested and blurred at the margins, sometimes a bit like a ring doughnut. This gives a serious indication of probable haemorrhage or tumour.

Periorbital oedema

Swelling around the eyes, or periorbital oedema, may result from allergies, local inflammation, fluid-retaining disorders or persistent crying. It should be observed closely and investigated promptly, as it may have an underlying infective cause which, if untreated, will lead to a periorbital or orbital cellulitis.

Ptosis

Ptosis, or a drooping upper eyelid, may be caused by an interruption in sympathetic innervation to the eyelid, muscle weakness or damage to the oculomotor nerve. (See *Recognising periorbital oedema and ptosis*, page 145.) People sometimes mistakenly think lid lag is another term for ptosis; it is in fact the opposite of ptosis.

Strabismus

In strabismus, the eyes deviate from their normal gazing position. This condition may result from extraocular weakness or paralysis as a result of poor vision in one eye. It may also result from thyroid disease. Although adults may develop strabismus, it most commonly occurs in children. Detected early, it can be corrected without *surgery*. (See *Strabismus in children*, page 135.)

Vision loss

Disorders of any structure of the eye can result in vision loss. Types of vision loss include central vision loss, peripheral vision loss or a

Recognising periorbital oedema and ptosis

During an eye examination, you may observe any of a number of abnormalities. These illustrations show periorbital oedema and ptosis.

Periorbital oedema

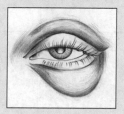

Ptosis

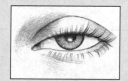

blind spot in the middle of an area of normal vision (scotoma). The degree and location of blindness depends on the disease which is causing the problem, as well as on the location of the lesion. Major causes of blindness include glaucoma, untreated cataracts, retinal disease and macular degeneration.

Visual floaters

Visual floaters are specks of varying shape and size that float through the visual field and disappear when the patient tries to look at them. Caused by small cells floating in the vitreous humour, one or two visual floaters seen occasionally when looking at the sky or a white wall are normal. A sudden onset of a larger number of visual floaters may signal vitreous haemorrhage, posterior uveitis (infection of the choroid) or retinal separation and therefore requires further investigation. A sudden large, black floater or curtain-like loss of vision occurring from above may indicate retinal detachment, and should be reviewed urgently to maximise the chances of preserving sight.

Floaters over 45

Many people over 45 years old will at some point experience a temporary sudden increase in floaters due to posterior vitreal detachment. This is a normal and generally harmless age-related detachment of part of the vitreous humour from the retina, although risk of retinal detachment or tearing is greater in the weeks following the posterior vitreal detachment. However, posterior vitreal detachment cannot be differentiated from more serious conditions without expert examination, so such patients should be referred for same-day assessment.

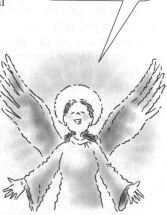

Visual halos may indicate glaucoma, corneal oedema or a fluctuation in blood glucose levels.

Visual halos

Increased intraocular pressure, which occurs in glaucoma, causes the patient to see halos and rainbows around bright lights. Other possible causes include corneal oedema as a result of prolonged contact lens wear or a fluctuation in blood glucose levels.

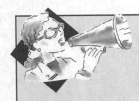

That's a wrap!

Eye review

Eye structures and functions

- Sclera – maintains the eye's size and shape
- Choroid – maintains blood supply to the eye
- Vitreous humour – maintains the placement of the retina and the eyeball's spherical shape
- Cornea – refracts, or bends, light rays entering the eye
- Iris – contains pigment granules that give the eye its colour; contains involuntary muscles that control pupil size
- Pupil – permits light to enter the eye
- Lens – refracts and focuses light onto the retina
- Retina – receives visual stimuli and transmits images to the brain for processing.

Health history

- Determine the patient's presenting complaint.
- Ask if the patient wears glasses or contact lenses.
- Obtain the patient's past medical history – be sure to ask about disorders that may affect vision, such as hypertension, diabetes or stroke.
- Ask about a family history of glaucoma, cataracts, diabetes, retinal detachment or vision loss.
- Obtain a medication history – some medications, such as digoxin (Lanoxin), can affect vision.
- Ask a patient with vision impairment how they manage activities of daily living, and assess support systems.

Assessment

- Note the position of the eyes.
- Check eyelids for closure, ptosis lid retraction, lid lag, redness, oedema, inflammation and lesions.
- Inspect for excessive tearing or dryness.
- Palpate the nasolacrimal sac if indicated by excessive tear production.
- Examine the conjunctiva.
- Inspect the cornea – only assess corneal sensitivity using a wisp of cotton wool, if necessary.
- Evaluate each iris for size, colour and shape.
- Examine the pupils for equal size, shape and reactivity.

Tests for visual acuity

- Test near and distance vision as indicated to measure visual acuity.
- Confrontation – tests peripheral vision and extraocular muscle function by assessing visual fields.
- Corneal light reflection – light should fall at the same spot on each cornea.
- Cardinal positions of gaze – eyes should remain parallel and move smoothly through the six cardinal positions.

Eye review *(continued)*

Ophthalmoscopic examination

- Patient and examiner remove glasses; darken the room.
- Check for the presence and depth of the red reflex.
- Examine the retina: note the characteristics of the blood vessels; identify the optic disc, noting colour, shape and borders; check for any opacities; locate the light-sensitive macula.
- Examine the lens for clouding, debris or opacities.

Abnormal findings

- Arteriolar narrowing – arterioles of the inner eye narrow to a width of about one-half that of vein width
- Decreased visual acuity – the inability to see clearly
- Diplopia – double vision
- Discharge – excretion of any substance other than tears
- Exudates and red dots – you may see these abnormalities as you look at the retina
- Lid retraction and lid lag – seeing the whites of the eyes above the iris when the patient is looking ahead (lid retraction) and when the patient looks down (lid lag)
- Pain – may be of varying degrees of acuity and severity
- Papiloedema – swelling of the disc due to raised intracranial pressure
- Periorbital oedema – swelling around the eyes
- Ptosis – a drooping upper eyelid
- Strabismus – eyes deviate from their normal gazing position
- Vision loss – may be central or peripheral
- Visual floaters – specks of varying shape and size that float through the visual field but disappear when the patient tries to look at them
- Visual halos – rings or halos seen when looking at bright lights.

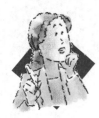

Quick quiz

1. The middle layer of the eyeball is called:
    A. the cornea.
    B. the sclera.
    C. the choroid.
    D. the retina.

2. A drooping eyelid is called:
    A. a strabismus.
    B. a ptosis.
    C. a lid lag.
    D. a stye.

3. Cone receptors are mainly responsible for sensing:
    A. light.
    B. colour.
    C. shapes.
    D. black and white.

4. To determine a patient's visual acuity, you would use:
    A. the Snellen chart.
    B. the near–far test.
    C. the corneal light reflex test.
    D. the cardinal positions of gaze.

5. The red reflex seen during an ophthalmoscope examination is the result of:
    A. an increase in intraocular pressure.
    B. incorrect adjustment of the diopter.
    C. light from the scope reflecting back from the choroid.
    D. arteriolar narrowing.

6. The red negative numbers on the ophthalmoscope are used for examining:
    A. the cornea.
    B. the eyes of a patient who is long-sighted.
    C. the red reflex.
    D. the eyes of a patient who is short-sighted.

For answers see page 399.

7 Ears, nose and throat

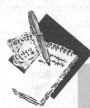

Just the facts

In this chapter, you'll learn:

♦ structures of the ears, nose and throat and their functions

♦ questions to ask about the ears, nose and throat during the health history

♦ techniques for assessing the ears, nose and throat

♦ ear, nose and throat abnormalities and their causes.

A look at the ears, nose and throat

The ability to hear, smell and taste allows us to communicate with others, connect with the world around us and take pleasure in life. Your assessment will not only enable you to identify problems with the ears, nose or throat, but may also uncover important clues to physical problems in the patient's other major body systems.

Anatomy and physiology of the ears, nose and throat

To perform an accurate physical assessment, you'll need to understand the anatomy and physiology of the ears, nose and throat.

Ears

The ear is divided into three parts: external, middle and inner. The anatomy and physiology of each part play separate but equally important roles in hearing. (See *A close look at the ear*, page 150.)

A close look at the ear

Use this illustration to review the structures of the ear.

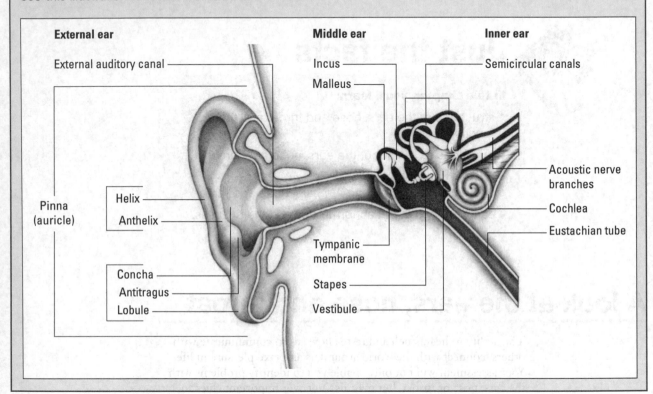

External ear

External auditory canal

Pinna (auricle)

Helix

Anthelix

Concha

Antitragus

Lobule

Middle ear

Incus

Malleus

Tympanic membrane

Stapes

Vestibule

Inner ear

Semicircular canals

Acoustic nerve branches

Cochlea

Eustachian tube

External ear

The flexible external ear consists mainly of elastic cartilage. This part of the ear consists of two parts; the pinna (the visible portion we refer to as the ear), which is also known as the auricle, and the external auditory (or ear) canal. The canal is lined with glands that secrete cerumen, or earwax. The cartilaginous, flap-like structure covering the ear canal is known as the tragus. The outer third of the canal has a bony framework, and its whole length is lined with skin. In men, coarse hair may be visible in the canal. The external ear and ear canal collect sounds and transmit them to the middle ear.

Middle ear

The tympanic membrane separates the external ear and middle ear. This pearl grey structure consists of three layers: skin, fibrous tissue and a mucous membrane. Its upper portion, the pars flaccida, has little support; its lower portion, the pars tensa, is held taut. The centre, or umbo, is attached to the tip of the long process of the malleus bone on the other side of the tympanic membrane.

A small, air-filled structure, the middle ear performs three vital functions:

• It transmits sound vibrations across the bony ossicle chain to the inner ear.
• It protects the auditory apparatus from intense vibrations.
• It equalises the air pressure on both sides of the tympanic membrane to prevent it from rupturing.

Hammer, anvil and stirrup

The middle ear contains the three small bones of the auditory ossicles: the malleus, or hammer; the incus, or anvil; and the stapes, or stirrup. These bones are linked like a chain, and vibration is passed from one to another. The long process of the malleus fits into the incus, forming a true joint, and allows the two structures to move as a single unit. The proximal end of the stapes fits into the oval window, an opening that joins the middle and inner ear.

A tube with connections

The eustachian tube connects the middle ear with the nasopharynx, equalising air pressure on either side of the tympanic membrane. This tube also connects the ear's sterile area to the nasopharynx. A normally functioning eustachian tube keeps the middle ear free from contaminants from the nasopharynx. It opens during yawning or swallowing. Upper respiratory tract infections and allergies can block the tube, obstructing middle ear drainage and possibly causing otitis media or effusion.

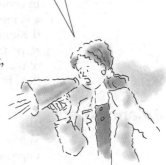

Did you hear me? The eustachian tube keeps contaminants away from the middle ear!

Earache explanation

Note that in infants and children the eustacian tube is shorter, wider and more horizontal, making the transmission of infection easier. This means that infants and children are particularly susceptible to ear infections as a complication of upper respiratory tract infections.

Inner ear

The inner ear consists of closed, fluid-filled spaces within the temporal bone. It contains the bony labyrinth, a series of cavities within the bone which form three connected structures: the vestibule, the semi-circular canals and the cochlea. The bony labyrinth is lined with the membranous labyrinth. Both compartments are fluid filled; the bony labyrinth with perilymph, and the membranous labyrinth with endolymph. These protect the sensitive structures of the ear.

The vestibule and semicircular canals help maintain equilibrium. The cochlea, a spiral chamber that resembles a snail shell, is the organ of hearing. The organ of Corti, part of the membranous labyrinth, contains about 16 000 hair cells which receive auditory sensations (Tortora 2005).

I heard it through the . . . sound waves

When sound waves reach the external ear, its structures transmit the waves through the auditory canal to the tympanic membrane, where they cause a chain reaction of vibrations along the structures of the middle and inner ear. Finally, the cochlear branch of the acoustic nerve (cranial nerve VIII) transmits the vibrations to the temporal lobe of the cerebral cortex, where the brain interprets the sound.

Double duty

In addition to controlling hearing, structures in the middle and inner ear also control balance. The semicircular canals of the inner ear contain cristae – hair-like structures that respond to body movements via the vestibular branch of the acoustic nerve (cranial nerve VIII). Endolymph fluid bathes the cristae.

The structures in my middle ear help me control my balance. Now that's an accomplishment!

Balancing act

When a person moves, the cristae bend, releasing impulses through the vestibular portion of the acoustic nerve to the brain, which controls balance. When a person is stationary, nerve impulses to the brain orient them to this position, and the pressure of gravity on the inner ear helps to maintain balance.

Nose

The nose is more than the sensory organ of smell. It also plays a key role in the respiratory system by filtering, warming and humidifying inhaled air. When you assess the nose, you'll commonly assess the paranasal sinuses too.

Inside and out

The lower two-thirds of the external nose consist of flexible cartilage and the upper one-third is rigid bone. Posteriorly, the internal nose merges with the pharynx. Anteriorly, it merges with the external nose.

Odour area

The sense of smell sits within a tiny area, about 5 centimetres square, in the upper part of the nasal cavity. It contains between 10 and 100 million receptors (Tortora 2005). Sensory messages are conveyed from here to the brain via the olfactory nerves, the first pair of cranial nerves.

Dividing line

The internal and external nose are divided vertically by the nasal septum, which is straight at birth and in early life, but becomes slightly deviated or deformed in many adults. Only the posterior end, which separates the posterior nares, remains constantly in the midline.

Nosebleed central

About nine out of ten nosebleeds occur in the Kiesselbach's plexus, in an area called Little's area, which contains all five arteries that supply the septum.

Just nosing around

Air entering the nose passes through the vestibule, which is lined with coarse hair that helps to filter dust. It then moves into the upper olfactory region which, in addition to containing the olfactory receptors, is also rich in capillaries and mucus-producing goblet cells which help warm, moisten and clean inhaled air.

Breathe easy

Within the nasal passage are the superior, middle and inferior turbinates. Separated by grooves called meatus, the curved bony turbinates and their mucosal covering increase surface area, and ease breathing by further warming, filtering and humidifying inhaled air. (See *A close look at the nose and mouth*, page 154.)

Singling out the sinuses

Four pairs of paranasal sinuses open into the internal nose, including the:
* maxillary sinuses, located in the cheeks below the eyes
* frontal sinuses, located above the eyebrows
* ethmoidal and sphenoidal sinuses, located behind the eyes and nose.

The sinuses serve as resonators for sound production and produce mucus. You'll be able to assess the maxillary and frontal sinuses, but the ethmoidal and sphenoidal sinuses aren't readily accessible.

The small openings between the sinuses and the nasal cavity can easily become obstructed because they're lined with mucous membranes which can become inflamed and swollen.

A close look at the nose and mouth

These illustrations show the anatomic structures of the nose and mouth.

Nose and mouth

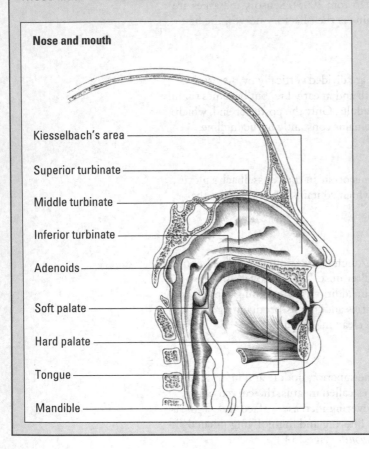

Kiesselbach's area

Superior turbinate

Middle turbinate

Inferior turbinate

Adenoids

Soft palate

Hard palate

Tongue

Mandible

Mouth and oropharynx

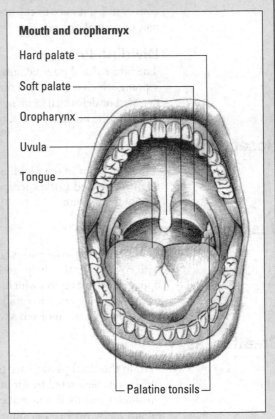

Hard palate

Soft palate

Oropharynx

Uvula

Tongue

Palatine tonsils

Mouth and throat

The mouth contains the teeth (32 in a full adult set, 20 the full temporary set in children) and the tongue.

Tongue tied?

The tongue should be rough on its anterior surface, and smooth with visible veins underneath. Note the frenulum, which is the midline attachment underneath the tongue. This can be overly tight in infants/toddlers, resulting in a 'tongue tie', which affects speech and chewing. The mouth also contains three pairs of salivary glands – the parotid, submandibular and sublingual.

Two palates

The hard palate forms the roof of the mouth, with the soft palate lying behind it. The uvula is the finger-like projection which should hang midline from the back of the soft palate; any deviation may indicate a problem with cranial nerve IX

Throat facts

The throat, or pharynx, is divided into the nasopharynx, oropharynx and laryngopharynx.

The mucous membrane lining the throat is usually smooth and bright pink to light red. The tonsils, which lie in the oropharynx (just behind the soft palate) are made of lymphoid tissue which swells in response to infection. Normally larger in infants and children, they tend to shrink somewhat during puberty. The nasopharynx sits above the oral pharynx at the back of the nose. It contains the adenoids and the opening of the eustacian tubes. The laryngopharynx runs from the oropharynx to join the oesophagus and the larynx.

Running neck and neck

The neck is formed by the cervical vertebrae, the muscles (the anterior sternomastoid and posterior trapezius) and their ligaments. Other important structures of the neck include the trachea, thyroid gland and chains of lymph nodes. (See *Locating lymph nodes*, page 170 for more detail regarding the cervical lymph nodes.)

Grand gland

The thyroid gland lies in the anterior neck, just below the larynx. Its two cone-shaped lobes are located on either side of the trachea and are connected by an isthmus below the cricoid cartilage, which gives the gland its butterfly shape. The largest endocrine gland, the thyroid produces the hormones triiodothyronine and thyroxine, which affect the metabolic reactions of every cell in the body.

Obtaining a health history

To investigate a presenting complaint relating to the ears, nose or throat, use the PQRSTU or OLD CART mnemonic (page 16) to systematically explore the problem.

Asking about the ears

The most common ear complaints include hearing loss, tinnitus, pain, discharge, 'blocked ears' (often due to cerumen), itching and dizziness. In addition to systematically exploring the presenting complaint, think about any other issues that might be important.

- Is there any history of a head injury?
- Has the patient previously had an ear or hearing problem?
- Is there a history of ear or hearing problems in the family?
- Has the patient had any recent illnesses that might help to explain the problem; for example, upper respiratory tract infection?
- Does the patient have any chronic illnesses or conditions? For example, diabetes can cause hearing loss, and hypertension can cause high-pitched tinnitus.
- Has the patient got any problems with balance, dizziness or vertigo (spinning)? If so, determine when the episodes occur, how frequently they occur and whether they're associated with nausea, vomiting or tinnitus.

Ask about current treatments and medications. Certain antibiotics and other medications can cause hearing loss and tinnitus.

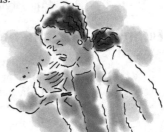

My seasonal allergies always seem to trigger an ear infection. Ah-choo!

Nothing to sneeze at

When you ask the patient about allergies, remember to include a prompt regarding hay fever. Serous otitis media, or inflammation of the middle ear, is common in people with environmental or seasonal allergies. Otitis externa, or inflammation of the external ear, can be caused by various factors including allergic reactions to toiletries, eczema, psoriasis or frequent exposure to water.

Asking about the nose

The most common complaints about the nose include loss of sense of smell (anosmia), nasal stuffiness, nasal discharge, epistaxis (or nosebleed) and sinusitis/sinus pain. Related problems might include frequent colds, hay fever and headaches. Remember sinus pain is often made worse when the patient leans forward. Determine whether certain conditions or places seem to cause or aggravate the patient's problem. Also note possible links with previous nose or head trauma; people who engage in boxing or other contact sports are particularly vulnerable to marked nasal septum deviation and its associated effects. Remember that illicit drug-taking nasally, notably cocaine, can cause serious damage to the internal nose.

Allergens all around

Environmental and seasonal allergies can cause hay fever, nasal stuffiness and discharge. Stagnant nasal discharge can act as a culture medium and lead to sinusitis and other infections. If present, ask about the colour and consistency of the discharge. Green or yellow discharge may suggest infection, whilst clear discharge is more typical of an allergic rhinitis (but remember it can also be cerebrospinal fluid if linked with a history of trauma). When enquiring about medication, explore whether there is prolonged use of nasal decongestant, which can cause 'rebound' rhinitis.

Asking about the mouth, throat and neck

Common complaints relating to the mouth, throat and neck include bleeding or sore gums, mouth or tongue ulcers, a bad taste in the mouth, bad breath, toothache, frequent sore throats, hoarseness or facial swelling. Be sure to recommend prompt referral to a dental surgeon for problems affecting the teeth and gums. Smoking history is important in relation to the risks of mouth and throat diseases, notably cancer. If the patient is having neck problems, explore neck pain or tenderness, neck swelling or trouble moving the neck. Remember that any history of trauma to the neck requires you to consider safety as an absolute priority – see Chapter 13.

Thyroid trouble?

As you take the history, be alert for responses that might indicate a thyroid disorder. Hyperthyroidism can cause heat intolerance, weight loss, palpitations, irritability, itching and a short menstrual pattern with scant flow. Hypothyroidism can cause cold intolerance, weight gain, heavy periods, tiredness, constipation and dry skin.

Get specific

Specific questions to assess the possibility of thyroid disorder include:
• Have you noticed changes in the way you tolerate heat and cold?
• Has your weight changed recently?
• Do you have breathing problems or feel as if your heart is skipping beats?
• Have you noticed a change in your menstrual pattern?
• Have you noticed any tremors, agitation or difficulty concentrating or sleeping?

Assessing the ears, nose and throat

Examining the ears, nose and throat mainly involves using the techniques of inspection and palpation. An ear assessment also requires the use of an auroscope and the administration of hearing acuity tests. Examination of the thyroid includes auscultation for thyroid bruits.

Examining the ears

To assess your patient's ears, you'll need to inspect and palpate the external structures, perform an examination of the ear canal with an auroscope and test hearing acuity.

External observations

Begin by observing the ears for position and symmetry. The top of the ear should line up with the outer corner of the eye, and the ears should look symmetrical. The face and ears should be the same shade and colour as each other.

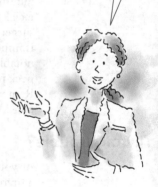

Low-set ears commonly accompany congenital disorders.

Ear-y situation

Pinna that don't lie flat against the head, sometimes known as 'bat ears', are fairly common and don't affect hearing ability. However, they can be a cause of teasing and bullying, leading many children/parents to consider corrective surgery. Low-set ears are of greater concern, commonly signifying congenital disorders such as chromosomal abnormalities.

Pin back the pinna

Inspect the pinna for lesions, drainage, nodules or redness. Gently palpate the tragus, and also pull gently on the helix (back part of the pinna). Note any tenderness with either, which might indicate otitis externa. Then inspect and palpate the mastoid area behind each pinna, noting tenderness, redness or warmth.

Conclude with the canal

Finally, inspect the opening of the ear canal, noting discharge, redness, odour or the presence of nodules or cysts. Patients normally have varying amounts and types of hair and cerumen (earwax) in the ear canal. (See *Cerumen variations*, page 161.)

Auroscopic examination

Next examine the patient's auditory canal, tympanic membrane and malleus with the auroscope. If you suspect otitis externa take great care with your auroscopic examination as it is likely to cause discomfort. Further guidance is given by the Rotherham Primary Ear Care Centre (2008) – a widely respected national ear care training centre.

Tell me if it hurts

Begin by asking the patient to tell you if they feel discomfort at any point during the examination. This occurs not only in infection, but also if the scope is inserted too far into the canal. Select a speculum that appears to be the largest that will fit comfortably into the ear canal.

Hold the scope

Hold the auroscope in a way that is comfortable for you – this should either be upright with the speculum/light source at the bottom (see *Using an Auroscope*, page 160) or at a right angle (3 o'clock or 9 o'clock position). In these positions, you can rest your little finger against the patient's head, so that if they jerk they will push your hand and the scope away from them. Don't hold the scope with the handle downward and the speculum uppermost, as if the patient jerks suddenly you are far more likely to push the scope further into the ear.

Insert speculum A into ear B

To insert the speculum of the auroscope, tilt the patient's head away from you. Hold the superior posterior part of the pinna (the upper part of the helix) with your thumb and index finger, and pull it up and back to straighten the canal. Because everyone's ear canal is shaped differently, you may need to pull the pinna in slightly different directions, slightly varying the angle of the speculum until you can see the tympanic membrane. You will find it easier to pull on the pinna if you hold the scope in your right hand to examine the right ear, and in your left hand to examine the left ear.

Children's ears are different

If your patient is a child younger than around 3-years-old the shape of the ear canal is different, meaning that you need to pull the ear lobe down to get a good view of the membrane.

Go gently

Insert the speculum gently to about one-third of its length; the inner two-thirds of the canal are more sensitive to pressure. Note the cerumen's colour and consistency. (See *Cerumen variations*, page 161.) An older patient may have harder, drier cerumen because of rigid cilia in the ear canal. The external canal should be free from inflammation and scaling.

Peak technique

Using an auroscope

Here's how to use an auroscope to examine the ears of an adult or older child.

Positioning the scope

To examine the ear's external canal, hold the auroscope with the handle parallel to the patient's head, as shown below, or in the 3 o'clock or 9 o'clock position. Bracing your hand firmly against the head keeps you from hitting the canal with the speculum and makes it more likely for the scope to be pushed away if the patient moves suddenly.

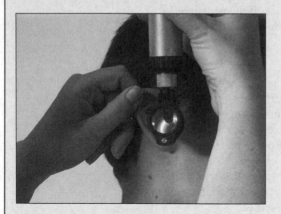

Viewing the structures

As you insert the auroscope, straighten the ear canal by grasping the auricle and pulling it up and back, as shown above, to allow a clear view down the ear canal. When the auroscope is positioned properly, you should see the tympanic membrane structures shown on the right.

Children are different

Remember that in infants and young children you will need to pull down on the pinna to straighten the ear canal.

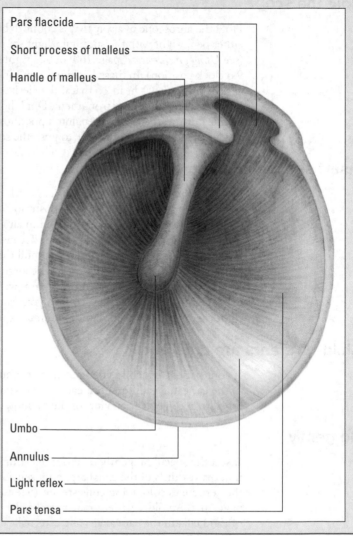

Pars flaccida

Short process of malleus

Handle of malleus

Umbo

Annulus

Light reflex

Pars tensa

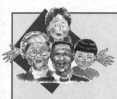

Bridging the gap

Cerumen variations

When examining your patient's ear canal, keep in mind that the presence of cerumen doesn't indicate poor hygiene, and is in fact a part of the ear's own self-cleaning and protection. The appearance and type of cerumen is genetically determined. There are two types of cerumen:

Dry cerumen – which is grey and flaky and is typically found in Asian people

Wet cerumen – which has a dark brown, moist appearance and is typically found in Afro-Caribbean and Caucasian people.

Blocked view

If your view of the tympanic membrane is obstructed by excessive cerumen, never try to remove it with an instrument. The traditional ear syringe is now also obsolete. Safe removal usually involves a procedure which requires specialist training (Rotherham Primary Ear Care Centre 2008). See also NHS Scotland (2006).

As the speculum turns

The membrane should be pearl grey, glistening and transparent. Identify both the pars flaccida and pars tensa. The annulus (edge) should be white and denser than the rest of the membrane. Inspect the membrane carefully for bulging (outward protrusion), retraction (pulling inwards), bleeding, lesions and perforations, especially at the periphery. The older patient's eardrum may appear cloudy.

'Timing' the light reflection?

Now, examine the membrane for the light reflection. This is sometimes called the 'cone of light' because of its cone shape extending from a point at the umbo to a wider base at the annulus. Imagine the membrane as a clock face; the light reflection should be at around 5 o'clock in the right ear, and around 7 o'clock in the left ear. If the reflection is displaced or absent, the patient's tympanic membrane may be bulging, inflamed or retracted. Finally, look for the bony landmarks. The handle of the malleus appears as a dense, white streak at the 12 o'clock position. At the top of the light reflection sits the umbo, the inferior point of the malleus.

No lesions, drainage, nodules or redness. Good!

Hearing acuity tests

The last part of an ear assessment involves testing the patient's hearing using the whisper test, Weber's test and the Rinne test. These tests assess conduction hearing loss (blocked sound transmission to the inner ear), and sensorineural hearing loss (pathology of the inner ear, cranial nerve VIII or auditory areas of the brain). (See also *Assessing hearing in young children*, page 163.)

Whisper test

To perform the whisper test, stand behind the patient at arm's length. With one hand, cover or distract hearing from one ear (rubbing the tragus is ideal). Then whisper a word or short phrase of at least two syllables, and ask the patient to repeat what you said. Repeat with the other ear using a different phrase. Make sure the patient can't guess the second side by word association; for example, if you say 'Cornflakes' on the first side, don't say 'Rice Krispies' on the second. In a quiet room, the patient should easily hear a true whisper if hearing is normal.

Weber's test

Weber's test should be performed in the following circumstances: when the patient reports diminished or lost hearing in one ear; when your findings on the whisper test are abnormal; when your auroscopic examination suggests a problem or as part of a cranial nerve examination. Note lateralisation can occasionally occur in patients with no underlying problem.

Choosing the right fork

This test uses a tuning fork, tuned to 512 cycles per second (about normal human speech). The test assesses conduction of sound through bone. To initiate the sound, strike the outer edge of one of the tines onto the back of your hand, your elbow or your knee. Be sure not to hold the fork anywhere other than the base or you will deaden the sound. Then place the base of the fork firmly on the patient's forehead at the midline or on the top of their head. Be sure the tines face to either side; like 'bunny ears'. (See *Positioning the tuning fork*, page 164.)

Do you hear what I hear?

Ask the patient if they can hear the sound, and if so whether it is *equal* in both ears. If so, record this as a normal Weber's test. If he/she hears the tone better in one ear, record the result as right or left lateralisation. This result helps you to determine whether the problem is conductive (for example, due to a foreign body, perforated ear drum or infection) or sensorineural.

That doesn't make sense!

If the sound isn't heard equally, it is likely that the patient will actually hear it better in their 'bad ear' than their 'good one' suggesting a conductive hearing loss. This may seem illogical! It happens because the test is transmitting the tuning fork sound via the bone of the skull. Normally this sound will be partially masked by the background room noise entering the ear via its normal route. But if normal sound transmission from the room to the inner ear is 'blocked' by the conductive problem (blocked ear canal, for example) then the transmission of sound via the bone won't be masked and will be heard better. In contrast, if the patient hears the sound better in their 'good' ear, it is probably a sensorineural hearing loss.

Rinne test

Perform the Rinne test after Weber's test to compare air conduction of sound with bone conduction of sound. (See *Positioning the tuning fork*, page 164.) Strike the tuning fork as before, and then place it on the patient's mastoid process (the bony area just behind the ear). Check the patient can hear the sound, and then ask them to tell you when the tone stops. When it does, quickly move the open end of the 'still ringing' tuning fork to the ear's opening without touching the ear. Ask the patient if they can still hear the sound. If so, record the finding as air conduction is greater than bone conduction; that is, AC > BC – a normal finding. Some texts suggest timing the sound, requiring air conduction to be twice as long as bone conduction for a normal finding (Jarvis 2008).

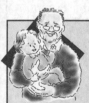

Ages and stages

Assessing hearing in young children

When assessing hearing in an infant or a young child, you can't use a tuning fork. Instead, for infants, stand behind them and clap your hands or squeeze a squeaky toy. A newborn will show the 'startle' or Moro reflex, and also blink. A slightly older infant will still blink, and is likely to appear to 'stop and listen', halting sucking or crying. After about 6 months old the infant will turn to localise the direction of the sound. If you have concerns, professional audiology assessment is required.

Note the history is very important here, as parents may have observed inattention to loud noises, the child not responding to their name or a delay in development of babbling, single-word utterances or speech development. The parents' input is vital here, as a shy child may be unresponsive in the clinical setting.

Because hearing disorders in children may lead to speech, language and learning problems, early identification and treatment is crucial. Undiagnosed hearing disorders can also cause behavioural problems or developmental delay, as well as inappropriate labelling with other possible causes of learning differences.

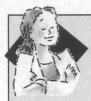

Peak technique

Positioning the tuning fork

These illustrations show how to hold a tuning fork to test a patient's hearing.

Weber's test

Position the base on the patient's forehead at the midline. Alternatively, place the tuning fork on the top of the patient's head, as shown in the left hand image. Be sure the fork is positioned with the U shape to the front; that is, the tines appear like 'bunny ears'.

Rinne test

To correctly position the tuning fork for the Rinne test, hold the base of the fork firmly on the mastoid process (central image) – the bony area immediately behind the ear.

When you move the fork in front of the ear to test air conduction, hold the open end (tines) close to the ear opening but take care not to actually touch the ear.

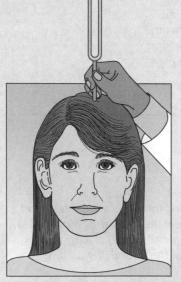
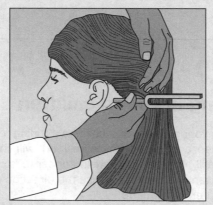
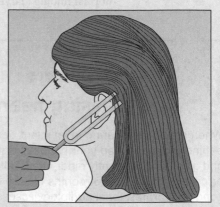

Willis, M.C. (2002) *Medical Terminology: A Programmed Learning Approach to the Language of Health Care*. Baltimore, MD: Lippincott Williams & Wilkins.

Air waves

If the patient can't hear the fork when you move it in front of the ear, it is likely that a conductive hearing loss is present. In sensorineural hearing loss, the air-conducted sound is typically still heard when bone-conducted sound has disappeared. But hearing in both may be very poor. In some cases the patient may simply hear neither sound.

Examining the nose and sinuses

A complete examination of the nose also includes checking the sinuses. To perform an examination of the nose and sinuses you will use the techniques of inspection and palpation.

Inspecting and palpating the nose

Begin by observing the patient's nose for signs of discoloration, swelling or deformity. Variations in size and shape are largely caused by differences in cartilage and in the amount of fibroadipose tissue, reflecting individual, age-related and cultural variations.

Also consider whether any of the following are present:
• Is there any flaring at the nostrils? If so, observe for other signs of respiratory distress.
• Are there any signs of discharge? If so, note the colour, quantity and consistency. If there is a history of head injury or trauma, remember a clear discharge could be cerebrospinal fluid; this requires urgent further evaluation.
• Is there a 'nasal salute', a horizontal crease below the bridge of the nose? It may be caused by habitual rubbing of the nose, especially in children, and can indicate the presence of allergy.

Name that smell . . .

Note that testing the patient's sense of smell is not practised routinely outside neurology clinics. If required, test the olfactory nerve (cranial nerve I) function by asking the patient to blow their nose, then block one nostril and inhale a familiar aromatic substance through the other. Possible substances include peppermint, coffee or lemon. Ask them to identify the aroma, and then repeat the process with the other nostril, using a different aroma. Note the reliability of this test can be questionable – a patient may recognise a smell but be unable to pinpoint it, so findings must be taken alongside other data from the history and examination.

Turn up the patient's nose

If indicated, inspect the nasal cavity. Ask the patient to tilt the head back slightly, and then push the tip of their nose up. Use the light from the auroscope or a pen torch to illuminate the nasal cavities. Check for severe deviation or perforation of the nasal septum. Examine the vestibule and turbinates for redness, swelling and discharge.

A light at the end of the speculum

Fuller examination of the nostrils can be conducted if indicated using a nasal speculum and a pen torch, or an auroscope with a short, wide-tip speculum. Sit the patient in front of you with the head tilted back. To use a nasal speculum, put on gloves and insert the tip of the closed nasal speculum into one nostril to the point where the blade widens. Gently open the speculum as wide as possible without causing discomfort, and then shine the torch into the nostril to illuminate the area. Or if using an auroscope, insert the speculum very gently into the nostril. Observe the colour and patency, and check for exudate. The mucosa should be moist, pink to light red and free from lesions and polyps. Repeat on the other side. (See *Inspecting the nostrils*, below.)

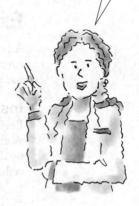

The mucosa should be moist, pink to light red and free from lesions and polyps.

Peak technique

Inspecting the nostrils

The illustration below shows the proper placement of the nasal speculum during direct inspection of the nostrils.

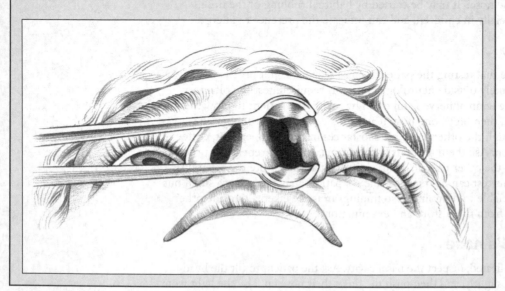

Examining the sinuses

Next examine the sinuses. Remember, only the frontal and maxillary sinuses are readily accessible; you can't directly palpate the ethmoidal and sphenoidal sinuses but can gather important data from the history. Also, if the frontal and maxillary sinuses are infected, it is likely that the other sinuses will be affected too.

Tell me if it hurts

Begin by checking for swelling around the eyes, especially over the sinus area. Then palpate the sinuses, checking for tenderness. To palpate the frontal sinuses, place your thumbs above the patient's eyes just under the bony ridges of the upper orbits, and place your fingertips on the forehead. Apply gentle pressure. Next palpate the maxillary sinuses. (See *Palpating the maxillary sinuses*, below.)

Examining the mouth and throat

Assessing the mouth and throat requires the techniques of inspection and palpation. Inspect the mouth and throat as indicated by the history. Sometimes a thorough inspection of all aspects will be needed, at other times just some elements (for example, just the tongue, uvula and soft palate if you are assessing the cranial nerves).

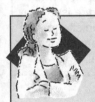

Peak technique

Palpating the maxillary sinuses

To palpate the maxillary sinuses, gently press your thumbs on each side of the nose just below the cheekbones, as shown. The illustration also shows the location of the frontal sinuses above the eyes.

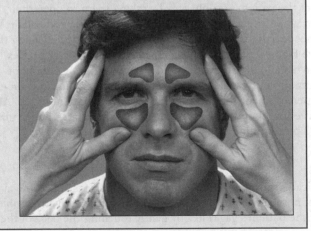

Moist mucosa?

First, inspect the patient's lips. They should be pink, moist, symmetrical and without lesions. Then use a pen torch to inspect the oral mucosa. This should be pink, smooth, moist, and free from lesions and unusual odours. Increased pigmentation is seen in dark-skinned patients.

Gums and then some

Next, observe the gingivae, or gums. They should be moist, and have clearly defined margins at each tooth. Colour varies from pale pink to darker shades, often in accordance with skin tone. They shouldn't be retracted (show too much of the base of the teeth). Inspect the teeth, noting condition, and whether any are missing or crowned. If the patient is wearing dentures, ask him/her to remove them if indicated, so you can inspect the gums underneath. This won't always be necessary, so be guided by your history as many patients will find this embarrassing. But do remember many oral lesions may be covered by dentures.

Give the tongue the once-over

The tongue should be midline, moist, pink and free from lesions. The back (posterior) should be fairly smooth, and the front (anterior) slightly rough with small fissures. It should move easily in all directions, and it should lie straight to the front at rest and when protruded. The underside (ventral surface) may appear darker – inspect for colour and lesions. (See *Checking the surface*, right.)

Say 'Ahhh'

Inspect the patient's oropharynx by asking them to open their mouth while you shine the pen torch on the uvula and palate. You may need to use a tongue depressor to aid your view. Placing the tongue blade slightly off centre may help to avoid a gag reflex. The uvula and oropharynx should be pink and moist, without inflammation or exudates. The tonsils should be pink and shouldn't be hypertrophied (shrunken looking). Ask the patient to say 'Ahhh'. Observe for an upward movement of the soft palate. The uvula should be central.

Gag order

If indicated (for example, other abnormal findings suggesting a cranial nerve problem, or history indicating a swallowing problem) assess the patient's gag reflex by gently touching the back of the

Ages and stages

Checking the surface

A number of oral abnormalities may affect older patients in particular. Inspect the tongue for cracks (which can indicate dehydration or mouth breathing) and the tongue, gums and oral mucosa for ulceration (which may disrupt eating) or non-healing lesions that could be malignant. Note the area underneath the tongue is a common site for the development of oral cancers.

pharynx with a tongue depressor. Note this is very uncomfortable, causing the patient to retch, hence not carrying this out routinely.

Examination of the neck

Examination of the neck is done for a variety of reasons, but it is rare to consider all aspects in one examination. Aspects of examination of the neck are therefore covered in a number of chapters. Remember any history of neck trauma requires urgent expert evaluation – see Chapter 13.

Assessment of tracheal position is covered in Chapter 8, and assessment of the carotid arteries and jugular venous pressure is covered in Chapter 9. Assessment of the sternomastoid and trapezius muscles, enervated by cranial nerve XI, is covered in Chapter 14. Other aspects of neck assessment are covered below.

Inspection of the neck

The neck should be symmetrical, and the skin should be intact. Note any scars; for example, a horizontal scar at the base suggesting thyroid surgery. Note any swelling, venous distension, thyroid or lymph node enlargement.

Palpation of the lymph nodes

Palpate the patient's head and neck to gather further data, particularly regarding the lymph nodes. Using the finger pads of both hands and a circling motion, bilaterally palpate the lymph nodes of the neck. (See *Locating lymph nodes*, page 170 and Chapter 10 for lymph node anatomy and physiology). The nodes to palpate are found:
- under the patient's chin (submental)
- in the areas under the jaw bones (submandibular)
- under the ears (tonsillar)
- in front of and behind the ears (preauricular and postauricular)
- at the base of the hairline (occipital)
- down the length of the neck (the anterior, posterior and deep cervical chains) – note that you have to work around the neck muscles to feel these, from both in front and behind
- above and below the clavicles (supra and infraclavicular).

One node or two?

Normally you shouldn't feel the nodes as you palpate the relevant areas. Document any nodes that are palpable, and assess size, shape, mobility, consistency (for example, hard like gunshot or rubbery), smoothness/roughness and tenderness, comparing one side with the other.

Peak technique

Locating lymph nodes

This illustration shows the location of the lymph nodes in the head and neck.

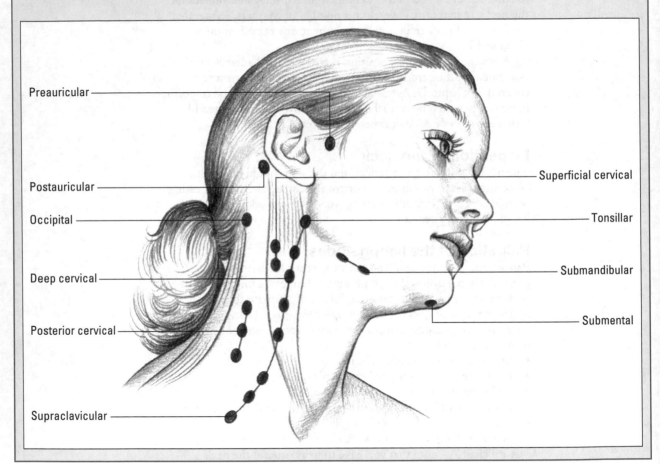

Preauricular

Postauricular

Occipital

Deep cervical

Posterior cervical

Supraclavicular

Superficial cervical

Tonsillar

Submandibular

Submental

Inspection and palpation of the thyroid gland

Firstly, inspect the thyroid by shining a torch across the neck to highlight any swelling. Ask the patient to do a dry swallow – or give a sip of water if you are sure there isn't a swallowing problem and risk of aspiration. Note the rising of the thyroid as they swallow. (See *A close look at the thyroid gland*, page 171.)

A close look at the thyroid gland

This illustration shows the structure and location of the thyroid gland.

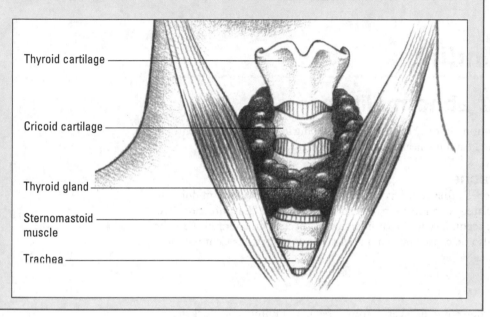

- Thyroid cartilage
- Cricoid cartilage
- Thyroid gland
- Sternomastoid muscle
- Trachea

Hard to swallow?

To palpate the thyroid, firstly explain to the patient what you plan to do, as it can be frightening. Remember, the normal thyroid is only palpable in about 50% of women and 25% of men (Bevan and Gawkrodger 2005) and also that this examination takes lots of practise. The patient should be sat up straight with their head slightly forward. Stand behind the patient, and then ask them to swallow while you put your hands around their neck, with the fingers of both hands over the lower trachea. Note whether you can feel the thyroid (along with the trachea and larynx) moving upwards under your fingers.

Side to side

Then push slightly with the fingers of the left hand and palpate with the right between the trachea and the sternomastoid muscle. Repeat on the other side. If you can feel the thyroid, assess for any nodules or tenderness, and assess to see if it feels enlarged. Turning the patient's head slightly toward the side you're palpating helps to relax the muscle and may help you palpate.

Auscultating the neck

If you detect an enlarged thyroid gland, also auscultate the thyroid area with the bell. Check for a bruit (a soft rushing or 'swooshing' sound), which indicates a hypermetabolic state.

Abnormal findings

Ear abnormalities

Common abnormalities you may find during an ear assessment include earache, hearing loss and discharge.

Earache

Earaches often result from disorders of the external and middle ear associated with infection, obstruction or trauma. Ear infections are often secondary to throat infections, especially in children. Earache can also be caused by pain in neighbouring areas, for example the throat.

An earful

Earaches range in severity from a feeling of fullness or blockage to deep, boring pain. At times, it may be difficult to determine the precise location of the earache. Earaches can be intermittent or continuous and may develop suddenly or gradually.

Hearing loss

Several factors can interfere with the ear's ability to conduct sound waves; that is, a conductive hearing loss. Cerumen, a foreign body or a polyp may be obstructing the ear canal. Otitis media may have thickened the fluid in the middle ear, which interferes with the vibrations that transmit sound. Otosclerosis, a hardening of the bones in the middle ear, also interferes with the transmission of sound vibrations. Trauma can disrupt the middle ear's bony chain.

Hear today, gone tomorrow

Sensorineural hearing loss also has several causes. The most common cause is loss of hair cells in the organ of Corti. In older people, presbycusis – or progressive hearing loss – results from atrophy of the organ of Corti and the auditory nerve. Hearing loss can also result from trauma to the hair cells caused by loud noise or ototoxicity. (See *Hearing loss*, page 173.)

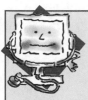

Interpretation station

Hearing loss

Use this chart to review the possible causes onset and associated signs and symptoms of hearing loss.

Cause	Likely onset	Possible signs and symptoms other than hearing loss
External ear		
Cerumen impaction	Sudden or gradual	Itching, fullness, tinnitus, pain
Foreign body	Sudden	Discharge, redness of the ear canal
Otitis externa	Sudden	Pain, discharge, itching
Middle ear		
Serous otitis media	Sudden or gradual	Fullness, possible earache
Acute otitis media	Sudden	Pain, fever, malaise, vomiting, frequent history of upper respiratory tract infection
Perforated tympanic membrane	Sudden	History of trauma or infection, possible discharge if infection is current
Inner ear		
Presbycusis (age-related hearing loss)	Gradual	Especially difficult to hear high-pitched sounds, possible tinnitus
Drug-induced loss	Sudden or gradual	Tinnitus, balance problems
Ménière's disease	Sudden	Vertigo (dizziness with a spinning sensation), tinnitus, fullness
Acoustic neuroma	Gradual	Vertigo, tinnitus, fullness, possible loss of sensation in the face

Drugs such as aspirin, aminoglycosides, loop diuretics, gentamicin and certain chemotherapeutic agents may cause rapid hearing loss.

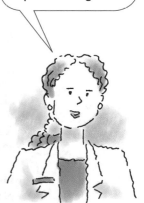

Now hear this!

A toxic reaction to a drug can cause a rapid loss of hearing. Drugs which may affect hearing include aspirin, aminoglycosides, loop diuretics, gentamicin and several chemotherapeutic agents. Urgent expert review is required to determine whether the drug should be stopped.

Discharge

Discharge may be bloodstained, purulent, clear or serous. It may occur alone or with other symptoms such as earache. Its onset, duration and severity provide clues to the underlying cause. It may result from disorders which affect the external ear canal or the middle ear, including allergies, infection, neoplasms, trauma and collagen disease. Note that clear fluid draining from the ear following a head injury could be cerebrospinal fluid, and must always be investigated urgently.

Tinnitus

Tinnitus is a perceived whistling, hissing, buzzing or roaring noise in the ear or head of the patient, which occurs internally rather than externally. It can be temporarily caused by a variety of factors including earwax, ear infection, anaemia, perforated ear drum or head injury. Alternatively, it can be permanent, especially if associated with ageing.

Nose, mouth and throat abnormalities

During a nose, mouth and throat assessment, you may note a variety of findings such as dysphagia, epistaxis, nasal flaring, nasal stuffiness, nasal discharge and sore throat.

Dysphagia

Dysphagia (difficulty swallowing) is a common symptom of oesophageal disorders. However, it may also result from oropharyngeal, respiratory, neurologic and collagen disorders or from the effects of toxins and treatments. Dysphagia increases the risk of choking and aspiration. It is an important finding which should always be investigated further. Specialist training is required to assess swallowing difficulties – in many instances referral to a speech and language therapist, who will have expertise in this area, is required.

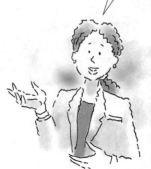

Swallow this: dysphagia is a common symptom of oesophageal disorders.

Epistaxis

A common event, epistaxis (nosebleed) can occur spontaneously or be induced from the front or back of the nose. A rich supply of fragile blood vessels makes the nose particularly vulnerable to bleeding. Dry, irritated mucous membranes bleed easily; they're also more susceptible to infection, which may trigger epistaxis. Additional causes include haematological, clotting, renal or gastrointestinal disorders, as well as trauma.

Nasal flaring

Nasal flaring, particularly in infants or young children, indicates respiratory distress. The patient requires urgent further assessment.

Nasal stuffiness and discharge

Obstruction of the nasal mucous membranes, along with a discharge of thin mucus, can signal systemic, nasal or sinus disorders. This could include trauma, nasal fracture, excessive use of nasal decongestant sprays/drops or nasal use of recreational drugs such as cocaine. Other common causes include allergies or exposure to irritants such as dust, tobacco smoke and fumes. Nasal drainage accompanied by sinus tenderness and fever suggests acute sinusitis, which usually involves the frontal or maxillary sinuses. Thick, white, yellow or greenish drainage suggests an infection.

Take a closer look

Be sure to evaluate clear, thin drainage closely. It may simply indicate rhinitis, or it may be cerebrospinal fluid leaking from a skull fracture or other defect.

Sore throat

Commonly known as a sore throat, throat pain refers to discomfort in any part of the pharynx. This common symptom ranges from a sensation of scratchiness to severe pain. Throat pain usually results from infection but can also be caused by trauma, allergy, cancer or a systemic disorder. It may also follow surgery and endotracheal intubation. Additional causes include mouth breathing, alcohol consumption, vocal strain and inhaling smoke or chemicals such as ammonia.

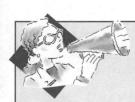

That's a wrap!

Ears, nose and throat review

Ear

External ear

- Consists mainly of elastic cartilage
- Collects sounds and transmits them to the middle ear.

Middle ear

- Separated from the external ear by the tympanic membrane
- Contains three small bones: the malleus, the incus and the stapes

- Connects to the nasopharynx via the eustachian tube
- Transmits sound vibrations to the inner ear, protects the auditory apparatus and equalises air pressure on both sides of the tympanic membrane.

Inner ear

- Consists of closed, fluid-filled spaces
- Contains the vestibule and semi-circular canals which help to maintain

(continued)

Ears, nose and throat review (continued)

equilibrium, and the cochlea, the organ of hearing (Cranial nerve VIII). Also controls balance.

Health history

- Explore common ear complaints, such as hearing loss, tinnitus, pain and dizziness using a mnemonic such as PQRSTU or OLD CART.
- Discuss past medical history, including allergies.
- Explore common nose complaints, such as nasal stuffiness, nasal discharge and nosebleed.
- Ask about colds, headaches and sinus problems.
- Explore common throat complaints, such as bleeding or sore gums, sore throat and tooth problems.
- Ask the patient whether he/she smokes or uses other types of tobacco.
- Explore neck problems, such as neck pain, swelling or trouble moving the neck.

Assessment

- Observe the ears for position and symmetry.
- Inspect the external ear for lesions, drainage, nodules or redness.
- Inspect and palpate the mastoid area behind each auricle.
- Perform an auroscopic examination: examine the external canal, noting the presence and colour of cerumen, and then advance the auroscope to view the tympanic membrane.
- Use the whisper test to evaluate hearing.
- Use Weber's test to evaluate a patient with diminished or lost hearing in one ear.
- Use the Rinne test to compare air conduction of sound with bone conduction of sound.

Abnormal findings

- Earache – severity ranges from a feeling of fullness or blockage to deep, boring pain
- Hearing loss – can be conductive or sensorineural
- Otorrhea – drainage from the ear
- Tinnitus – abnormal internally produced noises in the ears.

Nose

- Acts as sensory organ of smell
- Filters, warms and humidifies inhaled air
- Linked internally to four pairs of paranasal sinuses: maxillary (on the cheeks below the eyes), frontal (above the eyebrows) and ethmoidal and sphenoidal (behind the eyes and nose).

Assessment

- Observe the nose for position, symmetry, and colour. Note nasal flaring or discharge.
- Test nasal patency and the olfactory nerve (cranial nerve I) if indicated by asking the patient to obstruct one nostril and identify a smell with the other.
- Inspect the nasal cavity using the light from the auroscope, checking the vestibule, turbinates and nostrils.

Ears, nose and throat review *(continued)*

- Examine the frontal and maxillary sinuses (the only sinuses that are accessible for examination).
- Check for swelling around the eyes.
- Palpate the sinuses.

Abnormal findings

- Epistaxis – nosebleed; a common sign
- Nasal flaring – may be a sign of respiratory distress
- Nasal stuffiness and discharge – obstruction of the nasal mucous membranes along with a discharge of thin mucus.

Throat and neck

- Consists of nasopharynx, oropharynx and laryngopharynx
- Contains cervical vertebrae, the major neck muscles and their ligaments
- Contains trachea, thyroid gland and chains of lymph nodes.

Assessment

- Inspect the lips
- Inspect the oral mucosa, gingivae, gums and teeth using a torch
- Inspect the tongue and note the patient's ability to move it in all directions; also inspect underneath the tongue
- Inspect the throat using a torch, and a tongue depressor if indicated
- Inspect and palpate the neck
- Assess lymph nodes
- Palpate the thyroid gland
- Auscultate the neck by listening over thyroid gland (if it's enlarged).

Abnormal findings

- Dysphagia – difficulty swallowing
- Sore throat – discomfort in any part of the pharynx; may range from a scratchy sensation to severe pain.

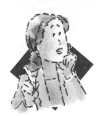

Quick quiz

1. When inspecting the tympanic membrane of a right ear via the auroscope, the light reflection should be at:

    A. 3 o'clock.
    B. 5 o'clock.
    C. 7 o'clock.
    D. 9 o'clock.

2. During an auroscope examination, pull the superior posterior auricle of an adult patient's ear:

    A. up and back.
    B. up and forward.
    C. down and back.
    D. straight back.

3. To assess the frontal sinuses, palpate:
   A. the forehead.
   B. below the cheekbones.
   C. over the temporal areas.
   D. below the ears.

4. A cerumen impaction may contribute to a form of hearing loss called:
   A. central hearing loss.
   B. conductive hearing loss.
   C. sensorineural hearing loss.
   D. cochlea hearing loss.

5. The patient's ability to identify a particular aroma depends on proper functioning of:
   A. cranial nerve I.
   B. cranial nerve II.
   C. cranial nerve IV.
   D. cranial nerve VI.

6. Clear, thin nasal drainage linked to trauma is a worrying finding because it may indicate:
   A. infection.
   B. cerebrospinal fluid leak.
   C. epistaxis.
   D. anosmia.

For answers see page 400.

8 Respiratory system

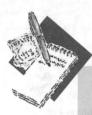

Just the facts

In this chapter, you'll learn:

♦ anatomy and physiology of the respiratory system

♦ methods for assessing the respiratory system

♦ abnormal respiratory system findings and their possible causes.

A look at the respiratory system

The respiratory system includes the airways, lungs, bony thorax and respiratory muscles. (See *A close look at the respiratory system*, page 180.) They work together to deliver oxygen to the bloodstream and remove excess carbon dioxide from the body. Knowing the basic structures and functions of the respiratory system will help you perform a comprehensive respiratory assessment and recognise any abnormalities.

Anatomy and physiology of the respiratory system

Airways

The airways are divided into the upper and lower airways. The upper airways include the nasopharynx (nose), oropharynx (mouth), laryngopharynx and larynx. Their purpose is to warm, filter and humidify inhaled air, and also to convey air to the lower airways.

A close look at the respiratory system

The major structures of the upper and lower airways are illustrated below. The alveolus, or acinus, is shown in the inset.

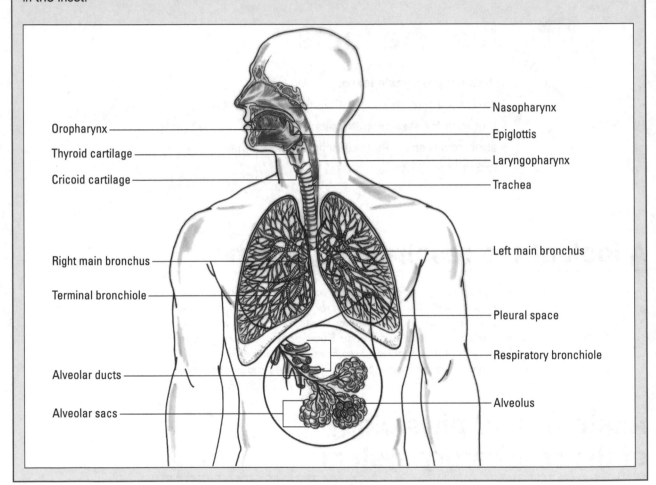

Oropharynx

Thyroid cartilage

Cricoid cartilage

Right main bronchus

Terminal bronchiole

Alveolar ducts

Alveolar sacs

Nasopharynx

Epiglottis

Laryngopharynx

Trachea

Left main bronchus

Pleural space

Respiratory bronchiole

Alveolus

Flapped for your protection

The epiglottis is a flap of tissue that closes over the top of the larynx when the patient swallows. It protects the patient from aspirating food or fluid into the lower airways.

Vocal point

The larynx is located at the top of the trachea and houses the vocal cords. It's the transition point between the upper and lower airways.

The lowdown on the lower airways

The lower airways begin with the trachea, which then divides into the right and left main bronchi. Note the right main bronchus is wider and more vertical than the left, hence the majority of inhaled foreign bodies (for example, peanuts) end up in the right lung.

   The main bronchi then further divide into the lobar bronchi, which are lined with mucus-producing ciliated epithelium, one of the lungs' major defence systems. The lobar bronchi then divide into secondary bronchi, tertiary bronchi, terminal bronchioles, respiratory bronchioles and alveolar ducts. They finally end in the alveoli, the gaseous exchange units of the lungs. An adult's lungs typically contain about 300 million alveoli (Tortora 2005).

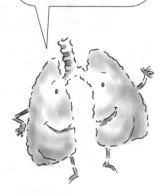

Now that I've taken time to get to know you, I see you have a lot going on underneath that smooth visceral pleura.

Lungs and lobes

Each lung is wrapped in a lining called the visceral pleura. The right lung is larger and has three lobes: upper, middle and lower. The left lung is slightly smaller to accommodate the heart, and has only an upper and a lower lobe.

Linking up the lobes

As you consider the diagram of the lung lobes note their positions, as this will help you to ensure that you have covered all the lobes in your examination. (See *A close look at the lung lobes*, page 182.) This is important because, although they are linked, each lobe is partially separate from its neighbour, so an infection may just affect one lobe (for example, lobar pneumonia). Most of the anterior (front) of the chest is made up of upper lobes and the right middle lobe, whereas the posterior (back) of the chest is mostly made up of the lower lobes. Note in particular the position of the right middle lobe. It doesn't appear at all on the back of the chest; it is only accessible to examine from the front and right side. It is particularly difficult to access in the adult female due to the overlying breast tissue.

A closer look at the lung lobes

Anterior view

- Note the position of the upper lobes, finishing at the fourth rib in the midsternal line on the right and the sixth rib on the left.
- Note the position of the triangular shaped right middle lobe extending from the fourth rib to the sixth rib in the midclavicular line. Note how it sits wholly within the anterior chest.
- Just a small segment of the lower lobes is accessible anteriorly.

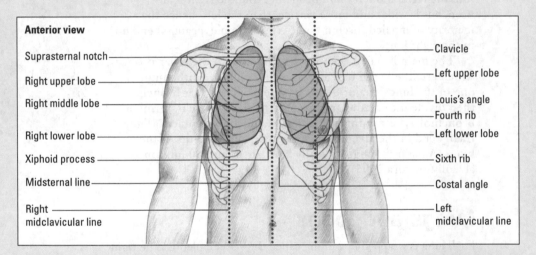

Anterior view

Suprasternal notch
Right upper lobe
Right middle lobe
Right lower lobe
Xiphoid process
Midsternal line
Right midclavicular line

Clavicle
Left upper lobe
Louis's angle
Fourth rib
Left lower lobe
Sixth rib
Costal angle
Left midclavicular line

Posterior view

- Note the position of the lower lobes, extending from vertebra T3 down to the lung bases.
- Only a small section of the upper back allows access to the upper lobes posteriorly.
- There is no access to the right middle lobe posteriorly.

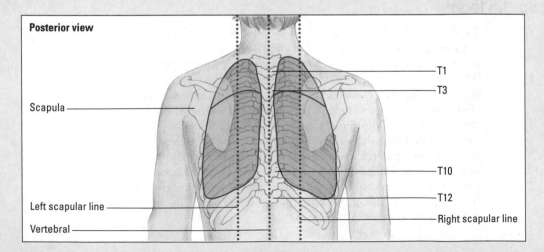

Posterior view

Scapula
Left scapular line
Vertebral

T1
T3
T10
T12
Right scapular line

A closer look at the lung lobes *(continued)*

Right lateral view

- Note the diagonal division between the upper and lower lobes.
- Note the triangular shape of the right middle lobe.
- Consider how you might assess this lobe in the presence of breast tissue.

Left lateral view

- Note the diagonal division between the upper and lower lobes.

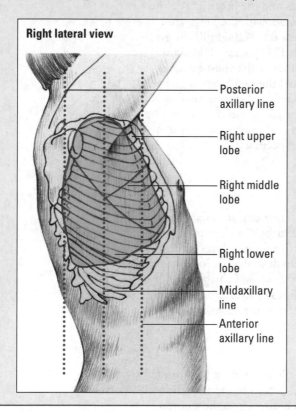

Right lateral view

- Posterior axillary line
- Right upper lobe
- Right middle lobe
- Right lower lobe
- Midaxillary line
- Anterior axillary line

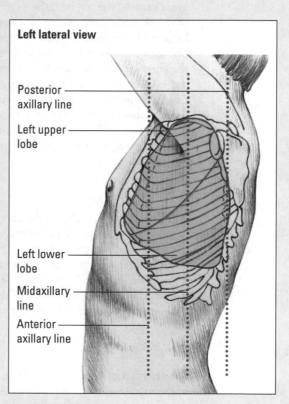

Left lateral view

- Posterior axillary line
- Left upper lobe
- Left lower lobe
- Midaxillary line
- Anterior axillary line

Higher at the front, lower at the back

Also note the position of the lungs in relation to the ribs.
(See *Respiratory assessment landmarks*, page 185.) On the front
of the chest (in the sternal line) the base of the lungs only extends
down to the level of the sixth rib, whereas at the sides (mid-

axilliary line) they extend to the eighth rib, and in the middle of the back adjacent to the spine (vertebral line) they extend to the tenth rib. This is important because the lung bases are an area where abnormalities often occur, and so you need to pay particular attention to them in your examination. When the patient takes a deep breath, the lungs extend down by a further two rib spaces all round the chest.

Smooth moves

The lungs share space in the thoracic cavity with the heart and great vessels, the trachea, the oesophagus and the bronchi. All areas of the thoracic cavity that come into contact with the lungs are lined with the parietal pleura. A small amount of fluid fills the area between the visceral and parietal pleura. This pleural fluid allows the layers to slide smoothly over each other as the chest expands and contracts. The fluid also helps to hold the two layers together, maintaining lung expansion. When this fails, substances such as air (pneumothorax), blood (haemothorax) or pus (pyothorax) enter the pleural space. The parietal pleura also contain nerve endings that transmit pain signals when inflammation occurs.

Thorax

The bony thorax includes the clavicles, sternum, scapula, 12 sets of ribs and 12 thoracic vertebrae. As described in Chapter 2, you can use the ribspaces and the anatomical reference lines (imaginary vertical lines drawn on the chest) to help describe the locations of your findings. (See *Respiratory assessment landmarks*, page 185.) It is important to learn the names of these lines as they are commonly referred to in respiratory, cardiac and abdominal assessment.

Rack of ribs

Ribs consist of bone and cartilage, and allow the chest to expand and contract during each breath. All ribs attach to the thoracic vertebrae. The first seven ribs also attach directly to the sternum. The eighth, ninth and tenth ribs each attach to the cartilage of the rib above them. The eleventh and twelfth ribs are the 'floating ribs' because they don't attach to anything in the anterior thorax. The intercostal spaces sit between the ribs, and are numbered according to the rib which sits directly above the space. Costal cartilages form the anterior ends of the ribs as they join the sternum.

Respiratory assessment landmarks

The illustrations below show common landmarks used in respiratory assessment.

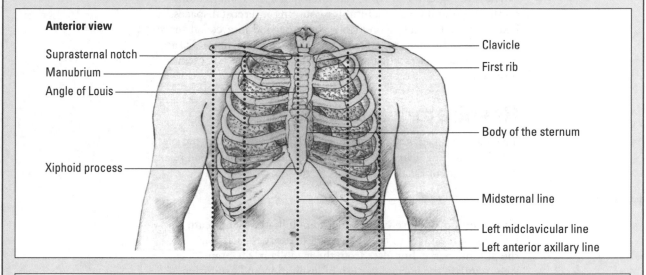

Anterior view

Suprasternal notch

Manubrium

Angle of Louis

Xiphoid process

Clavicle

First rib

Body of the sternum

Midsternal line

Left midclavicular line

Left anterior axillary line

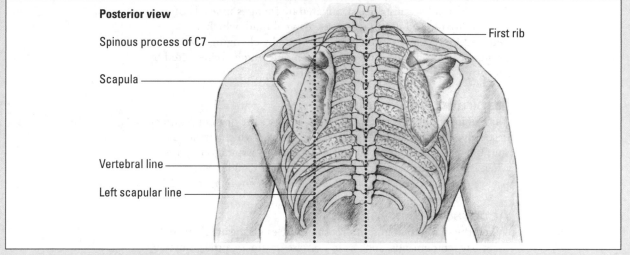

Posterior view

Spinous process of C7

Scapula

Vertebral line

Left scapular line

First rib

Study the sternum

The sternum is about 15 cm in length in the normal adult, and is shaped a bit like a tie. It comprises the upper manubrium (like the knot of the tie), the body and the pointed xiphoid process at the bottom. At the top of the manubrium sits the suprasternal notch, with a slightly hollow area immediately above it. Above this, the trachea can be easily palpated. About 3 to 5 cm down from the sternal notch lies the manubriosternal angle (sometimes called the Angle of Louis). It can often be felt as a small 'bump' on the chest and is very helpful for counting intercostal spaces, as it sits adjacent to the second rib with the second intercostal space just below. The manubriosternal angle is also approximately the point at which the trachea divides into the right and left main bronchus.

Respiratory muscles

The diaphragm and the intercostal muscles are the primary muscles used in breathing. They contract when the patient inhales and relax when the patient exhales.

Message in a nerve

The respiratory centre in the brain stem initiates each breath by sending messages to the primary respiratory muscles via the phrenic nerve. Impulses from the medulla in the brain stem regulate the normal pattern of inspiration and expiration. Alterations in breathing are stimulated by changes in levels of carbon dioxide and pH in the cerebrospinal fluid, which are detected by receptors in the medulla – and by changing levels of oxygen, carbon dioxide and pH in the blood which are detected by receptors in the aorta and carotid arteries.

Inspiration and expiration

Normal inspiration is an active process, and uses the diaphragm which descends and flattens, and the intercostal muscles which elevate the sternum and ribs, allowing air to enter the lungs. Expiration occurs when the diaphragm and intercostal muscles relax, and is essentially a passive process. (See *A close look at the mechanics of breathing*, page 187.)

Accessory to breathing

When the diaphragm and intercostal muscles are insufficient to meet oxygen demands, such as in exercise or illness, other muscles assist in breathing. Accessory inspiratory muscles include the trapezius, the sternomastoid and the scalenes, which combine to elevate the scapula, clavicle, sternum and upper ribs. This elevation further expands the front-to-back diameter of the chest. A forced expiration, on the other hand, uses the abdominal muscles to push the abdominal organs up against the diaphragm, squeezing air out of the lungs.

A close look at the mechanics of breathing

Inspiration and expiration occur as a result of changes in the pressure inside the lungs compared with atmospheric pressure outside the lungs.

Inspiration

- Intercostal muscles contract, moving the ribs upwards and outwards
- The diaphragm descends and flattens
- As a result of enlargement of the thorax, the lungs expand
- Negative alveolar pressure is created
- Air moves into the lungs until the pressures are equal.

Expiration

- Intercostal muscles relax
- The diaphragm ascends, returning to its resting position
- The lungs recoil to their resting size and position
- Positive alveolar pressure is created
- Air moves out of the lungs.

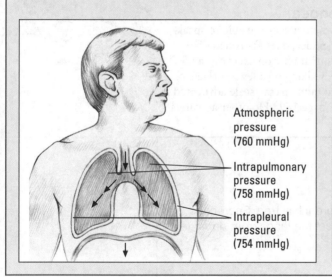

Atmospheric pressure (760 mmHg)

Intrapulmonary pressure (758 mmHg)

Intrapleural pressure (754 mmHg)

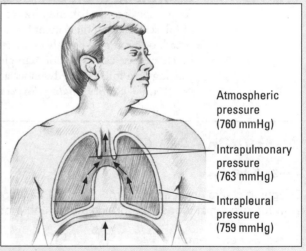

Atmospheric pressure (760 mmHg)

Intrapulmonary pressure (763 mmHg)

Intrapleural pressure (759 mmHg)

Obtaining a health history

In a respiratory examination, the timing of the history in relation to the physical examination will depend on the acuity of the presentation. In any assessment of respiratory symptoms an initial ABCDE assessment (airway, breathing, circulation, disability, exposure – Resuscitation Council UK 2006) is essential. It is also likely that pulse oximetry monitoring will be commenced at the beginning of the assessment process to inform the initial prioritisation of care, and provide ongoing monitoring. Assuming it is safe to take the history first, continue as follows.

When obtaining the health history of a patient with a respiratory disorder, it is important to follow the systematic approach described in Chapter 1. Use the PQRSTU or OLD CART mnemonic (page 16) to explore the patient's presenting problem. In addition, there are a number of focused questions that will help you learn more about the patient's respiratory system.

Questions about the respiratory system

Common symptoms reported by a patient with a respiratory disorder include shortness of breath, cough, sputum production, wheezing and/or chest pain. (See *Breathtaking facts*, below and *Listen and learn*, then *teach*, page 189.)

Shortness of breath (dyspnoea)

As you speak to the patient, observe whether they are able to speak in full sentences. If the patient has dyspnoea, does shortness of breath occur at rest, or only on exertion? If only on exertion, how much exercise causes it? For example, walking on a level surface, or walking up a hill? Grade dyspnoea according to the scale advocated by NICE (2007c). (See *Grading dyspnoea*, page 189.) Do other activities

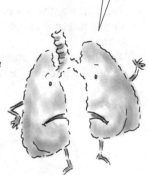

I always thought getting a high grade was a good thing – until I developed dyspnoea.

Breathtaking facts

Cough it up

Coughing clears unwanted material from the tracheobronchial tree. Secretions from the bronchial tubes trap foreign matter and protect the lungs from damage.

Game, set and match

The 300 million alveoli in each lung are important in providing a large enough surface area for gaseous exchange to take place. It is sometimes said that if all of the available surface area for gaseous exchange in an adult was laid out flat, it would be as large as a tennis court!

Oxygen and Chronic Obstructive Pulmonary Disease (COPD)

Patients with chronically high partial pressure of arterial carbon dioxide ($PaCO_2$), such as those with COPD, may be stimulated to breathe by a low oxygen level (the hypoxic drive) rather than by a slightly high $PaCO_2$ level, which is normal for them. For such patients, inappropriate oxygen therapy may cause respiratory depression. NICE (2004) recommends that short-burst oxygen therapy should only be given in severe breathlessness where other treatments have not been effective, and only continued if it improves breathlessness.

Listen and learn, *then* teach

Listening to what your patient says about their respiratory problems will help you to know when they need education. These typical responses indicate that the patient needs to know more about self-care techniques:

'Whenever I feel breathless, I just take a shot of my inhaler.'

This patient needs to know more about proper use of an inhaler and when to seek advice from a healthcare professional. Also be aware that incorrect inhaler technique is a common cause of poorly controlled asthma.

'If I feel all congested, I just smoke a cigarette, and then I can cough up that phlegm!'

This patient needs help to explore the dangers of cigarette smoking.

'None of the other guys wear a mask when we're working.'

This patient needs to know the importance of wearing an appropriate safety mask when working around heavy dust and particles in the air, such as sawdust or powders.

Grading dyspnoea

To assess dyspnoea as objectively as possible, particularly in patients with conditions such as COPD, NICE (2007c) recommends the practitioners ask patients to briefly describe how various activities affect his/her breathing. Then document their response using the following grading system.

Medical Research Council dyspnoea scale (NICE 2007c)

Grade	Degree of breathlessness related to activities
1	Not troubled by breathlessness except on strenuous exercise
2	Short of breath when hurrying or walking up a slight hill
3	Walks slower than contemporaries on level ground because of breathlessness, or has to stop for breath when walking at own pace
4	Stops for breath after walking about 100 metres or after a few minutes on level ground
5	Too breathless to leave the house, or breathless when dressing or undressing

cause shortness of breath? Is it worse at any particular time of day or night? Causes can include pulmonary embolism, asthma, emphysaema (overdistended alveoli), COPD, lung cancer and pneumothorax.

Orthopnoea

A patient with orthopnoea (shortness of breath when lying down) tends to sleep with the upper body elevated. Ask the patient how many pillows they use? One or two pillows are considered normal. Three or more (especially if the patient has started using more pillows recently) suggests orthopnoea. A patient who needs to use three pillows could be said to have 'three-pillow orthopnoea'.

Coughing or wheezing

If the patient has a cough or a wheeze is it a chronic or acute problem? If it's chronic, has anything changed recently? If so, how? If the patient has a wheeze, ask whether the wheezing is loud enough for others to hear it. Wheezing is especially common in asthma or bronchitis.

Sputum

When a patient produces sputum, try to find out the amount produced in a day in teaspoons or some other common measurement.

Now that you've brought it up . . .

Ask about the colour of sputum and whether it is frothy. Ask whether there is ever any blood in the sputum (haemoptysis), and if so, how much and whether there is any associated odour. If sputum is a chronic problem, find out if it has changed recently, and if so, how. If there is a sputum sample/pot available, examine it and note whether it is as the patient has described.

Chest pain

Chest pain should always be regarded as a severe symptom, but remember there are many potential causes, including cardiac and musculoskeletal as well as respiratory. Respiratory causes include pneumonia, pulmonary embolism or pleural inflammation. As you explore the symptoms, pay particular attention to the quality and severity of the pain; for example, is it sharp, stabbing, burning or aching?

Radiation red flag

Also be alert to any radiation, especially if the pain is left sided or central, and radiates to the shoulder, jaw or left arm. These are important 'red flags' for pain that is cardiac in origin.

Questions about general health

Remember to explore the patient's past medical history, paying particular attention to current or previous smoking, exposure to passive smoking and allergies. Ask about previous or current respiratory diseases such as pneumonia, asthma, bronchitis and tuberculosis. Family history of heart disease, COPD, lung cancer and asthma is also important. Also ask about environmental

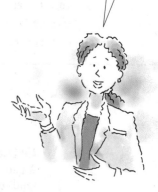

Let your patient's primary health problem, along with their risk of developing respiratory complications, determine the extent of your assessment.

or occupational hazards. People who work/worked in mining, construction or chemical manufacturing are commonly exposed to environmental irritants.

Assessing the respiratory system

By using a systematic assessment, you'll be able to detect subtle or obvious respiratory changes in your patients. The extent of your assessment will depend on several factors, including the patient's primary health problem and risk of developing respiratory complications. Your examination will follow the four key steps of inspection, palpation, percussion and auscultation. Before you begin, make sure the room is well lit and warm, and offer the patient a gown.

First impressions

Make a few initial observations about the patient – assess ABCDE at this point if you are meeting the patient for the first time. Is there any sign that the patient is short of breath? Also, are there any signs of pallor or cyanosis? Remember cyanosis is a late sign of hypoxaemia.

How many breaths a minute?

Count the patient's respiratory rate for 60 seconds. Consider disguising this by combining it with taking the pulse or listening to the heart, so that the patient doesn't alter their breathing. The normal adult respiratory rate is 12 to 20 breaths per minute (Resuscitation Council UK 2006). See Chapter 2 for more detail on respiratory rates in adults and in children of different ages. Also note the pulse rate, rhythm and volume. The respiratory depth and regularity should also be observed; breathing should be even, coordinated and regular, except in infants where gaps of 5 to 10 seconds are normal. Note obvious use of accessory muscles and any audible wheeze.

Pay attention to position

Note how the patient is seated, or positioned in the bed. They are likely to adopt a position that best aids their breathing. Sitting forward and leaning on outstretched arms is described as the 'tripod position', and is one which is commonly adopted by patients with severe shortness of breath. Look at the general appearance. Does the patient appear relaxed, or are they anxious or distressed?

Hands

Next examine the patient's hands, noting pallor or blue tinging, especially of the nails, associated with peripheral cyanosis. Also look for 'tell tale' signs of nicotine staining on the fingers. Note whether the

Ages and stages

Infants use the abdominal and diaphragmatic muscles to breathe, as the intercostal muscles are not fully developed. And although their respiratory rate is much higher, their breathing rhythm is often uneven, with several rapid breaths followed by gaps of 5 to 10 seconds. Also infants find it difficult to breathe through their mouth, so they really struggle when they have a blocked up nose, especially when feeding.

hands are warm or cool, paying attention to the physical environment and whether the hands are warmer or cooler than you would expect.

Nail it!

Now look more closely at the nails. Examine for signs of clubbing, which is a loss of the normal angle between the nail and the nail bed. (See *Evaluating clubbed fingers*, page 117.) Although no-one is sure exactly why this occurs, it is a sign found in many chronic respiratory disorders. Also check the patient's peripheral return, by holding the hand level with the patient's heart and compressing a fingertip firmly between your finger and thumb for 5 seconds. Initial blanching (pallor) will occur. At normal room temperature, normal colour should return within 2 seconds (Resuscitation Council UK 2006) – although McGee (2007) suggests that return up to 3 seconds can be normal in some individuals.

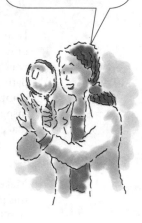

Blue is a great colour for the eyes, but not the nail beds!

In a flap?

Ask the patient to outstretch their arms and hands in front of them, and leave for around 20 to 30 seconds. Look for signs of fine tremor such as may occur if high doses of bronchodilator drugs have been taken. Now ask the patient to tip their hands back towards them, extending the wrists and spreading the fingers (they could pretend they are trying to push against a heavy object). Again observe for 20 to 30 seconds. A 'flapping tremor' can occur in patient's who are retaining carbon dioxide, and is a sign that requires urgent intervention.

Face and neck

Examine the conjunctiva (inner lining of the lower eyelids) for anaemia. Pay particular attention to the rim (nearest the eyelashes) as pallor here is particularly indicative of anaemia. If in doubt, request or suggest a haemoglobin check, if not recently done.

Open please

Now check the mouth and lips, looking for signs of cyanosis; a bluish tinge to the mucous membranes. Also check the tongue – a patient with breathing difficulties will often breathe through the mouth, making the tongue dry. Check for any signs of nasal (nostril) flaring or pursing of the lips when breathing, which can suggest a respiratory problem.

Check the neck

Then check the position of the trachea by gently palpating a centimetre or two above the suprasternal notch with your index finger, or finger and thumb. Tell the patient this may be a little uncomfortable. You should easily feel the tracheal rings in the centre and a space either side. If the trachea sits to one side, or you feel a hollow, this may indicate 'mediastinal shift' where the central mediastinal area of the chest containing the heart is shifted to one side by, for example, a pneumothorax (collapsed lung) or tumour.

Note the nodes

Finally, check the supraclavicular and infraclavicular lymph nodes which lie just above and just below the clavicles. Note that an enlarged supraclavicular node on one side may indicate respiratory pathology such as infection or malignancy on that side, although this sign is not specific to the lungs and could indicate pathology elsewhere in the body.

Examining the chest

The patient should be undressed from the waist up or clothed in an examination gown that allows you access to the chest.

Back to front or front to back?

You can examine either the back or the front of the chest first. If the patient is fairly well and mobile, it is often easier to examine the back first, including the sides. This is especially valuable on female patients where access to the front is often difficult/embarrassing. If feasible, ask the patient to sit on the edge of the bed and shuffle backwards so you can examine their back from the opposite side. Alternatively they could sit on a stool, or upright chair turned sideways.

A weaker patient will probably find it easier if you examine the front and sides first whilst they rest in a fairly upright position (if feasible) against a backrest and/or pillows. You can then sit them forwards with the help of another person for a minimal amount of time, whilst you examine the back.

Note that the four sections below describe how to examine the front and back within each section, but it makes sense to carry out a complete assessment on either the back or front, and then reposition the patient and examine the opposite side.

Inspecting the chest

First inspect the chest. Note any abnormal masses, scars, moles or lesions. Look for chest-wall symmetry. Both sides of chest should be equal at rest and expand equally as the patient inhales. The spine should appear straight. Inspect carefully from the side as well as the front and back.

Rugby or football?

With the exception of infants whose chest is normally round, the diameter of the chest from front to back (the anterior–posterior or A–P diameter) should be less than the width (lateral diameter). In other words, the patient's chest in cross-section (as might be viewed on a scan) should be 'rugby ball' shaped rather than 'football' shaped. The lateral diameter can be as much as twice the 'A–P' diameter.

A new angle

On the anterior chest, look at the angle between the ribs and the sternum at the point immediately below the xiphoid process. This angle – the costal angle – should be less than 90 degrees. The angle will be greater if the chest wall is chronically expanded because of an enlargement of the intercostal muscles, as can happen with chronic respiratory problems.

Muscles in motion

Accessory muscles are normally only used on exertion. If they are used frequently, they may hypertrophy. The examiner may notice this on inspection – for example, a loss of the normal angle between the neck and the shoulders (although note this occurs normally in Down's syndrome). Hypertrophy may be normal in some athletes, but for other patients it indicates a respiratory problem.

Raising a red flag

Watch for paradoxical, or uneven, movement of the chest wall. Paradoxical movement is where a segment of the chest wall moves in the opposite direction to the rest of the chest wall. It may appear as an abnormal 'pulling in' of part of the chest wall when the patient inhales or an abnormal expansion when the patient exhales, indicating loss of normal chest-wall function. Both require urgent referral.

Palpating the chest

Palpation of the chest provides important information about the respiratory system and the processes involved in breathing. (See *Palpating the chest*, page 195.) As you palpate, be sure to cover the sides of the chest as well as the front and back. The chest wall should feel smooth, warm and dry. Note any abnormal 'lumps or bumps', including their location, whether they are hard or soft and whether they feel smooth or rough. Note if the skin feels excessively dry, which could indicate dehydration, or moist, which can occur in conditions such as tuberculosis.

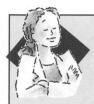

Peak technique

Palpating the chest

To palpate the chest, use the palms of your hands initially, and then the fingertips if needed. Use the palms of the hands to check for tenderness, and also to feel for warmth, moisture, crepitus and any possible 'lumps or bumps'. Then if required, feel with the fingertips to more carefully assess any lumps or bumps, and any crepitus, especially around drainage sites. Remember how important it is to assess the sides of the chest as well as the front and back.

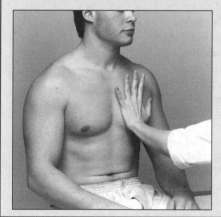 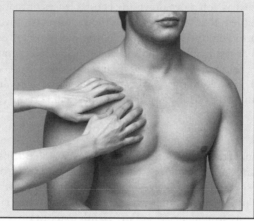

Snap, crackle, pop

Also look for abnormal sounds. Crepitus indicates subcutaneous air in the chest, an abnormal condition. Crepitus sounds like puffed-rice cereal crackling under the skin and indicates that air is leaking from the airways or lungs. If a patient has a chest drain, you may find a small amount of subcutaneous air around the insertion site. If the patient has no chest drain or the area of crepitus is getting larger, then the problem should be reported immediately.

Tender touch

Gentle palpation shouldn't cause the patient pain. As you palpate over the chest wall, ask the patient if there is any pain or tenderness. If the patient has noted chest pain in their history, try to determine whether there is a painful area on the chest wall. Painful costochondral joints are typically located at the midclavicular line or next to the sternum. Rib or vertebral fractures will be quite painful over the fracture, although pain may radiate around the chest as well. Tenderness may also be caused by sore muscles as a result of protracted coughing or physical activity.

Vibratin' fremitus

Although not always carried out routinely, palpation for tactile fremitus can be very useful. Tactile fremitus is the palpation of vibrations caused by the transmission of air through the bronchopulmonary system. (See *Checking for tactile fremitus*, page 197.)

Typically, fremitus is more easily felt in the upper parts of the chest, due to proximity to the trachea and main bronchi which cause more vibration, and is harder to feel lower down the chest where the airways are smaller. It is also more easily felt in thinner patients. Findings are abnormal if fremitus is not felt equally on both sides of the chest at the same level/position, or clearly increases (rather than decreases) as you move down the chest. Causes of reduced fremitus include pleural effusion, pneumothorax, atelectasis (overdistended alveoli) and emphysema. Increased fremitus occurs over consolidation (alveoli or tissue filled with fluid or blood) such as in pneumonia, or due to a tumour, because solid tissue transmits sound better than air or fluid. However, this only occurs if the abnormality lies close to the chest wall, so normal fremitus does not exclude these conditions.

Equal measure

To evaluate the patient's chest-wall symmetry and expansion, place your hands on the front or back of the chest wall with your hands/fingers spread like butterfly wings, and the thumbs touching or close to each other. To examine symmetry at the lung bases, aim to position your hands around the area of the eighth to tenth ribs on the back, or the fifth to sixth ribs (or just below the nipple line or breasts) on the front. As the patient inhales deeply, watch your hands/thumbs. They should separate simultaneously and equally, often several centimetres apart.

Repeat the measurement at the apices by placing your hands on the shoulders. This time you will see/feel your hands move upwards and outwards. Note that as these tests evaluate expansion of the upper/lower lungs as a whole, it is seldom necessary to repeat on the front and the back; do whichever is easiest for your patient. Note that the bases are much more easily examined on the back of the adult female patient if this is feasible. But if you suspect any abnormality, it is wise to repeat the tests on the front *and* back if this is possible.

There's no need for drums. The only percussion instruments you need in a respiratory assessment are your hands.

Warning signs

The patient's chest may expand asymmetrically in conditions such as pleural effusion, atelectasis, pneumonia or pneumothorax. Chest expansion may be decreased at the level of the diaphragm if the

Peak technique

Checking for tactile fremitus

What to do

Check for tactile fremitus by lightly placing either the bony part of your upper palm, or the 'ulnar edge' (little finger side) of your palms, on both sides of the patient's back in various positions. Ask the patient to repeat the phrase 'ninety-nine' loudly. Start with the upper back (over the apices), then move to the middle (around the fifth or sixth rib level) and lower back (around ninth or tenth rib level) and then finally place your hands at the sides. Palpate

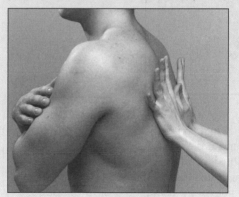

the front of the chest using similar hand positions (although remember, you can't feel the fremitus through breast tissue in an adult female and that the lung bases are higher anteriorly)

What the results mean

Vibrations that feel more intense on one side than the other may indicate tissue consolidation on that side with greater intensity, or emphysema, pneumothorax or pleural effusion on the side with less intensity. Faint or absent vibrations in the upper thorax may indicate bronchial obstruction or a fluid-filled pleural space, but remember vibrations may be faint in obese or muscular patients.

A helpful tip

When you check the back of the thorax for tactile fremitus, ask the patient to fold their arms across their chest. This movement shifts the scapulae out of the way. Try to position the hands between the scapulae when assessing the middle part of the back.

patient has a condition such as emphysema, diaphragmatic paralysis, atelectasis or ascites.

Percussing the chest

You'll percuss the chest to find the boundaries of the lungs and to determine whether the lungs are filled with air, fluid or solid material. (See *Percussing the chest*, page 198 and *Percussion and auscultation sequences*, page 200.)

Percuss in many places

On the back be sure to avoid percussing over the scapula, which will sound dull – asking the patient to cross their arms can help move

Peak technique

Percussing the chest

When you percuss the anterior chest, percuss in the ribspaces if you can, keeping your non-dominant finger horizontally positioned in the ribspaces. On the back the rib spaces are seldom visible, but remember to avoid the scapulae and the spine. Remember to keep your hand and finger firmly held; the percussion movement should come from the wrist of your dominant hand, not your elbow or upper arm. Keep the fingernail you use for tapping short so you won't hurt yourself. (See Chapter 2 for more detail regarding how to percuss.)

It's often helpful to use direct percussion (that is, tapping directly onto the bone with the percussing finger) when percussing over the patient's clavicle. This ensures that you start high enough up on the anterior chest to assess the apices of the lungs. The clavicle acts a bit like the non-dominant finger and normal resonance should be heard.

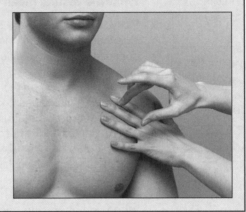

the scapula apart, making it easier to percuss between them. Percuss down, always moving from side to side to compare sound at the same level, until you find a change to dullness which marks the level of the diaphragm. Then pay particular attention to percussing round the bases to the mid axillary line. Also remember to percuss the sides of the chest, making sure on the right that you include the right middle lobe.

Follow a similar pattern on the front, working in the midclavicular line and then across the bases. For your first percussion position anteriorly, you may find it easier to directly percuss the clavicle to assess the apices. Then use indirect percussion as before, working side to side, using the rib spaces if you can see/feel them. Remember that on older girls and women you cannot percuss through breast tissue.

Significant sounds

Although you may hear some subtle variations in the percussion sound in different areas of the chest, the dominant sound you expect to hear in a normal adult chest is resonance – a low-pitched hollow sound. (See *Percussion sounds*, page 199.) You may hear slight dullness around the third and fourth rib spaces to the left of the sternum

Hyperresonance during percussion means there's increased air in the lungs or pleural space.

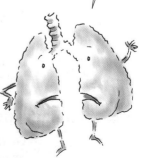

Interpretation station

Percussion sounds

Use this chart to help you become more comfortable with percussion and to interpret percussion sounds quickly. Learn the different percussion sounds by practising on yourself, your patients and other people willing to help.

Sound	Description	Examples of clinical significance
Flat	Short, soft, high pitched, extremely dull	Consolidation, as in atelectasis and extensive pleural effusion
Dull	Medium in intensity and pitch, moderate length, thud-like	Solid area, as in lobar pneumonia
Resonant	Long, loud, low pitched, hollow	Normal lung tissue; bronchitis
Hyperresonant	Very loud, lower pitched	Hyperinflated lung, as in emphysema or pneumothorax. Normal in infants
Tympanic	Loud, high pitched, moderate length, musical, drum-like	Air collection, as in a gastric air bubble, air in the intestines or a large pneumothorax

Peak technique

Double-check percussion findings

Use other assessment findings to verify the results of respiratory percussion. For example, if your history and examination leads you to suspect lobar pneumonia, a chest X-ray may also be indicated. Remember percussion only reaches 5 to 7 cm below the surface, so a patient could have a significant abnormality despite a normal percussion finding because a tumour or consolidation may not be close enough to the chest wall to yield dullness. So always use appropriate investigations to check out your findings.

due to the heart. In infants and younger children, hyperresonance is normal due to their thinner chest wall; for the same reason you may hear hyperresonance, especially at the apices and near the bronchi, in thin adults. Conversely, dullness may be found in obese or muscular patients due to the thicker underlying tissue; it may be very difficult to detect abnormal dullness in these patients.

Sounds other than these are abnormal sounds, suggesting underlying abnormalities. Pay particular attention to a different sound on one side of the chest when compared with the other, but remember an abnormality may be bilateral.

Sounds serious

When you hear abnormal hyperresonance during percussion, it may mean that you've found an area of increased air in the lung or pleural space. Expect hyperresonance with pneumothorax, acute asthma or emphysema. When you hear abnormal dullness, it may well mean that you've found areas of decreased air in the lungs. This can occur in the presence of consolidation, atelectasis or a tumour, or due to fluid in the pleural cavity.

On the move

Percussion also allows you to assess how much the diaphragm moves during inspiration; diaphragmatic excursion. Although rarely

Percussion and auscultation sequences

Follow these percussion and auscultation sequences to distinguish between normal and abnormal sounds in the patient's lungs. Remember to compare sound variations from one side with the other as you proceed. Remember on the back to work between the scapula (the patient folding his/her arms can help here); if you assess over the scapula you will hear a dull percussion sound or a muffled auscultatory sound, and may wrongly assume there is a problem. But also be careful not to percuss and auscultate too close to the spine. Carefully describe abnormal sounds you hear and include their locations.

Anterior

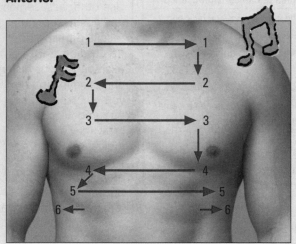

Posterior

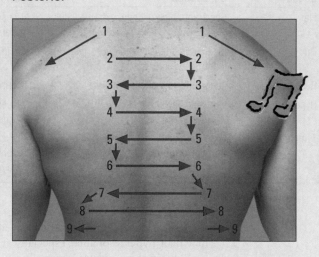

carried out routinely, it can be useful if the patient is well enough to comply and you suspect a condition such as diaphragmatic paralysis, emphysema or atelactasis. The test is based on the fact that the normal diaphragm descends 3 to 5 cm (up to two rib spaces) when the patient takes a deep breath. However, the diaphragm on one or both sides may move much less in a patient with one of these conditions. (See *Measuring diaphragm movement*, page 201.)

Auscultating the chest

As air moves through the bronchi, it creates sound waves that travel to the chest wall. The sounds produced by breathing are different when listening over the larger airways compared with the smaller airways. Sounds also change if they pass through fluid, mucous or narrowed airways. Auscultation of the chest therefore helps you to detect abnormalities in the lungs and pleura.

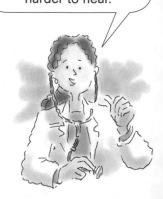

When auscultating the chest, ask the patient to breathe through their mouth; nose breathing alters the pitch of breath sounds and makes them harder to hear.

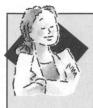

Peak technique

Measuring diaphragm movement – 'diaphragmatic excursion'

If your patient is well enough, and can sit forward unaided, you can measure how much the diaphragm moves. Start by asking the patient to inhale, then exhale and hold their breath. Then starting around the level of the bottom of the scapula, quickly percuss down on one side of the back to locate the diaphragm; the point at which normal lung resonance changes to dullness. Remember to tell the patient to start breathing again. Use a pen to mark the spot indicating the position of the diaphragm on that side of the back.

Then ask the patient to inhale as deeply as possible and hold their breath. Repeat the percussion as before until you locate the diaphragm. Use the pen to mark this spot as well. Repeat on the opposite side of the back.

Measure

Use a ruler or tape measure to determine the distance between the marks. The distance, normally around 3 to 5 cm, should be equal on both the right and left sides.

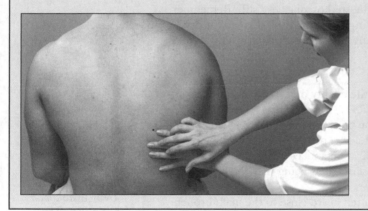
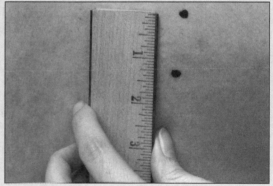

Familiar sites

Listen in the same positions as you used to percuss. (See *Percussion and auscultation sequences*, page 200.) Listen to a full inspiration and expiration at each site, using the diaphragm of the stethoscope, as this is better for hearing higher pitched sounds. On the front of the chest it is helpful to make your first listening position just above the clavicle; it is easier to use the bell here, as it tucks neatly into the space above the clavicle. As with percussion, it is difficult to hear breath sounds through breast tissue; work between the breasts and/or at the sides as appropriate, to maximise the listening areas available.

Breathe normally

Ask the patient to breathe normally through his/her mouth as you auscultate; this makes the sound more audible, and nose breathing alters the pitch of breath sounds. Ask the patient to wave at you if they feel dizzy or faint (you may not hear them if they just try to tell you).

Don't ask the patient to take deep breaths at the beginning of the examination, or they are likely to hyperventilate and become dizzy or short of breath. In fact, just asking them to breath through their mouth will usually be enough to make the patient breath a little more deeply than is usual. If you can't hear breath sounds properly, particularly as you come to the bases, you can then ask the patient to take a *few* deeper breaths for you. If a patient is very sick or breathless ask a second person to help you by keeping a close eye on the patient as you examine them, especially as you examine from the back where you can't see the patient's face.

Be firm

To auscultate for breath sounds, press the stethoscope firmly against the skin and keep the head of the stethoscope very still. Remember that if you listen through clothing (even the back of a bra) or dry chest hair, you may hear deceptive sounds, particularly 'crackles'.

Sounds perfectly normal!

As you listen, pay attention to the quality of the sound as well as its presence or absence. (See *Qualities of normal breath sounds,* page 203.)
• *Vesicular breath sounds* are the normal sounds heard when auscultating most of the lung fields. They are relatively quiet and low pitched, with a longer inspiration and a shorter, almost silent, expiration. Some examiners describe it as being like 'the wind blowing in the trees'.
• *Bronchovesicular sounds* are often heard close to the main bronchi, especially on the front of the chest and sometimes also on the back. They are characteristically more equal in length on inspiration and expiration, and a little louder/higher pitched. Note that these are also normally heard throughout the chest in infants, younger children and patients with very thin chest walls.
• *Bronchial breath sounds* are harsh and 'grating', with a short inspiration, a pause and then a longer expiration. They are only normal if heard over the trachea, an area that is not normally auscultated (although listening here can be a useful way of learning the sound).

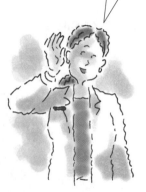

You might hear bronchial breath sounds over areas of consolidation.

Sounds in strange places

If you hear bronchial or bronchovesicular breath sounds in areas where you would expect to hear normal vesicular sounds, this is abnormal and may suggest consolidation. Also abnormal are what are

Qualities of normal breath sounds

Breath sound	Duration of sound	Intensity of sound	Pitch of sound	Location where normally heard
Vesicular	Inspiration longer than expiration	Soft	Low	Over most of the lung fields
Bronchovesicular	Inspiration and expiration of equal length	Intermediate	Intermediate	Over the lower trachea, left and right main bronchi. Sometimes between the upper scapula
Bronchial	Expiration longer than inspiration	Loud	Relatively high	Over the trachea in the neck

Adapted from *Breath Sounds Made Incredibly Easy* (2005:39).

known as 'added sounds' such as crackles, wheezes or a pleural friction rub. (See *Abnormal findings*, page 204.) As you listen to any abnormal sounds, consider their intensity, location, pitch and duration. Note whether the sound occurs when the patient inhales, exhales or both.

Sounds of silence

If you hear diminished vesicular breath sounds in both lungs, the patient may have a condition such as emphysema, atelectasis or severe bronchospasm. If you hear breath sounds in one lung only, the patient may have pleural effusion, pneumothorax, a tumour or mucous plugs in the airways. Complete absence of breath sounds in all or part of a lung requires urgent intervention.

Voicing complaints

Another test that can be undertaken, either as well as or instead of tactile fremitus, is checking the patient's vocal fremitus – voice sounds resulting from chest vibrations that occur as the patient speaks. Abnormal transmission of voice sounds – the most common of which are bronchophony, egophony and whispered pectoriloquy – may occur over consolidated areas. (See *Assessing vocal fremitus*, page 204.)

The next step

A patient with abnormal findings during a respiratory assessment may be further evaluated using diagnostic tests such as peak flow

Breath sounds in only one lung may indicate pleural effusion, pneumothorax, a tumour or mucous plugs in the airways.

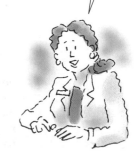

Assessing vocal fremitus

To assess for vocal fremitus, ask the patient to repeat the words below while you listen with a stethoscope. Auscultate over an area where you heard abnormally located bronchial breath sounds to check for abnormal voice sounds.

Bronchophony

Ask the patient to say 'ninety-nine' or 'blue moon'. Over normal lung tissue, the words sound muffled. Over consolidated areas, the words may sound unusually loud and clear.

Egophony

Ask the patient to say 'E'. Over normal lung tissue, the sound is muffled. Over consolidated lung tissue, it may sound like the letter 'A'.

Whispered pectoriloquy

Ask the patient to whisper '1, 2, 3'. Over normal lung tissue, the numbers will be almost indistinguishable. Over consolidated lung tissue, the numbers may be loud and clear.

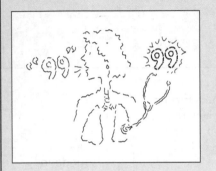
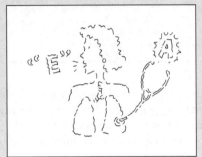
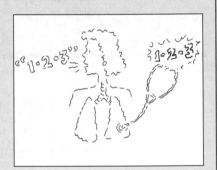

readings, arterial blood gas analysis and pulmonary function tests. (See *Further assessment of respiratory function*, page 205.)

Abnormal findings

Your assessment of the chest may reveal several abnormalities of the chest wall and lungs. In this section, we'll look at chest-wall abnormalities, abnormal respiratory patterns and abnormal breath sounds.

Chest-wall abnormalities

Chest-wall abnormalities may be congenital or acquired. Remember that a patient with a chest-wall deformity might have completely normal lungs, albeit that the lungs might be cramped within the chest. Alternatively the patient might have a smaller than normal lung capacity and limited exercise tolerance, and may develop respiratory difficulties from a respiratory tract infection. As such patients get older, they may fail to cope with chest-wall abnormalities

Further assessment of respiratory function

Peak flow testing

Peak flow, or peak expiratory flow rate, is a measurement of the peak (highest) rate of air expulsion from the mouth. It is measured using a peak flow meter. Normal readings vary due to age, gender and ethnic origin. Readings are therefore judged against a table of normal values or against a recording of the patient's best recorded measurement, and findings are quoted as a percentage of predicted value. In general terms a normal adult male value would be around 500 to 650 litres/minute and a female 400 to 500 litres/minute (Dougherty and Lister 2004a).

Pulse oximetry

Pulse oximetry uses a probe placed on a finger, toe or earlobe to detect an artery by pulsation. It then uses the colour difference between oxygenated and deoxygenated blood to calculate the oxygen saturation – the percentage of haemoglobin molecules that are fully saturated with oxygen. This is normally around 95% to 98%. Poor peripheral circulation may make the pulse difficult to detect and thus affects accuracy, as can bright fluorescent lights. It can also be inaccurate in severe cases of anaemia and carbon monoxide poisoning.

Arterial blood gases

Arterial blood gas analyses are used to explore respiratory symptoms and/or poor pulse oximetry readings, by establishing the partial pressure of oxygen (PaO_2), $PaCO_2$ and acid–base (pH) in the blood.

Chest X-ray

Chest X-ray is a valuable tool to evaluate respiratory symptoms, and may be used in a patient with an unexplained fever.

Pulmonary function tests

These tests measure the amount of air the lungs can inhale or exhale either per breath or per minute in a variety of different conditions. Tests commonly undertaken include:

- Tidal volume (VT) – amount of air inhaled or exhaled during normal breathing
- Minute volume (MV) – amount of air breathed per minute
- Inspiratory reserve volume (IRV) – amount of air that can be inhaled after normal inspiration
- Expiratory reserve volume (ERV) – amount of air that can be exhaled after normal expiration
- Vital capacity (VC) – amount of air that can be exhaled after maximum inspiration
- Inspiratory capacity (IC) – amount of air that can be inhaled after normal expiration
- Forced vital capacity (FVC) – amount of air that can be exhaled after maximum inspiration
- Forced expiratory volume (FEV) – volume of air exhaled in the first (FEV1), second (FEV2) or third (FEV3) second(s) of an FVC manoeuvre.

which they could cope with when they were younger. (See *Chest deformities*, page 207.)

Barrel chest

A barrel chest looks like its name implies. The chest is abnormally round and bulging, with a greater than normal A–P diameter. Barrel chest may be relatively normal/asymptomatic in some older patients, but can also occur as a result of chronic lung problems such as COPD. In such patients, barrel chest suggests that the lungs have lost their elasticity and that the diaphragm is flattened. Such patients typically use their accessory muscles and easily become breathless. You may well also note kyphosis (an outward curvature of the thoracic spine, which normally curves inwards), ribs that run horizontally rather than tangentially and a sternal angle greater than 90 degrees.

Pigeon chest

A patient with pigeon chest, or pectus carinatum, has a chest with a sternum that protrudes outward further than the ribs. The displaced sternum increases the front-to-back diameter of the chest. This may not cause the patient any respiratory problems, although it could restrict lung capacity, depending on the overall shape of the chest.

Funnel chest

A patient with funnel chest, or pectus excavatum, has a funnel-shaped depression on all or part of the sternum. The shape of the chest may interfere with respiratory and cardiac function. Compression of the heart and great vessels may cause murmurs.

Thoracic curvature

In thoracic curvature, the patient's spine curves outwards (kyphosis), sideways in an 'S' shape (scoliosis) or a combination of both (kyphoscoliosis). These abnormalities may make it more difficult to assess respiratory status. These deformities, which can be congenital, often worsen as the patient gets older and can significantly affect breathing in later life. Since routine screening of teenagers for this condition is now rare, your respiratory assessment offers opportunistic screening. A referral for further assessment if you suspect an abnormal curvature may save the patient from severe respiratory compromise in later years. (See also Chapter 13.)

Abnormal respiratory patterns

Identifying abnormal respiratory patterns can provide valuable clues about the patient's respiratory status and other health problems. (See *Abnormal respiratory patterns*, page 208.)

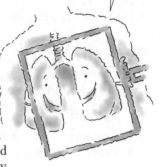

I may be normal, but a chest-wall abnormality may affect how I work.

Interpretation station

Chest deformities

As you inspect the patient's chest, note deviations in size and shape. The illustrations here show a normal adult chest and four common chest deformities.

Normal adult chest

Barrel chest

Funnel chest

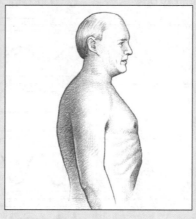

Increased A–P diameter.

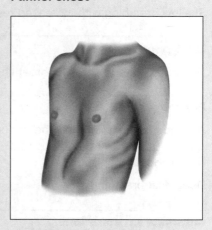

Depressed lower sternum. From Bickley, L.S. and Szilagyi, P. (2003) *Bates' Guide to Physical Examination and History Taking*. 8th edn. Philadelphia, PA: Lippincott Williams & Wilkins.

Pigeon chest

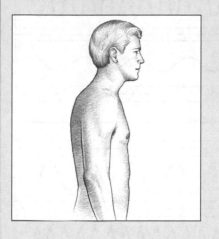

Depressed costal cartilages

Anteriorly displaced sternum

Anteriorly displaced sternum. From Bickley, L.S. and Szilagyi, P. (2003) *Bates' Guide to Physical Examination and History Taking*. 8th edn. Philadelphia, PA: Lippincott Williams & Wilkins.

Thoracic kyphoscoliosis

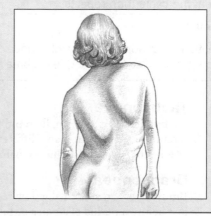

Raised shoulder and scapula, thoracic convexity and flared interspaces.

Interpretation station

Abnormal respiratory patterns

Here are typical characteristics of the most common abnormal respiratory patterns.

Tachypnoea

Shallow breathing with increased respiratory rate

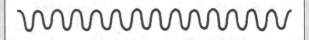

Bradypnoea

Decreased rate but regular breathing

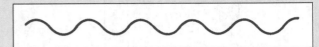

Apnoea

Absence of breathing; may be periodic

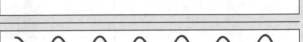

Hyperpnoea

Deep, fast breathing

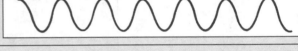

Kussmaul's respirations

Rapid, deep breathing without pauses; in adults, breathing usually sounds laboured with deep breaths that resemble sighs

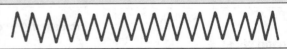

Cheyne–Stokes respirations

Regular periods of deep breathing alternated with periods of shallower breathing, usually ending in a period of apnoea; the cycle then repeats

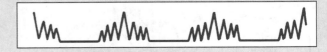

Biot's respirations

Rapid, deep breathing with abrupt periods of apnoea every three or four breaths; equal depth to each breath

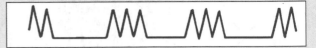

Tachypnoea

Tachypnoea, an abnormally rapid respiratory rate, is commonly seen in patients with many different lung diseases. It can also occur as a result of, and also due to, pain, sepsis, anxiety, obesity or fever.

Bradypnoea

Bradypnoea, an abnormally slow respiratory rate, is typically noted just before a period of apnoea or full respiratory arrest. Patients with bradypnoea might have central nervous system depression as a result of excessive sedation, excessive opiate analgesia, tissue damage or diabetic coma, which all depress the brain's respiratory control centre.

Apnoea

Apnoea is the absence of breathing. Periods of apnoea may be short, and occur sporadically during Cheyne–Stokes respirations, Biot's respirations or other abnormal respiratory patterns. Sleep apnoea is common in obese people. Apnoea may be life-threatening if periods last long enough.

Hyperpnoea

Characterised by deep, rapid breathing, hyperpnoea occurs in patients who have anxiety, pain, metabolic acidosis, hypoxia or hypoglycaemia.

Kussmaul's respirations

Kussmaul's respirations are rapid, deep, sighing breaths that occur in patients with metabolic acidosis, especially when associated with diabetic ketoacidosis.

Cheyne – Stokes respirations

Cheyne – Stokes respirations have a regular pattern of variations in the rate and depth of breathing. Deep breaths alternate with shallower breaths and short periods of apnoea. This respiratory pattern can occur in patients with heart failure, kidney failure or central nervous system damage, and is also commonly seen at the end of life.

Biot's respirations

Biot's respirations involve rapid, deep breaths (typically three or four breaths) that alternate with abrupt periods of apnoea. Biot's respirations are an ominous sign of severe central nervous system damage.

Abnormal breath sounds

In addition to hearing abnormal breath sounds in the form of bronchial or bronchovesicular sounds in the lung fields, you may also hear added (adventitious) sounds – crackles, wheezes, stridor and pleural friction rub. For more on breath sounds see *Breath Sounds Made Incredibly Easy* (2005).

Crackles

Crackles are intermittent, non-musical, brief crackling sounds that are caused by collapsed or fluid-filled alveoli popping open. They are heard primarily when the patient inhales. Crackles are classified as either fine or coarse. Fine crackles can be mimicked for learning purposes by rubbing the hair near the ear between the forefinger and thumb, whilst coarse crackles sound more like 'Velcro®' being pulled apart. Crackles

You need to do more than just count your patient's respiratory rate. Assessing the pattern of breathing can provide valuable clues about respiratory status and overall health.

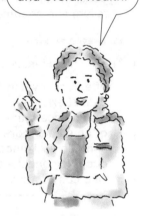

Types of crackles

Here's how to differentiate fine crackles from coarse crackles, a very helpful distinction when assessing the lungs.

Fine crackles

These characteristics distinguish fine crackles:

- usually heard first in the lung bases, spreading upwards as the condition worsens
- sound like a piece of hair being rubbed between the fingers
- may shift position as the patient moves; for example, may be found on the left side if the patient has just been sleeping on that side
- occur in conditions such as pulmonary fibrosis, asbestosis, silicosis, atelectasis, early congestive heart failure and pneumonia.

Coarse crackles

These characteristics distinguish coarse crackles:

- often occur when the patient starts to inhale and in the first half of inspiration; may be present when the patient exhales
- may be heard through the lungs and even at the mouth
- often sound more like bubbling or gurgling, as air moves through secretions in larger airways – sometimes likened to the sound of Velcro® being pulled apart
- occur in conditions such as COPD, bronchiectasis and pulmonary oedema, and in severely ill patients who can't cough.

are heard in a variety of conditions including pneumonia, bronchitis, heart failure and emphysaema. (See *Types of crackles*, above.)

Cough please!

Ask a patient with crackles to cough; if they clear with coughing, the problem is of less concern. Note that some practitioners and older texts use the term 'rales' to describe crackles, although use of this somewhat confusing term is now discouraged.

Wheezes

Wheezes are continuous sounds, often high pitched, and often heard first when a patient exhales. (See *When wheezing stops*, page 211.) The wheezing sounds occur when airflow is partially blocked or narrowed. As severity of the blockage increases, wheezes may also be heard when the patient inhales. The sound of a high-pitched wheeze tends not to change with coughing. Wheezes may occur as a result of a number of conditions including asthma, emphysaema, bronchitis or airway obstruction from a tumour or foreign body. (See *Signs and symptoms of upper airway obstruction*, page 211.)

When wheezing stops

If you no longer hear wheezing in a patient having an acute asthma attack, the attack may be far from over. When bronchospasm and mucosal swelling become severe, little air can move through the airways. As a result, you won't hear wheezing. This can be a very serious sign.

Other assessment criteria may also contribute to the suggestion that there is a serious problem – laboured breathing, prolonged expiratory time and accessory muscle use. As with the loss of audible wheeze, these signs are indicative of acute bronchial obstruction.

This is a medical emergency. Act to maintain the patient's airway and summon help. The patient may begin to wheeze again when the airways open.

Signs and symptoms of upper airway obstruction

If a patient can't maintain a patent airway, he/she may end up in respiratory arrest. Refer to this list of potential signs and symptoms when assessing a patient for partial or complete airway obstruction.

- Anxiety
- Dyspnoea
- Stridor
- Wheezing
- Decreased or absent breath sounds
- Use of accessory muscles
- See-saw movement between chest and abdomen
- Inability to speak, or severe difficulty in speaking
- Cyanosis.

Recognising rhonchi

Note that some practitioners use a different word for a lower pitched 'wheeze', describing this sound as a rhonchi. Rhonchi can be described as low-pitched, snoring, rattling sounds that occur primarily during exhalation, although they may also be heard on inhalation. The sound is more likely to change or disappear with coughing.

Stridor

Stridor is a loud, high-pitched crowing sound that is usually heard without a stethoscope, during inspiration. Stridor, which is caused by inflamed or obstructed upper airways, requires immediate attention. Causes include croup, epiglottitis and inhalation of a foreign body.

Pleural friction rub

Pleural friction rub is a low-pitched, grating, rubbing sound heard when the patient inhales and exhales; sometimes described as being like crunching leaves. Pleural inflammation causes the two layers of pleura to rub together. The patient may have pain in areas where the rub is heard.

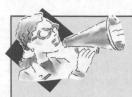

That's a wrap!

Respiratory system review

Structures and functions

Upper airways

- Include the nasopharynx, oropharynx, laryngopharynx and larynx
- Warm, filter and humidify inhaled air
- Transmits air to lower airways.

Lower airways

- Trachea – divides into the right and left main bronchi and continues to divide into smaller air passages
- Bronchioles – terminate in the alveolar ducts and the alveoli
- Alveoli – gaseous-exchange units of the lungs.

Lungs and lobes

- Left lung smaller than the right to accommodate the heart
- Left lung has two lobes – upper and lower
- Right lung has three lobes – upper, middle and lower
- Anterior chest mostly gives access to upper lobes and right middle lobes
- Posterior chest mostly gives access to lower lobes.

Thorax

- Includes the clavicles, sternum, scapulae, 12 sets of ribs (which allow the chest to expand and contract during each breath) and 12 thoracic vertebrae.

Respiratory muscles

- Diaphragm and external intercostal muscles (primary breathing muscles) – contract on inhalation and relax on exhalation
- Accessory inspiratory muscles (trapezius, sternomastoid and scalenes) – combine to elevate the scapulae, clavicle, sternum and upper ribs when primary breathing muscles aren't effective.

Health history

- Ask the patient about shortness of breath and its characteristics.
- Determine whether the patient has orthopnoea, and ask how many pillows he/she uses to sleep on at night.
- Ask the patient if they have a cough. If so, ask if it's productive or non-productive. If it's productive, ask them to describe the sputum.
- Ask the patient to describe any chest pain, including its location. Ask how it feels, if it radiates, what causes it and what makes it feel better.
- Ask about the patient's medical history, including smoking and exposure to irritants.

Assessment

Inspection

- Watch for chest-wall symmetry as the patient breathes. Note any paradoxical, or uneven, chest-wall movement. Note any use of accessory muscles.
- Count the patient's respiratory rate for a full minute. Normally 12 to 20 breaths per minute in an adult.
- Observe the patient's respiratory pattern; it should be even, coordinated and regular.
- Inspect the hands, fingers, nail beds, eyes, mouth and tongue, which can provide more information about the patient's respiratory status. Inspect the front and back of the chest for shape, scars, moles and lesions.

Palpation

- Palpate the front and back of the chest
- Palpate the chest for crepitus, tenderness, temperature and moisture as well as the presence of lumps
- Palpate for tactile fremitus
- Assess chest-wall symmetry and expansion.

Respiratory system review *(continued)*

Percussion

- Resonant sounds are heard over normal lung tissue
- Hyperresonance may be found over areas of increased air in the lung or pleural space (pneumothorax, emphysema)
- Dullness may be found over areas of decreased air in the lungs (atelectasis, pneumonia)
- Flatness may be found over highly consolidated areas (atelectasis, pleural effusion).

Auscultation

- Use the diaphragm of the stethoscope to listen to a full inspiration and a full expiration at each site.
- Ask the patient to breathe through their mouth.
- Hold the stethoscope firmly against the skin and avoid auscultating over clothing to prevent crackles.

Normal breath sounds

- Bronchial – loud, high-pitched and discontinuous (heard only over upper trachea)
- Bronchovesicular – medium-pitched and continuous (heard near the main bronchi)
- Vesicular – soft and low-pitched (heard in most of the lung fields).

Vocal fremitus

- Bronchophony – ask the patient to say 'ninety-nine'
- Egophony – ask the patient to say 'E'
- Whispered pectoriloquy – ask the patient to whisper '1, 2, 3'.

Abnormal findings

Chest-wall abnormalities

- Barrel chest – large front-to-back diameter
- Pigeon chest – sternum protrudes beyond front of abdomen; increased front-to-back diameter of chest

- Funnel chest – depression on all or part of the sternum
- Thoracic kyphoscoliosis – curvature of spine, rotation of vertebrae, distortion of lung tissues.

Abnormal respiratory patterns

- Tachypnoea – an abnormally rapid respiratory rate
- Bradypnoea – an abnormally slow respiratory rate
- Apnoea – the absence of breathing; may be life-threatening if it lasts too long
- Hyperpnoea – deep, rapid breathing
- Kussmaul's respirations – rapid, deep, sighing breaths
- Cheyne–Stokes respirations – deep breaths alternating with shallow breaths and periods of apnoea
- Biot's respirations – rapid, deep breaths that alternate with abrupt apnoeic periods.

Abnormal breath sounds

- Crackles – intermittent, non-musical, crackling sounds heard during inspiration; classified as fine or coarse
- Wheezes – high-pitched or low-pitched sounds caused by blocked airflow, heard on exhalation; low-pitched snoring or rattling sounds sometimes described as rhonchi
- Stridor – loud, high-pitched sound heard most commonly during inspiration, occasionally on expiration
- Pleural friction rub – low-pitched grating sound heard during inspiration and expiration; accompanied by pain.

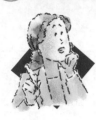

Quick quiz

1. Tactile fremitus would be considered abnormal if vibration was:
    A.   not equal on both sides of the chest at the same level.
    B.   greater at the apices than the bases.
    C.   absent at the bases and the patient was obese.
    D.   clearly felt throughout the chest and the patient was underweight.

2. The percussion sound usually heard over most of the lung fields in an adult is:
    A.   dullness.
    B.   resonance.
    C.   hyperresonance.
    D.   tympany.

3. When you auscultate the lower lobes of a healthy patient's lungs, you would expect to hear:
    A.   crackles.
    B.   bronchial breath sounds.
    C.   vesicular breath sounds.
    D.   bronchovesicular sounds.

4. If you percuss the chest of a normal infant the sound you are most likely to hear is:
    A.   hyperresonance.
    B.   dullness.
    C.   resonance.
    D.   flatness.

5. The anterior–posterior (A–P) diameter of the chest in an adult is:
    A.   normally the same as the transverse diameter.
    B.   sometimes less and sometimes more than the transverse diameter.
    C.   normally more than the transverse diameter.
    D.   normally less than the transverse diameter.

For answers see page 400.

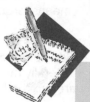

Just the facts

In this chapter, you'll learn:

♦ structures of the cardiovascular system and their functions
♦ the proper way to perform an assessment of the cardiovascular system
♦ normal and abnormal findings.

A look at the cardiovascular system

The cardiovascular system plays a vital role in the body. It delivers oxygenated blood, nutrients and other substances to the tissues and removes deoxygenated blood and waste products. The heart pumps blood to all the organs and tissues of the body. The autonomic nervous system controls how the heart pumps. The vascular network carries blood throughout the body, keeps the heart filled with blood and maintains blood pressure.

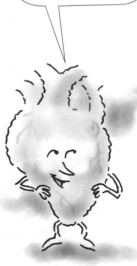

I don't want to brag too much, but pumping blood to all of the organs and tissues in the body is a big job!

Anatomy and physiology of the cardiovascular system

To make the most of your assessment of the cardiovascular system, you'll need to understand the anatomy and physiology of the heart and the vascular system.

Anatomy

The heart is a hollow, muscular organ located between the lungs in the mediastinum, behind and to the left of the sternum. In an adult it is about the size of a closed fist. The area of the chest overlying the heart is referred to as the precordium.

The heart spans the area from the second to the fifth intercostal space (spaces are numbered as those that sit below the corresponding rib). The right border of the heart aligns with the right border of the sternum. The left border lines up with the left midclavicular line. The upper, flatter part of the heart is known as the base, and sits around the second intercostal space, whilst the lower, more pointed part is known as the apex, and sits at the fifth intercostal space (fourth in an infant) in the midclavicular line. The exact position of the heart varies slightly with each patient.

> Remember: the prefix 'peri' means 'around', and 'cardium' means heart. So, 'pericardium' literally means 'around the heart'.

They'rrrrrre great!

Leading into and out of the heart are the great vessels: the inferior vena cava, the superior vena cava, the aorta, the pulmonary artery and four pulmonary veins.

Smooth sliding

The heart is protected by a thin sac called the pericardium, which has an inner, or visceral, layer that forms the epicardium and an outer, or parietal, layer. The space between the two layers normally contains a small amount of serous fluid, which prevents friction between the layers as the heart pumps.

Chamber made

The heart has four chambers (two atria and two ventricles) separated by a cardiac septum. The upper atria have thin walls and serve as reservoirs for receiving blood from the lungs (left side) and the body (right side). The thicker walled ventricles receive blood from the atria, and then push it into the lungs (right side) and out into the body (left side). (See *A close look at the heart*, page 217.)

Have blood, will travel

Blood moves to and from the heart through specific pathways. Deoxygenated venous blood is returned from the body to the right atrium via three different vessels; the superior vena cava returns blood from the upper body, the inferior vena cava returns blood from the lower body and blood from the heart muscle itself returns through the coronary sinus. All of the blood from those vessels empties into the right atrium.

A close look at the heart

This illustration details the internal structures of the heart.

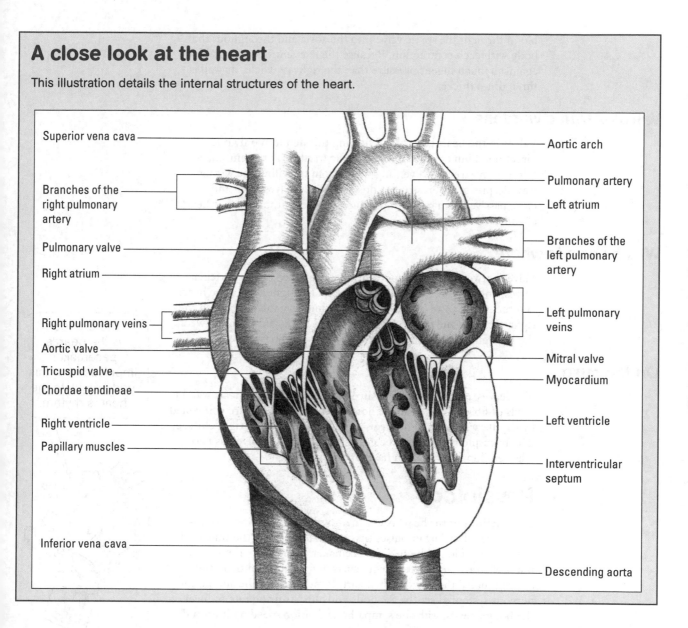

- Superior vena cava
- Branches of the right pulmonary artery
- Pulmonary valve
- Right atrium
- Right pulmonary veins
- Aortic valve
- Tricuspid valve
- Chordae tendineae
- Right ventricle
- Papillary muscles
- Inferior vena cava
- Aortic arch
- Pulmonary artery
- Left atrium
- Branches of the left pulmonary artery
- Left pulmonary veins
- Mitral valve
- Myocardium
- Left ventricle
- Interventricular septum
- Descending aorta

Travel plans

Blood in the right atrium is moved into the right ventricle, and from there it is ejected into the pulmonary artery when the ventricle contracts. The blood then travels to the lungs to be oxygenated.

From the lungs, blood travels to the left atrium. It then moves from the left atrium into the left ventricle, which then pumps the blood through the aortic valve into the aorta and throughout the body with each contraction. Because the left ventricle pumps blood against a much higher pressure than the right ventricle, its wall is three times thicker.

Valvular traffic wardens

Valves in the heart keep blood flowing through it in only one direction. Think of the valves as traffic wardens at the entrances to one-way streets, preventing blood from travelling the wrong way, despite great pressure to do so. Healthy valves open and close passively as a result of pressure changes within the four heart chambers and the great vessels.

Which valve is where?

Valves between the atria and ventricles are called atrioventricular valves, and include the tricuspid valve on the right side of the heart and the mitral valve on the left. The pulmonary valve (between the right ventricle and pulmonary artery) and the aortic valve (between the left ventricle and the aorta) are called semilunar valves.

On the cusp

The leaves, or cusps, of each valve are anchored to the heart wall by cords of fibrous tissue called chordae tendineae. They are controlled by papillary muscles. The cusps of the valves maintain tight closure. The tricuspid valve has three cusps, and the mitral valve has two. The semilunar valves each have three cusps.

Physiology

Contractions of the heart occur in a rhythm – the cardiac cycle – and are regulated by impulses that normally begin at the sinoatrial (SA) node, which is the heart's pacemaker. From here, these impulses travel to the atrioventricular node, and from there they are conducted throughout the heart. Impulses from the autonomic nervous system affect the SA node and alter its firing rate to meet the body's needs; with the sympathetic division speeding it up and the parasympathetic slowing it down.

The SA node is the heart's pacemaker. Impulses from this node regulate the heart's rhythm.

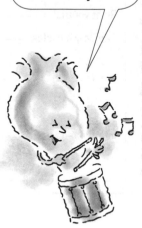

Contract, and then relax

The cardiac cycle consists of systole, the period when the heart contracts and sends blood on its outward journey, and diastole, the period when the heart relaxes and fills with blood. During diastole, the mitral and tricuspid valves are open, and the aortic and pulmonary valves are closed.

Diastole: parts I and II

Diastole consists of two parts, ventricular filling and atrial contraction. During the first part of diastole, about 75% of the blood in the atria drains into the ventricles as a result of the pressure in the atria being slightly higher than the pressure in the ventricles. This is a passive action.

The active period of diastole, atrial contraction (also called the atrial kick), accounts for the remaining 25% of blood that passes into the ventricles (Jarvis 2008). Diastole is also when the heart muscle receives its own supply of blood, which is transported by the coronary arteries.

Snap to it

Systole is the period of ventricular contraction. As pressure within the ventricles rises, the mitral and tricuspid valves snap closed. This closure leads to the first heart sound, S_1.

Open flow

When the pressure in the ventricles rises above the pressure in the aorta and pulmonary artery, the aortic and pulmonary valves open. Ventricular contraction then causes the blood to flow from the ventricles into the pulmonary artery to the lungs, and into the aorta for transport to the rest of the body.

Cycle of life

At the end of ventricular contraction, pressure in the ventricles drops below the pressure in the aorta and the pulmonary artery. This pressure difference – that is, the higher pressure in the aorta and pulmonary artery when compared with the ventricles – forces the blood back towards the ventricles, and thus causes the aortic and pulmonary valves to snap shut. This produces the second heart sound, S_2. As the valves shut, the atria fill with blood in preparation for the next period of diastolic filling, and the cycle begins again. (See *Cardiovascular changes with ageing*, page 220.)

Vascular system

The vascular system delivers oxygen, nutrients and other substances to the body's cells, and removes the waste products of cellular metabolism. The peripheral vascular system consists of a network of

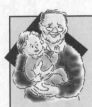

Ages and stages

Cardiovascular changes with ageing

Changes in the cardiovascular system occur as a natural part of the ageing process. These changes, however, place elderly patients at higher risk for cardiovascular disorders than younger patients. As you assess elderly patients, be aware of these changes which occur with ageing:

- slight decrease in heart size
- loss of cardiac contractile strength and efficiency
- gradual decrease in cardiac output
- thickening of heart valves, causing incomplete valve closure (as well as a possibility of a systolic murmur – but never assume this is normal)
- increase in left ventricular wall thickness

- fibrous tissue infiltration of the SA node and internodal atrial tracts, causing possible atrial fibrillation and flutter
- dilation and stretching of veins
- decline in coronary artery blood flow
- increased aortic rigidity
- increased amount of time necessary for heart rate to return to normal after exercise
- decreased strength and elasticity of blood vessels, contributing to arterial and venous insufficiency
- decreased ability to respond to physical and emotional stress.

arteries, arterioles, capillaries, venules and veins which, in an adult, is constantly filled with about 4 to 6 litres of blood – the circulating blood volume. (See *A close look at arteries and veins*, page 222.) In infants, the circulating blood volume is just a few hundred millilitres, making them especially vulnerable to blood or fluid loss.

Thick-skinned arteries

Arteries carry blood away from the heart. Nearly all arteries carry oxygen-rich blood from the heart throughout the rest of the body. The only exception is the pulmonary artery, which carries deoxygenated blood from the right ventricle to the lungs. Arteries are thick-walled because they transport blood under high pressure. Arterial walls contain a tough, elastic layer to help propel blood through the arterial system. Arteries then divide to become smaller arterioles, and eventually capillaries.

Thin-skinned capillaries

Capillaries enable oxygen to be delivered to the tissues of the body, and carbon dioxide to be returned to the lungs. They also enable the exchange of fluid, nutrients and metabolic waste between blood and cells. The exchange can occur because capillaries are thin-walled and highly permeable. Slightly more fluid tends to move out of the capillaries than is returned to them, with the remainder taken up by the lymphatic system. (See Chapter 10.)

Reservoir veins

Blood then flows from the capillaries into venules, which merge to form the larger veins. Venules and veins return blood to the heart. Nearly all veins carry deoxygenated blood – the sole exception being the pulmonary vein, which carries oxygenated blood from the lungs to the left atrium. Veins serve as a large reservoir for circulating blood.

The wall of a vein is thinner and more pliable than the wall of an artery. This pliability allows the vein to accommodate variations in blood volume. Veins contain valves at periodic intervals to prevent blood from flowing backwards.

Finger on the pulse

Arterial pulses are pressure waves of blood generated by the pumping action of the heart. All vessels in the arterial system have pulsations, but there are certain points in the body where peripheral pulses can be readily felt. These include the temporal, carotid, brachial, radial, femoral, popliteal, posterior tibial and dorsalis pedis. The precise location of these pulse points varies between individuals.

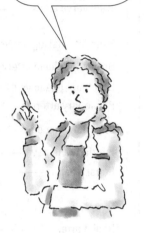

Veins are thin and pliable so they can accommodate variations in blood volume.

Obtaining a health history

In a cardiovascular examination, the timing of the history in relation to the physical examination will depend on the acuity of the presentation. In any assessment of cardiovascular symptoms an initial ABCDE assessment (airway, breathing, circulation, disability, exposure – Resuscitation Council UK 2006) is essential. In many settings/situations it is also likely that a continuous electrocardiogram recording will be commenced at the beginning of the assessment process, to inform the initial prioritisation of care and provide ongoing monitoring. (For more on electrocardiogram recording, see *ECG Interpretation Made Incredibly Easy* 2007.) Assuming it is safe to take the history first, continue as follows.

To obtain a health history of a patient's cardiovascular system, begin by introducing yourself and explaining what will occur during the health history and physical examination. Then obtain the following information.

A close look at arteries and veins

This illustration shows the major arteries and veins of the body.

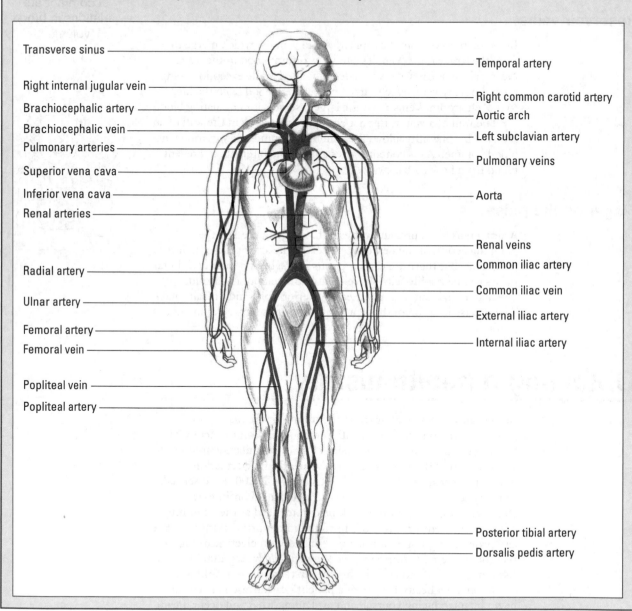

Transverse sinus

Right internal jugular vein

Brachiocephalic artery

Brachiocephalic vein

Pulmonary arteries

Superior vena cava

Inferior vena cava

Renal arteries

Radial artery

Ulnar artery

Femoral artery

Femoral vein

Popliteal vein

Popliteal artery

Temporal artery

Right common carotid artery

Aortic arch

Left subclavian artery

Pulmonary veins

Aorta

Renal veins

Common iliac artery

Common iliac vein

External iliac artery

Internal iliac artery

Posterior tibial artery

Dorsalis pedis artery

Asking about the reason for seeking care

You'll find that patients with a cardiovascular problem typically cite one or more specific complaints, such as:
- chest pain
- irregular heartbeat or palpitations
- shortness of breath on exertion, when lying down or at night
- cough
- weakness
- fatigue
- unexplained weight change
- swelling of the extremities
- dizziness
- headache
- changes to skin colour/appearance
- pain in the extremities, such as leg pain or cramps.

Explore each of these symptoms as reported using the PQRSTU, OLD CART or other mnemonic of your choice. (see page 16).

Rating the pain

Many patients with cardiovascular problems complain of chest pain at some point. As you use the mnemonic to assess pain, remember the 1 to 10 pain rating scale (1 = no pain, 10 = the worst pain imaginable). Compare ratings for when the pain was at its worst and currently. Continue to use the pain rating to assess improvement or deterioration.

Broadening the scope

A number of specific questions are useful in assessing a patient with cardiovascular disease. It is particularly helpful to also ask the patient these questions:
- Are you ever short of breath? If so, what makes you breathless?
- Do you feel dizzy or fatigued?
- Do your rings or shoes feel tight?
- Do your ankles swell? If so, at what part of the day?
- Have you noticed changes in colour or sensation in your legs? If so, what are those changes?
- If you have wounds or ulcers, how quickly do they heal?
- Do you ever wake up in the night feeling suddenly short of breath?

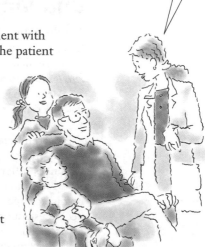

Does your family have a history of diabetes or lung, kidney or liver disease?

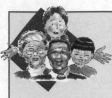

Bridging the gap

At risk for cardiovascular disease

As you analyse a patient's problems, remember that several factors increase a patient's risk of cardiovascular disease. These include:

- Hypertension
- Being male
- Being female and post menopausal
- Increasing age (see *Cardiovascular changes with ageing*, page 220)
- Ethnicity – Afro–Caribbean people have the highest prevalence of heart disease (Jarvis 2008)
- Smoking or history of having smoked
- Diabetes
- Family history of coronary heart disease
- High cholesterol
- Being overweight or having a large waist to hip ratio (see Chapter 4)
- Taking little or no exercise.

Explore any positive findings thoroughly to gain a clear picture of the problem.

Asking about personal and family health

Ask the patient for details about their past medical history and family history, including heart disease, raised cholesterol, high blood pressure, diabetes and diseases of the lungs, kidneys or liver. (See *At risk for cardiovascular disease*, above.)

Also, as per the guidelines for taking a comprehensive history discussed in Chapter 1, be sure to obtain information about:
- Stress and the patient's methods of coping with it
- Current health habits, such as smoking, alcohol intake, exercise, dietary intake of fat and salt and caffeine intake (especially if the patient is suffering from palpitations)
- Medication which the patient is taking, including over-the-counter medicines, recreational drugs and herbal preparations – remember, decongestant nasal sprays can cause palpitations
- Previous serious illnesses, hospitalisation or operations
- Environmental or occupational considerations.

Assessing the cardiovascular system

Cardiovascular disease affects people of all ages and can take many forms. A consistent, methodical approach to your assessment will help you identify abnormalities. As always, the key to accurate assessment is regular practise, which will help to improve technique and efficiency.

Before you begin your physical assessment, you'll need to obtain an appropriate stethoscope (see Chapter 2) and a pen torch.

Sitting comfortably

The heart is best examined with the patient undressed to the waist and lying on a bed or couch at about a 45 degree angle. Older girls and women will appreciate an examination gown and/or being able to keep their bra on until you need them to remove it. Examining the patient from the right, if feasible, will enable you to be in the best position to assess the jugular venous pressure (JVP).

In order to examine the heart you'll inspect, palpate and auscultate. Percussion of the heart is described in some texts, but is now seldom recommended as it is unreliable.

General inspection

First, take a moment to assess the patient's overall general appearance. Remember ABCDE and move on only if there is no need for immediate intervention in these areas. Also consider whether the patient appears alert or confused/aggressive.

Colour changes?

Consider the patient's skin colour – is there any sign of pallor, or peripheral or central cyanosis? Remember the variations to look for in darker-skinned patients. (See *Detecting colour variations in dark-skinned people* in Chapter 5, page 104.) Does the patient appear short of breath at rest? Is there any sign of excessive sweating (diaphoresis)?

Then move on to consider other factors. Is the patient overly thin or obese? Are they anxious or distressed? Are there any dysmorphic (abnormal) facial features? – remember many congenital conditions such as Down's syndrome are linked to a high incidence of congenital heart disease.

Inspection of the vital signs, hands and face

Now move on to inspect the vital signs, hands and face. These can give you a great deal of information about the cardiovascular system before you look at the chest.

How many beats a minute?

What is the radial pulse rate? Count for a minimum of 30 seconds, or a full minute if the patient is tachycardic, has an irregular pulse or is an infant/young child. Also note the rhythm and volume. Now feel the pulse in both wrists at the same time. Are both pulses the same? Also check the respiratory rate for a full minute. See Chapter 2 for normal values in adults and children.

Hands it to me

Inspect the hands for colour. Is there pallor or blue tinging suggesting peripheral cyanosis? Are they warm or cool? How do your findings compare with the temperature of the room?

Nail it!

Now look more closely at the nails. Is there any sign of clubbing, the loss of the normal angle between the nail and the nail bed? (See Chapter 5.) Also check for signs of splinter haemorrhages. These are fine vertical dark red lines in the nails and can be indicative of bacterial endocarditis.

Capillary check

Check the patient's peripheral capillary return, which helps to assess the status of circulation. Hold the hand level with the patient's heart and compress a fingertip firmly between your finger and thumb for 5 seconds, and then let go. Initial blanching (whitening) will occur. How long does it take colour to return? Initial blanching (pallor) will occur. At normal room temperature, colour should return within 2 seconds (Resuscitation Council UK 2006) – although note McGee (2007) suggests that return up to 3 seconds can be normal in some individuals.

What's the shape of it?

Next check the quality of the brachial pulses, which are found in the inner aspects of both elbows. Ask the patient to stretch their arms out in front of them, palms upwards. Some texts recommend palpating with the more sensitive thumb (Northridge *et al.* 2005), others suggest the index and middle fingers (Bickley and Szilagyi 2007). The brachial pulse is usually located on the medial side (closest to the body). In addition to rate, rhythm and volume, the brachial pulse allows you to assess the shape or 'wave form' of the pulse. (See *Pulse waveforms*, page 243.)

Under pressure?

What is the blood pressure? (See Chapter 2 for discussion of normal findings.) In a full cardiovascular examination this should be measured on both arms. A difference of more than 10 to 15 mmHg suggests arterial compression or obstruction (Jarvis 2008). If the patient is experiencing unexplained falls or blackouts, check their blood pressure in both lying and standing positions. A drop of more than 20 mmHg on standing suggests orthostatic hypotension, which may explain the problem (Jarvis 2008).

Eyes right?

Now look at the conjunctiva by pulling down the lower eyelids (or asking the patient to do this). Are there signs of pallor, especially on the outer edge nearest the eyelashes? This can suggest anaemia. Any suggestion of anaemia should be checked with a full blood count, which assesses the haemoglobin level in the red blood cells, as well as the number of red blood cells, white blood cells and platelets.

Cholesterol checks

Then look at the outer edge of the iris. A white ring, '*corneal arcus*', suggests raised cholesterol, and is particularly worrying in younger patients. Also look on the eyelids and around the eyes for small, irregular shaped, fatty deposits known as '*xanthalasmata*'. These sometimes indicate raised cholesterol. Either finding should prompt a cholesterol check.

Feeling blue?

Look at the lips, oral mucosa and tongue. Is there any sign of the bluish tinge of cyanosis? Are the teeth healthy? Untreated dental caries or gum disease increases the risk of bacterial endocarditis because bacteria can enter the bloodstream from the mouth. Patients with some heart conditions, such as valve replacements, must pay particular attention to dental hygiene, and may well require antibiotic 'cover' for any dental treatment.

Examination of the neck

Examination of the neck allows you to assess the carotid arteries and internal jugular vein.

Carotid arteries

As well as inspecting the carotid arteries you will also palpate and auscultate them. It makes good sense to complete the examination of the neck at this point, before moving on to the chest.

> Never palpate both carotid arteries at the same time. Doing so could cause the patient to faint or become bradycardic.

Peruse those pulsations

Inspect the neck for visible pulsations. Can you see the carotid arterial pulse – a brisk, localised pulsation medial to the sternomastoid muscle and lateral to the 'Adam's apple'? It is frequently, but not always, seen.

Feel the force

Now palpate the carotid pulse. You should be close to the middle of the neck, just lateral to the Adam's apple. Feeling too laterally is a common mistake. Some examiners suggest using the thumb, placing the fingers behind the neck and extending the thumb forward onto the artery (Northridge *et al*. 2005), others suggest using two or three fingers (Jarvis 2008). See which method works best for you. *Never* palpate both carotid arteries at the same time or press too firmly; the patient may faint or become bradycardic. Is the pulse weak or bounding?

Breath or bruit?

Auscultate the carotid arteries to listen for bruits. Bruit is a 'whooshing sound' caused by the turbulent blood flow through a narrowed artery, and should be investigated. However, many narrowed arteries don't produce a bruit, so their absence doesn't confirm that all is well. Listen on each side using the bell, as the sounds are often low-pitched. A breath sound may mimic a bruit, so if you are unsure repeat with the patient holding their breath. You will sometimes hear referred heart sounds when auscultating the carotids; this is quite normal.

Jugular venous pressure

The JVP provides information about blood volume and pressure in the right side of the heart. The internal jugular pulsation sits lateral to the carotid, has a softer pulsation and beats at double the rate. Unlike the carotid, the internal jugular pulsation changes in response to positioning (rising higher in the neck as the patient lies down, falling as the patient sits up). Also, it can't normally be palpated.

Pressure from the right

The JVP is always assessed on the right-hand side of the neck, and usually the internal, as opposed to external, jugular vein is used. Ask the patient to lie back at an angle of around 30 to 45 degrees (assuming flat is 0 degrees and upright 90 degrees) and to turn their head slightly to the left. Use a torch or overhead light to help create shadows and ease your view. The internal jugular vein runs from behind the ear, down the neck towards the clavicle, mostly lying under the sternomastoid muscle. You can sometimes confuse it with the external jugular vein, which lies lateral to it (the external jugular is sometimes more obvious because it doesn't sit under the sternomastoid muscle). If you are unsure which vein you can see, don't worry. Although the internal jugular is traditionally used for JVP measurement, McGee (2007) suggests that either the internal or external jugular can be used.

Double take

Start looking for the JVP above the clavicle (the area known as the supraclavicular fossa) and then look upwards at the side of the neck, until you spot its characteristic 'double pulsation'. If it helps, feel the carotid or radial pulse to confirm that the pulsation you can see is twice as fast. The JVP is the highest pulsation point you can see.

Scale the heights

To measure the JVP, place a ruler vertically up from the sternal angle ('bump' on the sternum, see Chapter 8), and a straight edge horizontally across from the highest point of pulsation to the ruler. What is the height in cm? Pulsation above 3 to 4 cm indicates an elevation in central venous pressure (Bickley and Szilagyi 2007). This may be due to problems with the right side of the heart and/or fluid overload. A very low JVP may suggest dehydration. Note: more experienced examiners estimate the JVP height visually, but this takes lots of practise.

Can't see it?

If you can't see a JVP it may be low or very high. Check again with the patient lying flatter, which may make a low JVP visible just above the collar bone, and again with the patient sat more upright, which may make a very high JVP visible below the ear. Note JVP is difficult to see in children younger than about 12 years of age.

Peak technique

Identifying cardiovascular landmarks

These views show where to find critical landmarks used in cardiovascular assessment.

Anterior thorax

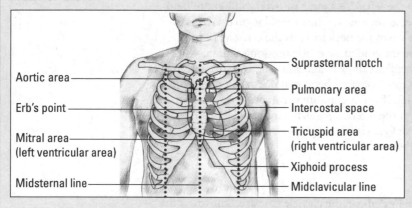

Aortic area

Erb's point

Mitral area
(left ventricular area)

Midsternal line

Suprasternal notch

Pulmonary area

Intercostal space

Tricuspid area
(right ventricular area)

Xiphoid process

Midclavicular line

Lateral thorax

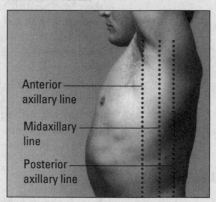

Anterior
axillary line

Midaxillary
line

Posterior
axillary line

Inspection of the chest (precordium)

The last part of inspection looks at the area of the chest over the heart, the precordium. Remember the landmarks you can use to describe your findings. (See *Identifying cardiovascular landmarks*, above.)

Heave ho!

Look for pulsations, symmetry of movement, retractions (pulling in of the chest) or heaves. A heave is a strong outwards movement of the chest wall that moves with the heartbeat. Are there any other abnormalities of the chest as you inspect it?

On impulse

Lastly look for the apical impulse – use a torch or tangential light to help. This is also sometimes known as the 'point of maximal impulse'. It is only visible in some patients; its presence and absence are both normal findings. If seen it should be located in the fifth intercostal space (fourth in an infant) at, or just medial to, the left midclavicular line. To find the apical impulse in a woman, ask her to hold her breast up out of the way during this part of the examination.

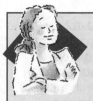

Peak technique

Assessing the apical impulse

The apical impulse is associated with the first heart sound and is sometimes described as the point of maximal impulse. As you palpate the apical impulse, note the following features:

- Location – the pulsation should be at the fifth intercostal space in or just medial to the mid-clavicular line, except in an infant where it sits in the fourth intercostal space
- Amplitude – the pulsation should feel like it is gently 'tapping' or 'kissing' your fingertips; it should not feel overly strong or forceful
- Size – the pulsation should be no bigger than 2.5 cm, or two fingertips in diameter
- Duration – the pulsation should be no more than a third of the total cardiac cycle
- Rate, rhythm, volume and shape.

Note: if you are unsure whether you are palpating the apical impulse, it should match the carotid pulse, so feeling both together might be helpful.

Palpation

Now palpate to feel the apical impulse. Place two fingertips over the impulse you can see, or over the fifth intercostal space in the mid-clavicular line if you can't see it. Move your fingers around slightly if you don't feel it. The apical impulse may be difficult to palpate in overweight patients or those with muscular chests. If so, try asking the patient to lie on their left side and palpate again, although this will displace the impulse towards the anterior axillary line. (To interpret your findings, see *Assessing the apical impulse*, above.)

Tender touch

Now generally palpate over the whole chest with your finger-tips, paying particular attention to the area either side of the sternum. Is there any tenderness? Musculoskeletal pain is more likely than cardiac pain to be induced or made worse by palpation, although never rely on this finding alone to determine the cause of pain.

Plentiful places to palpate

Palpate again using the flat of your hand. Note pulsation in any areas other than the apical impulse. Pulsation in other areas is generally abnormal, although may be normal in very thin patients. You may also feel heaves that you didn't notice on inspection.

Feel a thrill

Thrills are vibrations felt under the skin, sometimes described as feeling like the 'purr of a cat'. They are best felt with the bony part of the upper palm, or the edge of the hand adjacent to the little finger. They are most often associated with a loud murmur, so some experienced examiners only feel for thrills if they hear a murmur on auscultation. Feel for thrills over the aortic, pulmonary, tricuspid and mitral areas. (See *Sites for heart sounds*, page C5.)

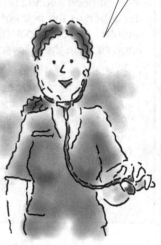

Cardiac auscultation requires a methodological approach and lots of practise.

Auscultation

Cardiac auscultation tells you a lot about the heart, but it requires a methodical approach and lots of practise. Warm the stethoscope in your hands if it's cold. Use the bell to hear lower-pitched sounds and the diaphragm to hear higher-pitched sounds. It is really important to listen in all areas with both the diaphragm *and* the bell, as some abnormalities will only be heard with one or the other. (See *Sites for heart sounds*, page C5.)

Have a plan

Auscultate for heart sounds with the patient lying on his/her back with the head of the bed/couch raised to around 45 degrees.

The main positions where you should listen *as a minimum* are as follows:

• Second intercostal space, right sternal border – aortic area (remember, the sternal angle is adjacent to the second rib, with the second intercostal space just below; this is a good way to find your starting point)

• Second intercostal space, left sternal border – pulmonary area

• Third intercostal space, left sternal border – Erb's point; this is the midpoint between the four heart valves

• Fourth/fifth intercostal space, left sternal border – tricuspid area (it is often useful also to listen in the same position on the right sternal border – sometimes tricuspid is heard better there)

• Fifth intercostal space, midclavicular line – mitral area (remember, if the heart is enlarged the apex will be positioned more laterally, so it is useful to listen in the anterior axillary line to check the sound is quieter rather than louder).

Note that some experts now discourage the use of the terms aortic, pulmonary, tricuspid and mitral areas. Although they describe the listening points where the valves are typically heard, sounds from an abnormal valve may actually be heard in the 'area' of a different valve – for example, aortic stenosis may be heard loudest in the mitral area (McGee 2007). So take care not to jump to any conclusions.

Inching around

Although these are the minimum positions, sounds may radiate in different directions, so if you hear any abnormal sounds you should 'inch' the stethoscope around, making small movements, to follow them where they go. Also 'inch' the stethoscope if the sound is quiet to ensure you are listening in the best place for that valve.

Repositioning request

Two other positions can provide very helpful information in a complete cardiac examination – the left lateral position and the upright, forward leaning position. (See *Additional positioning of the patient for auscultation*, page 236.)

Interpreting your findings

At each listening position, note the heart rate and rhythm. Always identify S_1 and S_2, and then listen for adventitious (added) sounds between and either side of them, such as third and fourth heart sounds (S_3 and S_4) and murmurs. (See *Cycle of heart sounds*, pages C6–C7.)

Listen for the 'dub'

Start auscultating at the aortic area where S_2, the second heart sound, is loudest. The sound corresponds to closure of the pulmonary and aortic valves, and is generally described as sounding like 'dub'. It tends to be a shorter, higher pitched and louder sound than S_1. In some situations, particularly in children, you here a 'double dub' – a split S_2. This occurs because the pulmonary valve closes fractionally later that the aortic valve, so both closing sounds are heard separately. If it occurs in children during inspiration only, it is regarded as normal. In adults, or if present all the time or only on expiration, it should be investigated further, although it may turn out to be of no clinical significance.

> The 'lub' of the S_1 is loudest at the mitral area.

> The 'dub' of the S_2 is loudest at the aortic area.

Listen for the 'lub'

From the aortic area of the heart, move to the pulmonary area (S_2 will also be loudest here) and then down via Erb's point to the tricuspid area. Then move to the mitral area, where S_1 is the loudest. This sound corresponds to closure of the mitral and tricuspid valves and is generally described as sounding like 'lub'. It's low-pitched and dull. If heard as a 'lub-lub', a split S_1, it should be further investigated.

'Sloshing in . . .'

A third, low-pitched heart sound, S_3, may be heard immediately after S_2. It may be a normal finding in children and young adults, but is usually abnormal after the age of 40. Commonest causes include left ventricular failure and mitral valve regurgitation. The sound of S_1, S_2 and S_3 is often compared with the sound when you say '*slosh-ing in*', with the S_3 sound made by the 'in'. This also helps you remember that S_3 typically occurs as a result of vibration during early diastole, when the ventricles are filling rapidly.

. . . or 'a stiff wall'

The rarer abnormal sound S_4, occurs just before S_1, at the end of diastole. Causes include left ventricular hypertrophy, hypertension and aortic stenosis. It is often likened to the sound when saying '*A stiff wall*', with the S_4 being the 'A' sound. This also helps remind you that the abnormal sound is caused by vibrations that occur as the atria contract and try to push blood into resistant ventricles that are enlarged or hypertrophied and don't expand as much as they should.

Auscultating for murmurs

Murmurs occur when structural defects in the heart's chambers or valves cause turbulent blood flow. (See *Understanding murmurs*, page C8.) Turbulence may also be caused by changes in the viscosity of blood or the speed of blood flow. Murmurs are typically described as a 'whooshing sound', although the sound varies depending on the cause. Remember, detecting murmurs, especially mild ones, takes lots and lots of practise listening to both normal and abnormal hearts.

Auscultation tips

Follow these tips when you auscultate a patient's heart:

- Concentrate as you listen for each sound.
- Avoid auscultating through clothing, or wound dressings (if possible), because they can block sound.
- Avoid picking up extraneous sounds by keeping the stethoscope tubing off the patient's body and other surfaces.
- Until you become proficient at auscultation and can examine a patient quickly, explain that even though you may listen to the chest for a long period, it doesn't mean anything is wrong.
- The patient should just breathe normally, but it may be helpful to ask them to hold their breath briefly if you are trying to listen to a particular sound that is difficult to hear. Always remember to remind them to start breathing again after a few seconds. If you think you'll forget, hold your own breath at the same time.

Tips for learning to recognise and describe murmurs

Describing murmurs can be tricky. Try to gain experience with patients in your clinical area who have a murmur. After you've auscultated a murmur, list the terms you would use to describe it. Then check the patient's notes to see how others have described it, or ask an experienced colleague to listen and describe the murmur. Compare the descriptions and then auscultate for the murmur again, if necessary, to confirm the description.

Murmur variations

Murmurs can occur during systole or diastole and are described by several criteria. (See *Tips for learning to recognise and describe murmurs*, above.) They are graded primarily according to intensity on a scale from 1 to 6. (See *Grading murmurs*, below.) Their pitch can be high, medium or low. They can vary in intensity during the cardiac cycle, growing louder or softer, or louder and then softer. They can vary by location, sound pattern (blowing, harsh or musical) and radiation pattern (to the neck or axillae). They are also described by their duration and timing during the cardiac cycle; for example, pansystolic, midsystolic or diastolic.

Grading murmurs

Use the system outlined here to describe the intensity of a murmur. When recording the findings, note that some practitioners use Roman numerals. All murmurs are graded out of 6, so use this as your denominator. For example, a grade 3 murmur would be recorded as 'grade 3/6'.

- Grade 1 is a barely audible murmur
- Grade 2 is audible but quiet and soft
- Grade 3 is moderately loud, without a palpable thrill
- Grade 4 is loud, with a palpable thrill
- Grade 5 is very loud, with a palpable thrill
- Grade 6 is loud enough to be heard before the stethoscope comes into contact with the chest.

This standardised grading system for all murmurs is sometimes described as Levine's grading system, after its inventors Freeman and Levine (McGee 2007).

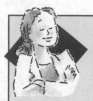

Peak technique

Additional positioning of the patient for auscultation

In addition to examining all of the key positions with the patient lying at about 45 degrees, for a comprehensive cardiac examination listen in the following positions:

Left lateral position

Place the patient lying down in the left lateral position. Listen again to the tricuspid and mitral using the bell. This is the best position to hear the abnormal sounds of S_3 and S_4, or mitral valve problems.

Sitting up and leaning forward

Then ask the patient to sit up, lean forward and hold their breath. Listen over the aortic and pulmonary valves, and down the left sternal border, using the diaphragm. Allow the patient to take one or more breaths part way through as they require. This examination is particularly helpful to assess aortic and pulmonary valve problems.

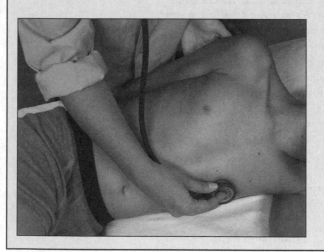

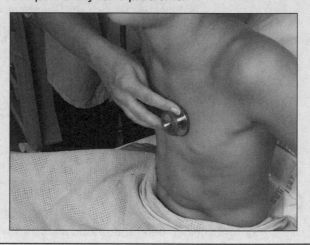

Sit up, please

Sometimes the best way to hear murmurs is with the patient sitting up and leaning forward, so it is important to do this if you suspect a murmur. Also listen with the patient on his/her left side. (See *Additional positioning of the patient for auscultation*, above.)

Normal or not?

Not all murmurs are abnormal. Some murmurs, especially in children or pregnant women, can be normal. But expert assessment is needed to judge which murmurs are a cause for concern, so newly identified murmurs should always be referred for further investigation.

Auscultating for pericardial friction rub

A pericardial friction rub is a high-pitched scratchy sound. It can be heard anywhere in the precordium but is often heard best at the lower left sternal border and/or the apex, with the patient sitting up and leaning forwards. You may hear it more easily if the patient holds their breath.

Auscultating the lung bases

To complete cardiac auscultation, listen to the lung bases for 'crackles'. This is because left-sided heart failure may cause fluid congestion in the lungs, particularly the lung bases.

For more information on assessing heart sounds see *Heart Sounds Made Incrediby Easy* (2005).

Completing the cardiovascular examination

Completing the cardiovascular examination requires the examiner to consider the lower part of the vascular system and also to examine for any signs of oedema.

Swell scale

Whilst left-sided heart failure causes back pressure on the lungs, right-sided failure causes back pressure on the venous system. So examine the sacral area (perhaps whilst the patient is sitting forward for lung auscultation, or whilst they are rolled on their left side) for signs of sacral oedema. Also check the abdomen for ascites. (See Chapter 11.) Also examine the legs and ankles for signs of oedema – if you press for 5 seconds and then release, you shouldn't see an indentation.

Artery check!

Palpate the lower pulses, including:
• Femoral (in the groin)
• Popliteal (behind the knee, difficult to feel so don't worry if you can't feel it provided the dorsalis pedis and posterior tibial pulses are normal)
• Posterior tibial (just behind the medial malleoulus)
• Dorsalis pedis (in the middle of the top of the foot, often felt about 3 to 5 cm up from the second toe).

Palpate for the pulse on each side, comparing pulse volume and symmetry. If you haven't put on gloves for the examination, do so when you palpate the femoral arteries. All pulses should be regular in rhythm and equal in strength. (See *Assessing arterial pulses*, page 239.)

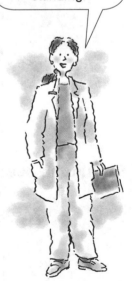

Leg veins should be evaluated while the patient is standing.

Vascular verification

Note finally the importance of examination of the abdomen for signs of abdominal aortic aneurysm, or arterial stenosis of the aorta and other major arteries. See Chapter 11 for these techniques.

Abnormal findings

This section outlines some of the most common cardiovascular abnormalities and their causes.

Chest pain

Chest pain can arise suddenly or gradually, and its cause may be difficult to ascertain initially. The pain can radiate to the arms, neck, jaw or back. It can be steady or intermittent, mild or acute. In addition, the pain can range in character from a sharp, shooting sensation to a feeling of heaviness, fullness or even indigestion – so check a history of severe or current indigestion carefully. Cardiac pain may also be the cause of pain in the shoulder, left upper quadrant of the abdomen or the epigastric region.

Common culprits

Chest pain may be caused by various disorders. Common cardiovascular causes include angina, myocardial infarction and cardiomyopathy. Chest pain may be provoked or aggravated by stress, anxiety, exertion, deep breathing or eating certain foods. Or it may have no apparent cause.

Palpitations

Palpitations – defined as a conscious awareness of one's heartbeat – are usually felt over the precordium or in the throat or neck. The patient may describe them as pounding, jumping, turning, fluttering or flopping or as missed or skipped beats. Palpitations may be regular or irregular, fast or slow, paroxysmal (intermittent) or sustained.

Behind the beat

Although sometimes insignificant, palpitations may result from a cardiac or metabolic disorder or from the effects of certain drugs. A key factor determining severity is whether or not the patient's cardiac function is affected. Transient palpitations may accompany emotional stress (such as fright, anger or anxiety) or physical stress (such as exercise or fever). Stimulants such as tobacco and caffeine may also cause palpitations.

Peak technique

Assessing arterial pulses

To assess arterial pulses, apply pressure with your index and middle fingers. Note some authors suggest carotid and brachial pulse quality may be better felt with the thumb (Northridge *et al*. 2005). These illustrations show where to position your fingers or thumb when palpating for various pulses.

Carotid pulse

Lightly place your fingers or thumb just lateral to the trachea and below the jaw angle. Never palpate both carotid arteries at the same time.

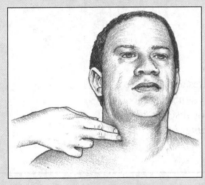

Brachial pulse

With the patient's arm outstretched and palm upwards, position your fingers or thumb on the medial (inner) aspect of the elbow crease.

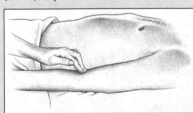

Radial pulse

Apply gentle pressure to the area of the wrist that sits just below and slightly inward from the base of the thumb.

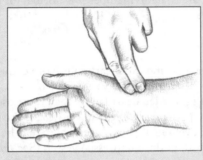

Femoral pulse

Palpate in the crease of the groin, approximately halfway between the pubic bone and the hip bone.

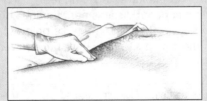

Popliteal pulse

Press firmly in the popliteal fossa at the back of the knee. Note this pulse is particularly difficult to feel, and thus if pulses in the feet are normal, not being able to palpate it should not be regarded as a cause for concern.

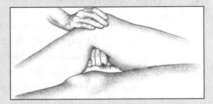

Posterior tibial pulse

Apply pressure behind and slightly below the medial malleolus of the ankle.

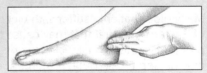

Dorsalis pedis pulse

Place your fingers on the medial dorsum (top) of the foot. The pulse is typically felt about 3 to 5 cm down from the base of the second toe – but if not felt, feel in adjacent toe to look for it.

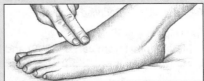

Fatigue

Fatigue is a feeling of excessive tiredness, lack of energy or exhaustion accompanied by a strong desire to rest or sleep. Fatigue is a normal response to physical overexertion, emotional stress and sleep deprivation. However, it can also be a non-specific symptom of cardiovascular disease, especially heart failure and valvular heart disease.

Skin and hair abnormalities

Cyanosis, pallor or cool skin may indicate poor cardiac output and tissue perfusion. Conditions causing fever or increased cardiac output may make the skin warmer than is normal. Absence or loss of body hair on the arms or legs may indicate diminished arterial blood flow to those areas, but remember it is normal for body hair to decrease with age.

That's just swell

Swelling, or oedema, may indicate heart failure or venous insufficiency. It may also result from varicosities or thrombophlebitis. Right-sided heart failure may cause ascites and/or generalised oedema, particularly in the lower legs. If the patient has compression of a vein in a specific area, there may be localised swelling along the path of the compressed vessel. (See *Findings in arterial and venous insufficiency*, below.)

Findings in arterial and venous insufficiency

Many older patients suffer with ulceration of the lower legs and feet, pain in the lower legs and other symptoms of the legs and feet that may cause them concern. Assessment findings differ depending on whether the problem is arterial insufficiency or venous insufficiency. The table below shows some of the differences that may be seen – although remember some patients will have arterial *and* venous disease.

Assessment	Arterial	Venous
Skin	Pale and cool. Patient may have noticed hair loss on legs and toes	May be cyanotic
Pain	Likely to be in the calf. May radiate to the foot or thigh. Often caused, or made worse, by walking	Whole leg. Often only relieved by elevation
Temperature	Normal or cool	Normal or warm
Pulses	Reduced or absent	Present but may be difficult to feel due to oedema
Swelling	No	Yes

Table compiled from Jarvis (2008) and Northridge *et al.* (2005).

Sites for heart sounds

When auscultating for heart sounds, the examination will include auscultation over the sites illustrated below. Normal heart sounds indicate events in the cardiac cycle, such as the closing of heart valves, and are reflected to specific areas of the chest wall. Auscultation sites are identified by the names of heart valves but aren't located directly over the valves. Rather, these sites are located along the pathway blood takes as it flows through the heart's chambers and valves.

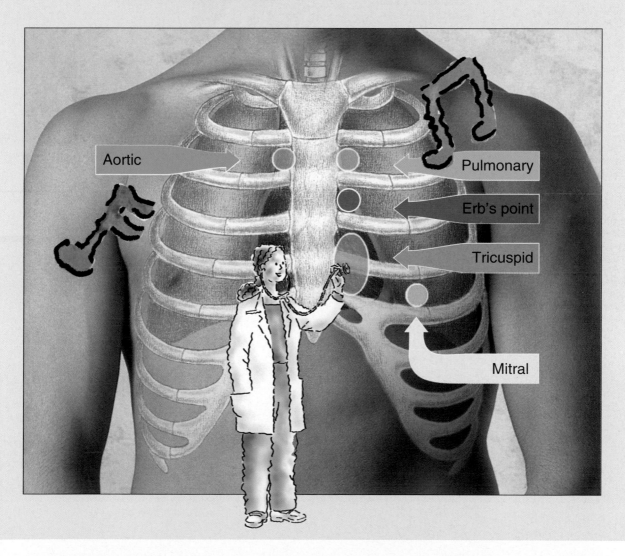

Cycle of heart sounds

When you auscultate a patient's chest and hear that familiar 'lub-dub', you're hearing the first and second heart sounds, S_1 and S_2. At times, two other abnormal sounds may occur: S_3 and S_4. Heart sounds are generated by events in the cardiac cycle. When valves close or blood fills the ventricles, vibrations of the heart muscle can be heard through the chest wall.

Varying sound patterns

The phonogram on the right shows how heart sounds vary in duration and intensity. For instance, S_2 (which occurs when the semilunar valves snap shut) is a fractionally shorter-lasting sound than S1 because the semilunar valves take less time to close than the atrioventricular valves, which cause S_1. Note that the two valves don't shut at exactly the same time, but the gap is normally too small to hear. If the gap gets larger, then two sounds are heard, known as 'splitting' of S_1 or S_2.

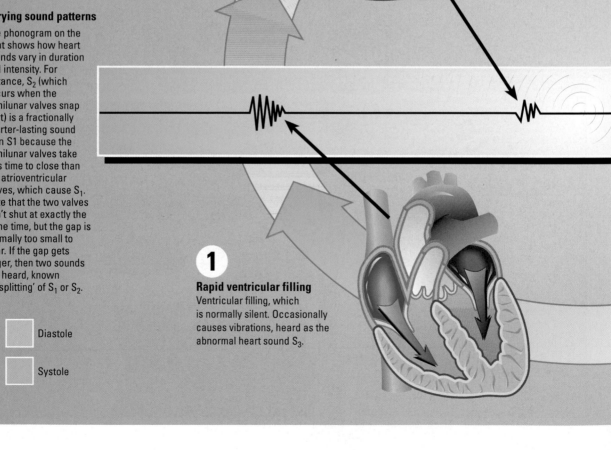

2

Slow ventricular filling
Atria contract and eject remaining blood into the ventricles. Occasionally, ventricular resistance causes vibrations heard as the abnormal heart sound S_4.

1

Rapid ventricular filling
Ventricular filling, which is normally silent. Occasionally causes vibrations, heard as the abnormal heart sound S_3.

Diastole

Systole

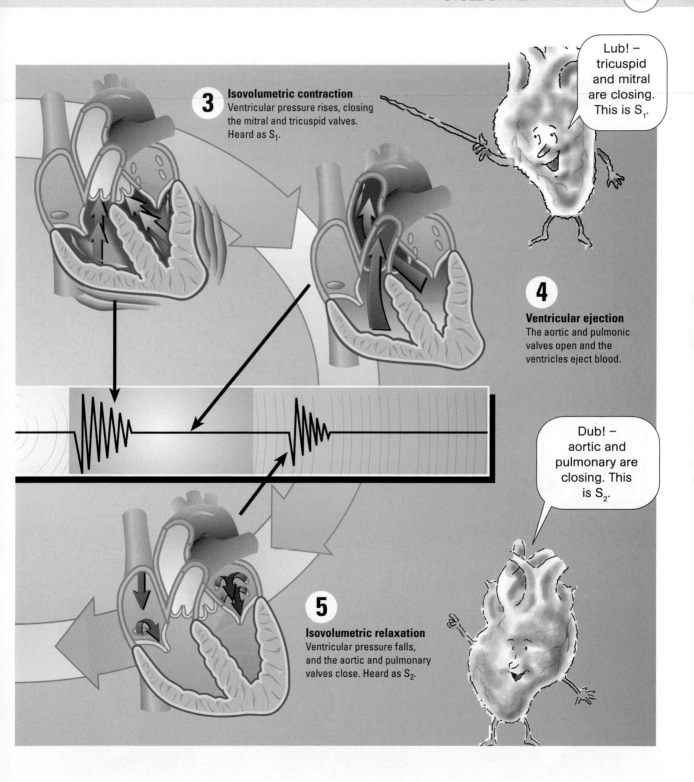

Understanding murmurs

Normally, heart valves close tightly and then open completely to let blood flow through. However, various conditions may alter blood flow through the valves, causing murmurs. In many cases this increases the workload of the heart.

The first two illustrations show a normal valve open and closed. The other illustrations portray three common reasons for the development of murmurs.

Valve closure is normally an open-and-shut case.

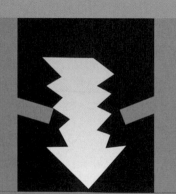

Normal valve open

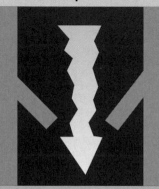

Normal valve closed

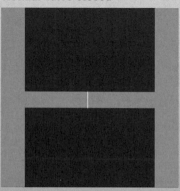

High blood flow

High blood flow through a normal valve may cause a murmur. Examples include an aortic systolic murmur, which can be caused by anaemia and a subsequent compensatory increase in cardiac output.

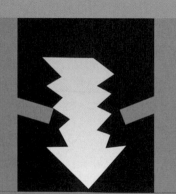

Decreased blood flow

Low blood flow through a stenotic valve can cause a murmur. The valves can't open or close properly because they're thickened, fibrotic or calcified. Common examples include aortic and mitral stenosis.

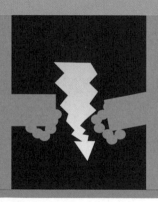

Backflow of blood

A backflow of blood through an insufficient or incompetent valve can cause a murmur. Because the valve can't close properly, blood can leak back or regurgitate into the heart chamber from which it came. Common examples include aortic and mitral insufficiency.

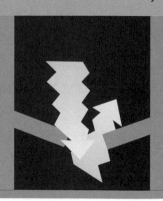

Abnormal pulsations

Abnormalities of the apical impulse include it being bigger than 2.5 centimetres in diameter, displaced, forceful or of prolonged duration.

Pulses here, there, everywhere

Pulsation in the patient's aortic, pulmonary or tricuspid area may indicate heart disease. Other causes include anaemia and anxiety. It may be normal if the patient has a thin chest wall.

Weak ones, strong ones

A weak arterial pulse may indicate decreased cardiac output or increased peripheral vascular resistance, both suggesting possible atherosclerotic disease. Strong or bounding pulsations usually occur during/after exercise, but also occur due to increased cardiac output in conditions such as hypertension, hypoxia, anaemia or anxiety. (See *Pulse waveforms*, page 243.)

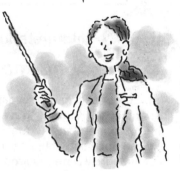

A weak arterial pulse points to arterial atherosclerotic disease.

Thrills and heaves

A thrill, which is a palpable vibration, usually suggests a valvular dysfunction. A heave or lifting of the chest wall, found on inspection or palpation, may indicate ventricular hypertrophy.

Abnormal sounds

Abnormal auscultation findings include abnormal heart sounds (see *Abnormal heart sounds*, page 242), heart murmurs and bruits.

Murmurs

Murmurs can occur as a result of a number of conditions and have widely varied characteristics.

They are divided into six grades (see *Grading murmurs*, page 235), which relate to their intensity.

Murmurs are also described by:
• pitch – a murmur can be described as high, medium and low-pitched
• sound quality – a murmur may be described as soft, harsh, rumbling or blowing
• point in systole and diastole – a murmur may be described as systolic or diastolic depending when in the cardiac cycle it's heard; more precise terms are also used such as pansystolic (all of systole),

midsystolic (in the middle of systole) or early diastolic (at the beginning of diastole)

- position on the chest – described in relation to the sternum, rib spaces and anatomical reference lines
- crescendo or decrescendo – crescendo means increasing in intensity and decrescendo means decreasing intensity; one or both may occur within a particular presentation of a murmur.

Interpretation station

Abnormal heart sounds

Whenever auscultation reveals an abnormal heart sound, try to identify the sound and its timing in the cardiac cycle. Knowing those characteristics can help you identify the possible cause for the sound. Use this chart to put all that information together. Note though, learning to distinguish these different abnormalities and their position in the cardiac cycle takes lots of experience, and considerable feedback from more senior practitioners will be required as you develop the skill.

Abnormal heart sound	Timing	Possible causes
Accentuated S_1	Beginning of systole	Mitral stenosis, fever or anaemia
Diminished S_1	Beginning of systole	Mitral insufficiency, heart block or severe hypertension
Split S_1	Beginning of systole	Right bundle-branch block or premature ventricular contractions. May be a normal finding
Accentuated S_2	End of systole	Hypertension; mitral, aortic or pulmonary stenosis
Diminished or inaudible S_2	End of systole	Aortic or pulmonic stenosis, shock
Persistent S_2 split	End of systole	Right ventricular failure, atrial septal defect ('hole' in the heart)
Reversed or paradoxical S_2 split that appears during exhalation and disappears during inspiration	End of systole	Patent ductus arteriosis, aortic stenosis, left bundle branch block
S_3	Early diastole	Mitral, aortic or tricuspid regurgitation, heart failure, increased cardiac output, fluid overload. (May be a normal finding in children and young adults; invariably abnormal over age 40)
S_4	Late diastole	Pulmonic or aortic stenosis, hypertension, coronary artery disease, left ventricular hypertrophy
Pericardial friction rub (grating or leathery sound at the left sternal border; usually muffled, high-pitched and transient)	Throughout systole and diastole	Pericardial inflammation

Pulse waveforms

If you feel an abnormal pulse waveform, check to see if it matches any of these abnormal pulse waveform patterns.

Weak, thready pulse

A weak pulse is difficult to feel. It has a decreased amplitude with a slower upstroke and downstroke. Possible causes of a weak pulse include decreased cardiac output, heart failure, hypovolaemia and aortic stenosis.

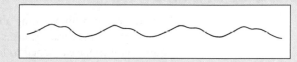

Bounding pulse

A bounding pulse is easily palpable. It has a sharp upstroke and downstroke with a pointed peak. The amplitude is elevated. Possible causes of a bounding pulse include exercise, anxiety and fever. Warter–Hammer pulse, linked to aortic valve regurgitation, feels similar, but after the forceful pulse it suddenly seems to 'collapse'.

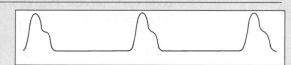

Pulsus alternans

Pulsus alternans has a regular, alternating pattern of a weak and a strong pulse. This pulse is associated with heart failure.

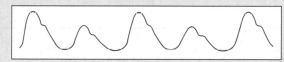

Pulsus bigeminus

Pulsus bigeminus is similar to pulsus alternans but alternate pulses seem to occur early, with a reduced force in the premature beat. This pulse associated with premature atrial or ventricular contraction.

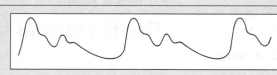

Pulsus paradoxus

Pulsus paradoxus is when there are increases and decreases in amplitude associated with the respiratory cycle. Marked decreases occur when the patient inhales. Pulsus paradoxus is associated with pericardial tamponade, advanced heart failure and pulmonary embolism.

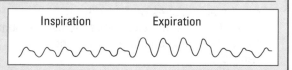
Inspiration   Expiration

Pulsus biferiens

Pulsus biferiens appears to have two 'mini beats' within the same pulse beat. Pulsus biferiens is associated with aortic stenosis and aortic insufficiency.

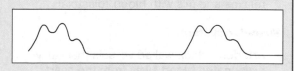

Several terms will be applied to the same murmur. For example, an aortic stenosis, caused by calcification of the aortic valve, typically causes a murmur that is loud, harsh, midsystolic, crescendo – decrescendo and heard best at the second right intercostal space.

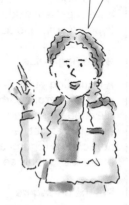

A murmur is never just a murmur. Variations in sound provide clues about the patient's underlying heart condition.

One step at a time

Remember that distinguishing abnormal heart sounds, and describing them accurately, takes a great deal of experience and requires you to have listened to lots of normal and abnormal hearts. Initially focus on learning to distinguish normal heart sounds from abnormal ones. Then gradually develop other skills as you continue to practise. (See also *Tips for learning to recognise and describe murmurs*, page 235.)

Bruits

A murmur-like sound of vascular (rather than cardiac) origin is called a bruit. If you hear a bruit during arterial auscultation, the patient may have occlusive arterial disease or an aneurysm. Various high cardiac output conditions – such as anaemia, hyperthyroidism and pheochromocytoma – may also cause bruits.

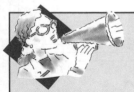

That's a wrap!

Cardiovascular system review

Structures

Heart

- A hollow, muscular organ that pumps blood to all organs and tissues of the body
- Protected by a thin sac called the pericardium
- Consists of four chambers: two atria and two ventricles
- Contains valves to keep blood flowing in only one direction
- Contracts to send blood out (systole), then relaxes and fills with blood (diastole).

Vascular system

- Arteries – thick-walled vessels that carry oxygenated blood away from the heart (except the pulmonary artery, which carries deoxygenated blood to the lungs)
- Veins – thinner-walled vessels that carry deoxygenated blood toward the heart (except the pulmonary vein, which carries oxygenated blood to the heart)
- Pulses – pressure waves of blood generated by the pumping action of the heart.

Blood circulation

- Deoxygenated venous blood flows from the superior vena cava, inferior vena cava and coronary sinus into the right atrium.
- Blood flows from the right atrium through the tricuspid valve and into the right ventricle.
- Blood is ejected through the pulmonary valve into the pulmonary artery, where it travels to the lungs for oxygenation.

(continued)

Cardiovascular system review *(continued)*

- Oxygenated blood then flows through the pulmonary veins and returns to the left atrium.
- Blood passes through the mitral valve and into the left ventricle.
- Blood is pumped through the aortic valve and into the aorta for delivery to the rest of the body.

Obtaining a health history

- Ask about current problems, including chest pain, palpitations, shortness of breath, peripheral skin changes and changes in extremities.
- Ask patient to rate chest pain on a scale of 1 to 10, with 1 being no pain and 10 being the worst pain imaginable.
- Ask about a family history of cardiovascular disease, raised cholesterol, high blood pressure, diabetes and chronic diseases of the lungs or kidneys.

Assessing the cardiovascular system

- Inspect the patient's general appearance, noting skin colour, signs of distress, sweating or dysmorphia
- Inspect the hands for colour, warmth, clubbing, splinter haemorrhages and peripheral return
- Assess brachial and radial pulses, and bilateral blood pressures
- Inspect the eyes for anaemia, corneal arcus and xanthalasmata
- Inspect the mouth for cyanosis and the teeth/gums for disease
- Inspect and auscultate carotid artery pulsations, and inspect the jugular venous pulse
- Inspect the chest, noting any heaves and the location of the apical impulse
- Palpate the apical impulse
- Palpate the chest for tenderness
- Palpate the aortic, pulmonary, tricuspid and mitral areas for thrills
- Auscultate for heart sounds with the patient lying on their back at around 45 degrees; assess additionally with patient sitting up, and then lying on their left side.

Heart sounds

- S_1 – best heard at the apex of the heart; corresponds to closure of the mitral and tricuspid valves
- S_2 – best heard at the base of the heart; corresponds to closure of the pulmonary and aortic valves
- S_3 – abnormal sound commonly heard in patients with high cardiac output or heart failure; can be a normal finding in children and young adults
- S_4 – abnormal sound heard in patients with hypertension, pulmonary or aortic stenosis or coronary artery disease.

Completing the cardiovascular examination

- Auscultate the lung bases for signs of crackles
- Inspect the sacrum, abdomen and legs/ankles for signs of oedema
- Palpate femoral, popliteal, posterior tibial and dorsalis pedis pulsation
- Inspect the abdomen for signs of abnormal aortic pulsation
- Auscultate the aortic, renal, iliac and femoral arteries. (See Chapter 11.).

Abnormal findings

- Chest pain – a sensation that varies in severity and presentation depending on the cause
- Palpitations – a conscious awareness of one's heartbeat
- Fatigue – a feeling of excessive tiredness, lack of energy or exhaustion accompanied by a strong desire to rest or sleep
- Thrill – palpable vibration indicating valvular dysfunction
- Heave – lifting of the chest wall seen during inspection or felt during palpation
- Abnormal S_1 or S_2
- Extra heart sounds – S_3, S_4, pericardial friction rub
- Murmur – sound made by turbulent blood flow
- Bruit – a murmur-like sound heard over blood vessels.

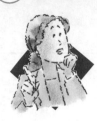

Quick quiz

1. When listening to heart sounds, you can hear S_1 loudest at:
   A. the base of the heart.
   B. the apex of the heart.
   C. the second intercostal space to the right of the sternum.
   D. Erb's point.

2. You're auscultating for heart sounds in a 3-year-old girl and hear an S_3. You assess this sound to be:
   A. probably a normal finding.
   B. probably a sign of heart failure.
   C. possibly a sign of atrial septal defect.
   D. possibly a sign of patent ductus arteriosus.

3. Capillary refill time is normally:
   A. less than 3 seconds.
   B. 4 to 6 seconds.
   C. 7 to 10 seconds.
   D. 11 to 15 seconds.

4. S_2 is the closing of which of the following two valves:
   A. Tricuspid and mitral
   B. Aortic and mitral
   C. Aortic and pulmonary
   D. Tricuspid and pulmonary

5. In an adult or older child the apical impulse is normally:
   A. smaller than 2.5 cm in diameter.
   B. visible on inspection in about 50% of patients.
   C. located at the fifth intercostal space in the midclavicular line.
   D. all of the above.

For answers see page 400.

10 Breasts and lymphatics

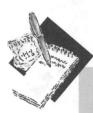

Just the facts

In this chapter, you'll learn:

♦ structures that make up the breasts

♦ how to interpret findings in respect of breast abnormalities which are recognised when taking the patient history or when examining the patient's chest

♦ the correct referral processes for a patient with a breast abnormality

♦ how to examine the lymph nodes in the axillae

♦ causes of breast and axillae abnormalities and how to recognise them.

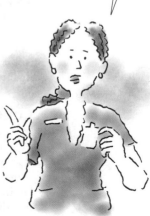

Breast awareness empowers the patient to take control of her own health.

A look at the breasts

Breast cancer has become increasingly prominent in the news in recent years, and around one in nine women will experience breast cancer in their lifetime (Cancer Research UK 2008a). By staying informed and being breast aware, women can take control of their health and seek medical care when they notice a change in their breasts.

A delicate matter

No matter how informed a woman is, she can still feel anxious and embarrassed when talking about a breast problem or during chest examinations. That's because the social and psychological significance of female breasts goes far beyond their biological function. The breast is more than just a delicate structure; it's a delicate subject. Keep this in mind during your assessment. It will let you proceed carefully and professionally, helping your patient feel more at ease.

Not just women . . .

It is also important to remember that breast cancer can also affect men. Although rare (less than 1% of cases), around 300 men in the UK develop breast cancer each year (Cancer Research UK 2007a). Many people don't even realise that this can happen. And for men it can be a particularly embarrassing condition to have or to discuss. (See *Male concerns*, page 253.)

Anatomy of the breasts

The breasts, also called mammary glands in women, lie on the anterior chest wall. (See *The female breast*, page 249.) They're located vertically between the second or third and the sixth or seventh ribs over the pectoralis major muscle and the serratus anterior muscle, and horizontally between the sternal border and the midaxillary line.

Breast structures

Each breast has a centrally located nipple of pigmented erectile tissue ringed by an areola that's darker than the adjacent tissue. (See *Differences in areola pigmentation*, page 249.) Sebaceous glands, also called Montgomery's tubercles, are scattered on the areola surface, along with hair follicles.

Support structures

Beneath the skin are glandular, fibrous and fatty tissues that vary in proportion with age, weight, gender and breast size. A small triangle of tissue, called the tail of Spence, projects into the axilla. Attached to the chest wall musculature are fibrous bands, called Cooper's ligaments, that support each breast.

Lobes and ducts

In women, each breast contains 15 to 25 glandular lobes surrounded by adipose (fatty) tissue. Each lobe contains several smaller lobules that produce milk in lactating women. Ducts from each lobe transport milk to the nipple, sometimes via storage areas called lactiferous sinuses. In men, the breast has a nipple, an areola, and mostly flat tissue bordering the chest wall.

The breasts have four lymph node chains that drain various areas, including the chest wall and arms.

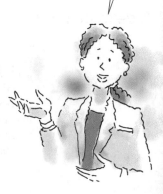

The female breast

This illustration shows a lateral cross-section of the female breast.

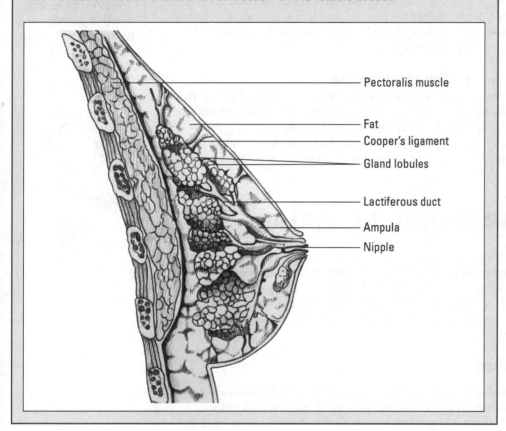

- Pectoralis muscle
- Fat
- Cooper's ligament
- Gland lobules
- Lactiferous duct
- Ampula
- Nipple

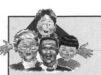

Bridging the gap

Differences in areola pigmentation

The pigment of the nipple and areola varies according to skin tone, getting darker as skin tone darkens. Fair-skinned people tend to have lighter-coloured nipples and areolae, usually pink or light beige. People with darker skin have medium brown to dark brown nipples and areolae. Fair-skinned people will see a darkening of the areolar area during pregnancy, and this pigment change is likely to remain to some extent.

How the breasts change with age

The appearance of a woman's breasts starts changing at puberty and continues changing during the reproductive years, pregnancy and menopause.

Changes during puberty

Breast development is an early sign of puberty in girls. It usually occurs between 8 and 13 years of age. Menarche, the start of the menstrual cycle, typically occurs about 2 years of age later. Development of breast tissue in girls younger than 8-years-old is abnormal, and the patient should be referred for further investigations. During puberty, breast development is commonly asymmetrical.

Changes during the reproductive years

During the reproductive years, a woman's breasts may become cyclically full or tender in response to hormonal fluctuations during the menstrual cycle. During pregnancy the breasts and nipples become larger, and other changes take place as a result of hormonal influences. Some changes, such as darkening of the areolar area, tend to remain after pregnancy.

Changes after menopause

After menopause, oestrogen levels decrease, causing glandular tissue to atrophy and be replaced with fatty deposits. The breasts become flabbier and smaller than they were before menopause, with less dense tissue. As the ligaments relax, the breasts hang loosely from the chest. The nipples flatten, losing some of their erectile quality.

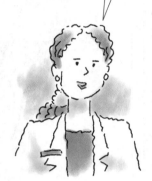

After menopause, decreased oestrogen levels cause glandular tissue in the breast to atrophy.

A look at the lymphatic system

The lymphatic system works closely with the vascular system to promote fluid drainage from the body back to the heart. It runs in parallel to the venous system. It also plays a very important part in the prevention of infection. Its third function is to transport lipids and fat soluble vitamins from the gastrointestinal tract to the blood.

Relieving the pressure

As fluid moves between the blood capillaries and the tissues, an imbalance in the various pressures which allow this to happen means that slightly more fluid leaves the arterial circulation than can re-enter the venous circulation. The remainder is taken up by blind ended lymphatic capillaries. These then merge to form the lymphatic vessels and ducts which conduct the fluid back to the heart via this alternative route. The fluid moves more slowly here than it does in the venous system.

Notable nodes

Along the way this fluid, which is now called lymph, encounters groups of lymph nodes. There are about 600 in the average adult (Tortora 2005). These nodes filter out microorganisms, pathogens and other unwanted items such as tumour cells. Lymph nodes that are actively 'fighting' tend to get inflamed and become palpable.

One-quarter and three-quarters

It is important to remember that the drainage patterns of the lymphatic system are not symmetrical. Lymph from the right side of the head, right arm, right side of the chest and right upper portion of the liver drains back via the right lymphatic duct. In contrast, the thoracic duct on the left drains all the remaining lymph, not only from the left side of the head, left arm and chest, but also from all of the abdomen and both legs.

This means that pathology in the abdomen and legs would tend to cause swelling of the supraclavicular nodes (one of the last points in the drainage system) on the left, rather than on the right, irrespective of which side of the body the problem occurs.

Where to feel?

Not all lymph nodes are palpable when enlarged; those in the abdomen and some in the chest are generally too deep to palpate. Others such as those in the head and neck, axilla, groin and limbs are readily palpable when enlarged, and give you important information about the possibility of infection or tumour.

Examination of the axillary lymph nodes is explained within this chapter. Examination of other lymph nodes is covered alongside the relevant body systems. For examination of the nodes of the head and neck see Chapter 7, for nodes in the groin see Chapter 12 and for nodes in the limbs see Chapter 13.

Axillary lymph nodes

Within the axilla there are four distinct chains of lymph nodes, each serving different areas.
• The pectoral (anterior axillary) lymph nodes drain lymph fluid from most of the breast and anterior chest wall.
• The brachial (lateral) nodes drain most of the arm.
• The subscapular (posterior axillary) nodes drain the posterior chest wall and part of the arm.
• The midaxillary (or central axillary) nodes, located near the ribs and the serratus anterior muscle high in the axilla, are the central draining nodes for the pectoral, brachial and subscapular nodes.

Lymph then drains from the central axillary nodes to the supraclavicular and infraclavicular nodes. In addition to these nodes, the superficial lymphatic vessels drain the skin. In women, the internal mammary nodes drain the mammary lobes.

Lymph node chains

This illustration shows the different lymph node chains in the breast, axilla, and upper arm.

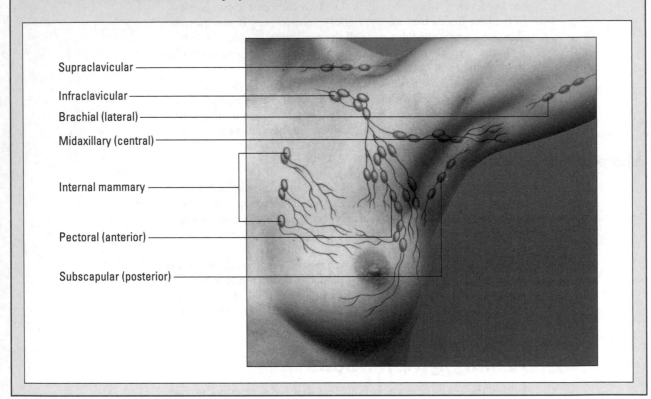

Supraclavicular

Infraclavicular

Brachial (lateral)

Midaxillary (central)

Internal mammary

Pectoral (anterior)

Subscapular (posterior)

Cancer route

In both men and women, the lymphatic system is a key route by which breast cancer cells spread to other parts of the body. (See *Lymph node chains*, above.)

Obtaining a health history

You'll typically begin your health history by asking the patient about their reason for seeking care. You'll then want to ask the patient questions about their personal and family medical history as well as their current health.

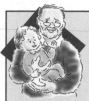

Ages and stages
Male concerns

Men with breast disorders may feel uneasy or embarrassed about their condition and its association with women and the breast. In addition to the small risk of breast cancer, other conditions can also affect the male breast.

chronic liver disease and some adrenal tumours. Adolescent boys may have temporary stimulation of breast tissue caused by the hormone oestrogen; it usually stops when they begin producing adequate amounts of the male sex hormone testosterone.

Gynecomastia

Gynecomastia is abnormal glandular enlargement of the male breast. It may be caused by a variety of factors, including hormonal imbalance, taking steroids, taking prescribed oestrogens, recreational drug use, thyrotoxicosis,

Obesity

Some men develop breast enlargement due simply to excessive subcutaneous fat, although on palpation this will feel soft. In contrast, gynecomastia presents with a palpable firm disc of glandular enlargement.

Asking about the reason for seeking care

Common concerns about the breasts include breast pain, nipple discharge, rashes, lumps, masses, lesions and other changes. Concerns such as these from either women or men warrant further investigation. (See *Male concerns*, above.)

Dig deeper

To explore further, use the PQRSTU or OLD CART mnemonic (page 16) to learn more about the symptoms. Establish whether changes such as discharge, pain or rashes are affecting one breast or both. Remember to ask if there have been any other breast symptoms as well as the one initially mentioned, or any changes in the axillae. It may be helpful to offer prompts regarding particular changes the patient might have noticed, such as rashes or other skin changes, pain, dimpling or recent nipple inversion.

Asking about medical history

Ask the patient if they have ever had any breast lumps, a biopsy or breast surgery, including enlargement or reduction. Ask about

Mammography screening

Currently in the UK all women should be invited for mammography screening every 3 years from age 50 to 70 (64 in Northern Ireland). However, plans are currently being phased in to extend screening to all women aged between 47 and 73-years-old.

Younger women are not routinely called for breast screening, partly because breast cancer is less likely in this age group, partly because of the risk of radiation exposure in younger women, and partly because younger women tend to have 'denser' breast tissue, making mammography less reliable. However, screening is offered to younger women who are at higher risk of breast cancer as a result of family history or previous breast cancer; the frequency and type of scan will depend on the individual risk assessment.

Older women are entitled to 3-yearly breast screening but are not invited routinely, so it is helpful to remind older women of this and encourage them to ask for further appointments.

(Source: Cancer Backup 2008a.)

breast cancer, fibroadenoma or fibrocystic disease or any other type of cancer. Have they ever had a mammography or an ultrasound examination of the breasts? If so, when and what were the findings? If a woman is over 50-years-old and has not been called for routine mammography screening, check that she hasn't been overlooked in the system. (See *mammography screening*, above.)

Periods and pregnancies

Inquire about a woman's menstrual cycle and record the date of her last period or date of onset of the menopause. When did her periods first start? Find out about previous pregnancies and whether she breastfed.

All in the family

Ask the patient if any family members have had breast disorders, especially breast cancer. Although most breast cancers are not genetically linked, having a first-degree relative (mother or sister) with breast cancer significantly increases a woman's risk. If two or more first-degree relatives are affected, the risk increases further (Cancer Research UK 2008b). Also ask about breast cancer in other relatives including grandparents and aunts. Women with a strong family history can be referred for genetic screening to allow more precise estimation of their risk. Also ask about any other types of cancer in the family.

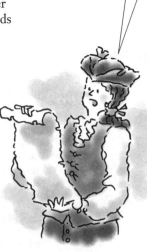

Hear ye! Hear ye! Let it be known that hormonal birth control methods can make the breasts swollen and tender!

Down on the pharm

Ask the patient what drugs they take regularly, including oral and other forms of hormonal contraception, and hormone replacement therapy. Oral contraceptive pills can cause breast swelling and tenderness. Several drugs can cause discharge.

Reducing the risk

Several risk factors have been linked to increased risk of breast cancer. Many factors which increase the risk of breast cancer are not under the individual's control, such as increasing age, increasing height and late menopause. Modifiable risk factors (factors which increase risk of breast cancer and are under individual control) offer opportunities for health promotion. These include:

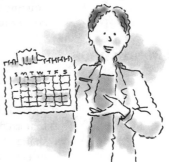

Note that symptoms may change in relation to the menstrual cycle.

* Obesity
* Alcohol consumption
* Hormone replacement therapy (notably greater risk if used for more than 5 years)
* Oral contraceptive pill (slight risk)
* Obesity
* Lack of exercise
* Not breast-feeding.

For more information on risk factors, including the degree of risk and the evidence, see Cancer Research UK (2008b).

Assessing the breasts and axillae

As a result of a number of women being given 'false reassurance' in the past, UK healthcare practitioners are given very specific guidance when it comes to breast examination. The Royal College of Nursing (2002: page 4) recommend that 'nurses should not undertake the practice of routine breast palpation. The only exception would be breast care nurses with specialist training who include breast palpation as a significant part of their role'.

Other healthcare professionals, unless they are clinical experts, should be similarly cautious. NICE (2002: page 21) states that all primary care teams should have at least one practitioner who is specifically trained in the clinical breast examination of women who have breast symptoms. So any concerns you identify, either in the patient history, or when inspecting the chest, should be reviewed as soon as possible by a practitioner with these skills.

Triple assessment

Patients with worrying signs or symptoms, including a breast lump, skin nodule, ulceration, skin distortion, nipple eczema, recent nipple retraction or unilateral nipple discharge, should be *urgently* referred for triple assessment which should take place within 2 weeks (NICE 2002: 20). This includes:

- Mammography or ultrasound
- Fine needle aspiration or core biopsy
- Expert clinical assessment.

No information gained from breast palpation by a non-expert should change a 'triple assessment' referral decision in any situation where the history or inspection raises a possible concern.

Inspection

Although you should not carry out routine breast examination unless you are a clinical expert, you may notice abnormalities when you undertake a heart or lung examination that causes you to be concerned.

Chest check

Breast skin should be smooth, undimpled, and the same colour as the rest of the skin. Check for any signs of swelling in the breast or surrounding area, which may suggest lymphatic obstruction. Note that asymmetry occurs normally in some adult women. Notice the shape of the breasts, and whether the nipples point in the same direction. Notice any dimples or creases. If a nipple is inverted, ask the patient when she first noticed the abnormality; long-standing nipple inversion would not be a concern, but a recent change would be. Note any indication of discharge on skin or clothing. If you have any concerns, seek expert advice as previously discussed.

Breast aware

A few years ago, women were encouraged to undertake regular, systematic breast self-examination. But advice has changed (NICE 2002) as 'self-examination' focuses too narrowly on 'feeling' the breasts, when many abnormalities are in fact 'seen' rather than 'felt'. Instead, current advice, such as that produced by the NHS Cancer Screening Programme (2006), emphasises the importance of being 'breast aware' as part of a woman's general body awareness. It stresses the importance of 'looking at' as well as 'feeling' the breasts; for example, looking for rashes, dimpling or changes in shape, size or nipple direction. Pain is also an important factor to consider. Breakthrough Breast Cancer (see page 420 for patient support and breast cancer research website) suggests the mnemonic **TLC**:

- **T**ouch – feel for anything unusual
- **L**ook – for changes, and be aware of their shape and texture
- **C**heck – anything unusual with your general practitioner.

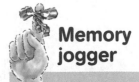

Memory jogger

To remember abnormalities of concern in the nipple, think of the word **DISC**:

Discharge

Inversion

Skin changes

Compare with the other side.

Examining the axillae

There are a number of causes of enlargement of the axillary lymph nodes. They may suggest infection or malignancy in the breast, arm or chest wall or be part of a generalised lymphadenopathy (having swollen lymph glands in different parts of the body at the same time). Because localised swollen axilliary lymph nodes can be a first sign of breast cancer, seek further advice urgently if an alternative infective isn't immediately apparent.

Look before you leap

To examine the axillae, use the techniques of inspection and palpation. With the patient sitting or standing, firstly inspect the skin of the axillae for rashes, infections or unusual pigmentation.

Assessing the axillary nodes

Before palpating, ask the patient to relax their arm on the side you're examining. Keep the arm at the patient's side, and support their elbow with one of your hands. Use the slightly cupped fingers of your other hand to reach high into the axilla.

It's the pits

It is helpful to think of the axilla as a pyramid.
• Palpate the *central nodes* by pressing your fingers upward and inward toward the chest wall. You should be able to feel the bones of the ribcage against your fingers.
• To palpate the *pectoral (or anterior) nodes*, grasp the anterior axillary fold between your thumb and fingers with your fingers on the axillary side, and palpate inside the borders of the pectoral muscles.
• To palpate the *subscapular (or posterior) nodes*, stand behind the patient and feel inside the muscle of the posterior axillary fold.
• Palpate the *lateral nodes* by pressing your fingers along the upper, inner arm. Try to compress these nodes against the humerus.
Remember to keep the arm down at all times to relax the axilla and have the best chance of feeling the nodes.

What are you feeling for?

Note that although the nodes are usually non-palpable, you may occasionally feel one or more normal, small, soft, non-tender nodes when you palpate centrally (Jarvis 2008). But differentiating between normal and abnormal takes a great deal of experience, so always seek

Identifying locations of breast abnormalities

Mentally divide the breast into four quadrants and a fifth segment, the tail of Spence. Describe your findings according to the appropriate quadrant or segment. You can also think of the breast as a clock, with the nipple in the centre. Then specify locations according to the time (2 o'clock, for example). Either way, specify the location of an abnormality by the distance in centimetres from the nipple and remember to make clear which breast you are referring to.

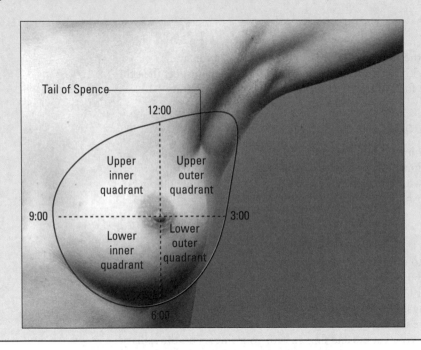

expert advice. Any hard, large or tender lesion will be a cause for concern and should be further investigated urgently.

Assessing the clavicular nodes

It is also important to assess the nodes in the clavicular area. To do this, ask the patient to relax their neck muscles by flexing their head slightly forward. Stand in front of them and hook your fingers over the clavicle beside the sternomastoid muscle. Rotate your fingers deeply into this area to feel the supraclavicular nodes. Then, again using a circling motion, palpate the area just underneath the clavicle to check for infraclavicular nodes. Do both sides together to get a good comparison, and work along the line of the clavicle both above and below to be sure you have checked thoroughly.

Abnormal findings

This section describes some of the abnormal breast findings that you might encounter.

Breast lump

A breast lump may occur in any part of the breast, including the axilla. Remember that patients may describe an area of thickening or nodularity; there is not always a clearly defined lump. As noted above, such findings should *always* be referred for 'triple assessment'. However, there are many causes of breast lumps other than cancer. These include fibroadenoma, cysts and fat necrosis, all of which are benign. Overall, around 90% of breast lumps are benign (Cancer Research 2007b). In younger women under 30 years old breast cancer is rare, but this should *never* be used as a reason for non-referral.

Dimpling

Breast dimpling – the puckering or retraction of skin on the breast – results from abnormal attachment of the skin to underlying tissue, often 'pulled in' by attachment to the Cooper's ligaments. It suggests an inflammatory or malignant mass beneath the skin's surface and may well be indicative of breast cancer which could be quite far advanced. (See *Dimpling and peau d'orange*, page 260.)

Peau d'orange and other skin changes

Often a late sign of breast cancer, peau d'orange (orange peel skin) is the oedematous thickening and pitting of breast skin. Remember that nipple eczema and ulceration also require urgent referral.

Nipple retraction

Nipple retraction, the inward displacement of the nipple below the level of surrounding areolar tissue, may indicate an inflammatory process, lesion or cancer. It results from scar tissue formation within a lesion or a large mammary duct. As the scar tissue shortens, it pulls adjacent tissue inward, causing nipple deviation, flattening and finally retraction. Importantly though, many women have nipple retraction which has always been present; this would not be a cause for referral.

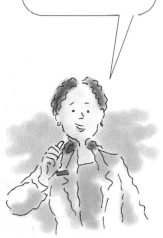

'Orange' you glad you know how to spot breast abnormalities such as peau d'orange?

Dimpling and peau d'orange

These illustrations show two common abnormalities in breast tissue: dimpling and peau d'orange.

Dimpling

Dimpling usually suggests an inflammatory or malignant mass beneath the skin's surface. The illustration shows breast dimpling and nipple inversion caused by a malignant mass above the areola.

Peau d'orange

Peau d'orange is usually a late sign of breast cancer, but it can also occur with breast or axillary lymph node infection. The skin's orange-peel appearance comes from lymphatic oedema around deepened hair follicles.

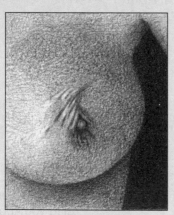
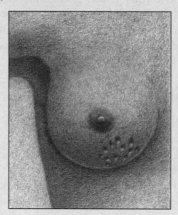

Nipple discharge

Nipple discharge is characterised as intermittent or constant, and unilateral or bilateral. It is also classified by colour, consistency and composition, and by whether it comes from one duct or multiple ducts of the nipple. Nipple discharge can signal serious underlying disease, particularly when accompanied by other breast changes. Significant causes include endocrine disorders (for example, pituatory tumour), cancer, certain drugs and blocked lactiferous ducts. Therefore, apart from the normal lactation of breast-feeding, nipple discharge should always be investigated; urgently via 'triple assessment' if it is unilateral.

Breast pain

Breast pain commonly results from benign breast disease, such as mastitis or fibrocystic breast disease, but it can signify a malignancy. The myth that if pain is part of a problem it 'can't be cancer' has in the past led to a number of delayed diagnoses. It may occur during rest or movement and may be aggravated by manipulation or palpation. Breast pain that is bilateral and cyclic, particularly when occurring just before a period, is considered a normal finding. Any unilateral or non-cyclic pain should be investigated.

Visible veins

Prominent veins in the breast may indicate cancer in some patients; however, they are considered normal in pregnant women because of engorgement.

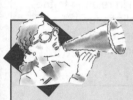

That's a wrap!

Breasts and axillae review

Structures – breast

- Nipple: pigmented erectile tissue located in the centre of each breast
- Areola: ringed area that surrounds the nipple, darker in colour than adjacent tissue
- Cooper's ligaments: fibrous bands that support each breast
- Glandular lobes: contain the alveoli that produce milk
- Lactiferous ducts: transport milk from each lobe to the nipple.

Structures – lymphatics

- Alternative route to the venous system for return of fluid from the capillaries back to the heart
- Lymph drains via lymphatic vessels, passing through lymph nodes on its journey
- Lymph nodes act as filters for unwanted organisms
- Drainage of lymph from right side of the head, right side of the chest, the right arm and top of the liver passes into the right lymphatic duct
- Drainage of lymph from left side of the head, left side of the chest, the left arm and all of the abdomen and legs passes into the thoracic duct (on the left side of the chest)

- Breast/chest/arm drainage via four sets of axillary nodes – pectoral (anterior), supscapular (posterior), midaxillary (central) and brachial (lateral).

Health history

- Be alert in the patient history to any concerns in relation to breast lumps, breast pain, dimpling, unusual skin appearance, lesions, eczema, abnormal contours, nipple asymmetry, nipple inversion, non-cyclic breast pain, discharge or any other breast disorders.
- Ask about the patient's menstrual and pregnancy history.
- Ask about a family history of breast disorders, especially breast cancer.
- Ask about history of mammography.
- Ask patient about their understanding of breast awareness.

Assessment

- Remember that routine inspection and palpation of the breasts is not recommended in the UK, except by specialist breast practitioners.
- Seek expert opinion or refer for screening if the history indicates a concern.

(continued)

Breasts and axillae review (continued)

- Also seek expert opinion or refer any abnormalities noted on chest inspection.
- Inspect the axilla for rashes and lesions.
- Remember there are four lymph node chains to palpate in each axilla.
- Palpate the supraclavicular and infraclavicular nodes.

Abnormal findings

- Breast lump – lump, thickening or nodularity reported by the patient, or observed on inspection
- Breast dimpling – the puckering or retraction of skin on the breast
- Peau d'orange (orange peel skin) – the oedematous thickening and pitting of breast skin. Nipple eczema and ulceration are also causes for concern.
- Nipple retraction – inward displacement of the nipple below the level of surrounding breast tissue; probably a normal finding if long-standing but of concern if a recent change
- Nipple discharge – can signal serious disease
- Pain – may occur during rest or movement; consider duration of the pain, whether it is unilateral or bilateral and timing in relation to the menstrual cycle. Can signify malignancy
- Visible veins – may indicate abnormality but also occur normally in pregnant women.

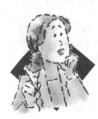

Quick quiz

1.   The lymph nodes that drain the arm are called:
  A.   the pectoral.
  B.   the central.
  C.   the subscapular.
  D.   the brachial.

2.   Normal changes in the breasts of a premenstrual woman include:
  A.   a single hard, fixed mass.
  B.   nipple inversion and skin dimpling.
  C.   bilateral tenderness before the menstrual cycle.
  D.   redness and scaling over a portion of the breast.

3.   The following would be considered a normal finding and does not require referral:
  A.   Unilateral nipple retraction that has always been present
  B.   A painful lump
  C.   Bilateral discharge from the nipples
  D.   A small sore area that isn't healing.

4.   The tail of Spence is located:
  A.   above the nipple at the midclavicular line.
  B.   in the upper outer quadrant, toward the axilla.
  C.   in the upper inner quadrant, near the sternum.
  D.   in the lower outer quadrant, close to the ribs.

For answers see page 401.

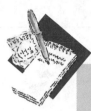 11 Gastrointestinal system

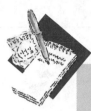

Just the facts

In this chapter, you'll learn:

♦ organs and structures that make up the gastrointestinal system

♦ methods to obtain a patient history of the gastrointestinal system

♦ techniques for performing a physical assessment of the gastrointestinal system

♦ causes and characteristics of abnormalities in the gastrointestinal system.

A look at the gastrointestinal system

The gastrointestinal (GI) system's major functions include ingestion and digestion of food, and elimination of waste products. When these processes are interrupted the patient can experience problems ranging from loss of appetite to severe malnutrition or dehydration.

Anatomy and physiology of the GI system

The GI system consists of two major divisions: the GI tract and the accessory organs. (See *Parts of the GI system*, page 264.)

GI tract

The GI tract is a hollow tube which begins at the mouth and ends at the anus. If stretched out fully it would measure around 9 metres in

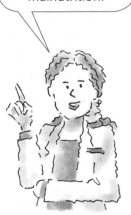

A disruption of the function of the GI system can cause problems ranging from loss of appetite to severe malnutrition.

Parts of the GI system

This illustration shows the GI system's major anatomic structures. Knowing these structures will help you conduct an accurate physical assessment.

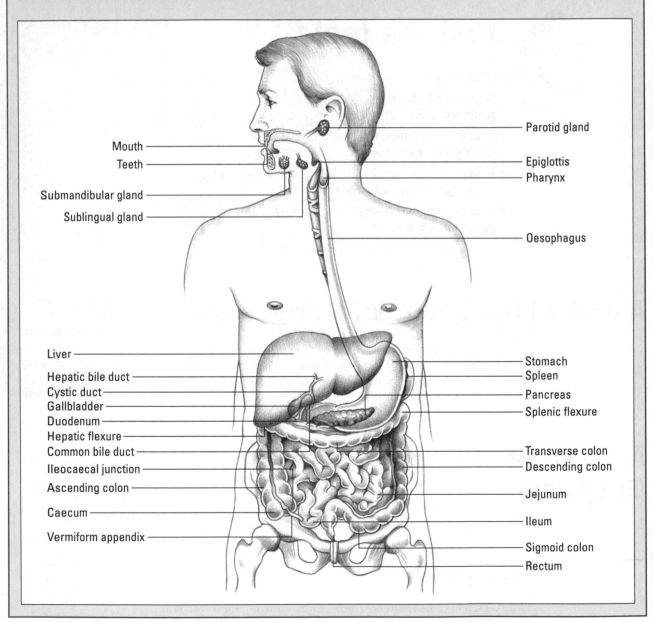

Mouth
Teeth
Submandibular gland
Sublingual gland

Liver
Hepatic bile duct
Cystic duct
Gallbladder
Duodenum
Hepatic flexure
Common bile duct
Ileocaecal junction
Ascending colon
Caecum
Vermiform appendix

Parotid gland
Epiglottis
Pharynx
Oesophagus

Stomach
Spleen
Pancreas
Splenic flexure
Transverse colon
Descending colon
Jejunum
Ileum
Sigmoid colon
Rectum

length (Tortora 2005). It consists of smooth muscle alternating with blood vessels and nerve tissue. Specialised circular and longitudinal fibres contract along most of its length, causing peristalsis, which aids in propelling food through the GI tract. The GI tract includes the mouth, pharynx, oesophagus, stomach, small intestine and large intestine.

Start at the mouth

Digestive processes begin in the mouth (sometimes called the buccal cavity) with chewing, salivating and swallowing. The tongue provides the sense of taste. Saliva is produced by three pairs of glands: the parotid, submandibular and sublingual. Saliva keeps the mouth moist, lubricates and dissolves food and begins the process of digestion. Food, once chewed and mixed with saliva, forms a soft mass called the bolus.

Proceed to the pharynx

The pharynx, or throat, allows the passage of food from the mouth to the oesophagus. The pharynx assists in the swallowing process, and secretes mucous that aids the passage of the bolus. The epiglottis – a thin, leaf-shaped structure made of fibrocartilage – is directly behind the root of the tongue. When food is swallowed, the epiglottis closes over the larynx, and the soft palate lifts to block the nasal cavity. These actions keep food and fluid from being aspirated into the airway.

Down the oesophagus

The oesophagus is a muscular, hollow tube about 25 cm long which moves food from the pharynx to the stomach. When food is swallowed, the upper oesophageal sphincter relaxes and the food moves into the oesophagus. Peristalsis then propels the food towards the stomach. The cardiac sphincter (sometimes called the lower oesophageal sphincter or gastro-oesophageal sphincter) is formed by a narrowing at the lower end of the oesophagus. It normally remains closed to prevent the reflux of gastric contents. The sphincter opens during swallowing, belching and vomiting.

Stay awhile in the stomach

The stomach, a reservoir for food, is a dilated, sac-like structure that lies obliquely in the left upper quadrant of the abdomen. It sits below the oesophagus and diaphragm, to the right of the spleen, and partly under the liver. The rounded upper portion of the stomach is known as the fundus. The main body of the stomach leads to the lower pylorus, which connects the stomach to the duodenum. The pyloric sphincter guards the exit of the stomach.

The stomach has three major functions:
- storing food
- mixing food with gastric juices (including hydrochloric acid and enzymes which aid digestion)
- passing chyme – a watery mixture of partly digested food and digestive juices – into the small intestine for further digestion and absorption.

An average meal can remain in the stomach for 2 to 4 hours, with a fatty meal taking longest to digest. Rugae, accordion-like folds in the stomach lining, allow the stomach to expand when large amounts of food and fluid are ingested; at full capacity it can hold around 1.5 litres.

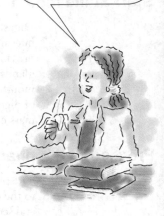

Once this food reaches my stomach, it could remain there for up to 4 hours before moving on to the small intestine.

Slip through the small intestine

The small intestine is about 6 m long and is named for its diameter, not its length. It has three sections: the upper duodenum which comprises only the first 25 cm, the middle jejunum which is around 2.5 m in length, and finally the ileum which makes up the remaining 3.5 m.

As chyme passes into the small intestine, carbohydrates, fats and proteins are broken down. Enzymes secreted from the pancreas and the small intestine itself, together with bile from the liver, aid digestion. These secretions mix with the chyme as it moves through the intestines by peristalsis. The end products of digestion are absorbed through its thin mucous membrane lining into the bloodstream.

And finally head through the large intestine

The small intestine joins the large intestine, or colon, at the ileocaecal junction in the right lower quadrant of the abdomen. (See *Abdominal quadrants*, page 267.) The large intestine is about 1.5 metres long. It includes the caecum, the colon (including the ascending, transverse, descending and sigmoid sections), the rectum and the anus – in that order. The appendix, a finger-like projection, is attached to the caecum. The large intestine is responsible for:
- completion of digestion through bacterial activity (which also produces flatus)
- absorbing excess water and electrolytes
- storing food residue
- eliminating waste products.

Abdominal quadrants

To perform a systematic GI assessment, try to visualise the abdominal structures by dividing the abdomen into four quadrants, as shown here.

Right upper quadrant

- Right lobe of liver
- Gallbladder
- Pylorus
- Duodenum
- Head of the pancreas
- Hepatic flexure of the colon
- Portions of the ascending and transverse colon.

Right lower quadrant

- Caecum and appendix
- Lower portion of the ascending colon
- Ileocaecal junction.

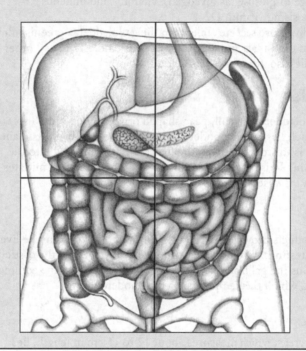

Left upper quadrant

- Left lobe of the liver
- Stomach
- Body and tail of the pancreas
- Splenic flexure of the colon
- Portions of the transverse and descending colon.

Left lower quadrant

- Lower portion of the descending colon
- Sigmoid colon.

Passage of the digestive substances through the large intestine is a slow process; it typically takes several hours before the chyme becomes solid or semi-solid. This end product of digestion is known as faeces, and comprises waste products ready to be eliminated.

Accessory organs

Accessory GI organs include the liver, pancreas, gallbladder, bile ducts and spleen. The abdominal aorta and parts of the venous system also aid the GI system.

Look at the liver

The liver is located in the right upper quadrant under the diaphragm. It has two major lobes, divided by the falciform ligament, and two smaller lobes. The liver is the largest and heaviest internal organ in the body, weighing about 1.4 kilograms in an adult (Tortora 2005).

The liver's functions include:
- metabolising carbohydrates, fats, and proteins
- detoxifying blood (for example, toxins in alcohol and some drugs)
- storage of glucose (as glycogen), vitamins and minerals
- synthesising vitamin D.

The liver also secretes bile from the gallbladder, a greenish fluid that helps digest fats and absorb fatty acids, cholesterol and other lipids. Bile also gives faeces its colour.

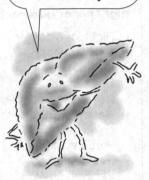

You'd think with all my functions I'd lose a little weight, but I'm the heaviest organ in the body!

Gape at the gallbladder

The gallbladder is a small, pear-shaped organ, about 7 to 10 cm long, which lies halfway under the right lobe of the liver. Its main function is to store bile from the liver until it is emptied into the duodenum. This process occurs when the small intestine initiates chemical impulses that cause the gallbladder to contract.

Behold the bile ducts

The bile ducts provide passageways for bile to travel from the liver to the intestines. Two hepatic ducts drain the liver, and the cystic duct drains the gallbladder. These ducts converge into the common bile duct, which then empties into the duodenum.

Probe the pancreas

The pancreas, which measures about 12 to 15 cm in length, lies horizontally in the abdomen, behind the stomach. It consists of a head, body and tail. The head of the pancreas is located in the right upper quadrant, attached to the duodenum and the tail is in the left upper quadrant.

The pancreas has two sets of functions. As part of the endocrine system it releases insulin and glycogen into the bloodstream. In addition, it produces pancreatic enzymes which are released into the duodenum for digestion.

Spectacular spleen

The spleen is located at about the level of the ninth to 11th ribs behind the midaxillary line. This is further back than most people think because on anatomical diagrams it often looks like it sits anteriorly. It is normally only about 13 cm long, but has the capacity to enlarge to several times this size. It isn't technically part of the GI system but is closely linked to it, due to its position in the abdominal cavity. It is a large mass of lymphatic tissue, responsible for filtering bacteria and other debris from the blood, removing damaged or worn out red blood cells and platelets, and platelet storage.

Amazing arteries

The abdominal aorta supplies blood to the GI tract. It enters the abdomen through the diaphragm. Numerous vessels lead off it, including the renal arteries at the level of the second lumbar vertebrae (anteriorly about level with the costal margins).

It then continues downward and separates into the common iliac arteries at about the level of the fourth lumbar vertebrae (anteriorly just below the umbilicus). The common iliac arteries are continuous with the femoral arteries, supplying blood to the legs. In addition, many branches off the common iliac arteries supply blood to the length of the GI tract.

Visualise the veins

Veins from the GI tract, spleen, pancreas and gallbladder drain into the hepatic portal vein which takes blood to the liver. After processing in the liver, the venous blood exits the liver through the hepatic veins, emptying into the inferior vena cava.

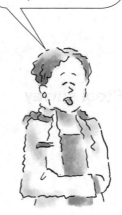

Stomach pain, nausea and vomiting strongly suggest a GI problem.

Obtaining a health history

If your patient has a GI problem, symptoms may include pain, heartburn, indigestion, nausea, vomiting, bloating or altered bowel habits. To investigate these or any other signs and symptoms, use the PQRSTU or OLD CART mnemonic (see page 16).

Cardiac alert

It is really important to recognise that reports of upper GI pain must be differentiated from possible cardiac causes. So also carefully explore any history of chest pain, pain on exertion, palpitations or shortness of breath. (See Chapter 9 for more details regarding the cardiac history.)

Asking about current health

In addition to using the mnemonic to explore the presenting complaint(s), consider these points:

Pain perspectives

If the patient has pain associated with eating, does eating make it better or worse? If worse, how long after eating does the pain occur?

Various vomits

If the patient is vomiting, find out what they have eaten and drunk in the last 24 hours? Is there any sign of blood in the vomit? Is there any sign of bile? (Remember, if infants or toddlers vomit bile this is always a serious finding.) Have they passed urine recently and what colour was it? Having not passed urine for several hours, or passing very concentrated (dark) urine, may suggest dehydration.

Gnawing problems

Ask the patient about recent weight loss or gain, changes in appetite and difficulty chewing or swallowing. Is there any change in taste? Remember the sense of taste and also salivation may diminish in older people as a part of ageing. Is there any excessive belching or passing of gas? Recurrent indigestion is often seen as 'normal' by patients and may need further investigation.

Stool survey

Asking about the patient's bowels may be something they (and you) find embarrassing, but it is important to ask. Ask firstly how frequently they have their bowels open, and document frequency in days, not just as 'regularly'. Remember there is wide normal variation in frequency – some patients normally only have their bowels open every 2 or 3 days, whereas for others this may suggest constipation. So ask if stool is hard or soft, and easy or difficult to pass.

A key question is whether there is a change in bowel habit, or in the colour, amount and/or appearance of their stool? Also, is there ever any blood in the stool, and if so is it dark or bright red? Change in bowel habit or stool may indicate bowel cancer, although there are many alternative explanations.

A national occult blood screening programme for bowel cancer is currently being 'rolled out' across the UK, inviting people over 60-years-old (50 years in Scotland) for screening every 2 years. Upper age limits and dates when the scheme will be fully operational vary across the four UK countries. For further details see Cancer Backup (2008b). Ask eligible patients if they have been invited to take part, and to encourage them to do so. Also encourage 'self-testing' in non-eligible older patients.

Travel plans

Find out if the patient has recently travelled abroad. Diarrhoea, hepatitis and parasitic infections can result from ingesting contaminated food or water.

Illness or irritation?

Many patients say they have an irritable bowel. If so, find out more about how they were given this diagnosis and what investigations they have had; patients have sometimes 'self-diagnosed' this condition and need further investigation.

Asking about past health

To determine if your patient's problem is new or recurring, ask about past GI illnesses, such as an ulcer. Also consider previous liver, pancreatic or gallbladder disease; inflammatory bowel disease; rectal or GI bleeding; hiatus hernia; diverticulitis; gastro-oesophageal reflux disease or cancer. Also ask about any abdominal surgery or trauma, especially appendicectomy.

Asking about medication and allergies

Ask the patient if they are taking any medications. Several medicines have GI side-effects – for example, gastric irritation (aspirin, non-steroidal anti-inflammatory drugs (NSAIDs)), diarrhoea (antibiotics) or constipation (analgesics such as morphine and codeine). Be sure to ask about laxative use; habitual use may cause constipation. Also ask the patient if they are allergic to medications or foods. Such allergies commonly cause GI symptoms.

Asking about family health

Because some GI disorders are hereditary, ask the patient whether anyone in his/her family has had a GI disorder.

Disorders with a familial link include:
- ulcerative colitis
- colorectal cancer
- gastric and duodenal ulcers
- gastric cancer
- diabetes
- alcoholism
- Crohn's disease.

Asking about social and lifestyle history

Inquire about your patient's social history as discussed in Chapter 1. Remember that stress has been linked to some types of GI condition, such as irritable bowel syndrome. Be sure to ask about alcohol, smoking and caffeine, which all have links with upper digestive disorders.

Explore diet carefully by asking the patient to describe what they ate yesterday, or in a typical day. Consider possible links with the symptoms described. If indicated, ask the patient to construct a food diary over a 7-day period.

Assessing the GI system

A comprehensive physical assessment of the GI system includes examination of the mouth, abdomen and rectum, although in reality the examination is often more selective.

Order! Order!

The usual sequence of examination is often modified when examining the GI system, to the order: inspection, auscultation, percussion and palpation. This is because there is a suggestion that palpating the abdomen before you auscultate can change the bowel sounds and lead to inaccurate assessment. Also, percussing before palpating may help you make more informed decisions about where to palpate. However, some texts and practitioners retain the traditional order of inspection, palpation, percussion and auscultation – this is an acceptable approach if you prefer it. Also, the GI examination is often combined with a urinary or genitourinary examination (see Chapter 12).

Be prepared

Before beginning your examination, explain the techniques you'll be using and warn the patient that some procedures might be uncomfortable. Make sure you have a stethoscope to hand, and perform the examination in a private, quiet, warm and well-lit room. Have access to a light source which you can shine across the abdomen (anglepoise lamp or torch).

Hands first

As with most major body system examinations, start with the hands. Look for clubbing (see Chapter 5) which has been linked to some

GI disorders. Also look for reddening on the palms of the hands (palmar erythema), or white nails (Terry's nails – see Chapter 5), both of which are linked with liver disease. Also note whether the patient has signs of Dupytron's contracture (pulling in of the ring and little fingers – see Chapter 13). Patients with this condition sometimes have an alcohol-related liver problem.

In a flap?

Asking patients to hold their hands out in front of them may reveal a tremor which could suggest alcohol dependency. In patients with liver disease, ask the patient to hold their hands out in front for 30 seconds with wrists bent back and fingers apart. This could reveal a 'liver flap', a jerky hand movement indicative of hepatic encephalopathy, which is a serious finding.

Skin survey

Look at the patient's skin for any signs of jaundice (yellowing of the skin) or any spider naevi (see Chapter 5). More than five or six spider naevi and/or signs of jaundice both have strong associations with liver disease, although remember spider naevi also occur in pregnancy.

Eyes right?

Check the conjunctiva of the eyes for any signs of anaemia (see Chapter 9). Look at the sclera for yellowing, a sign of jaundice. Remember, jaundice may show here before being evident in the skin, and it's a good place to inspect for jaundice in darker-skinned patients.

Open wide

Inspect the patient's mouth and jaw for any abnormalities. Inspect the lips, teeth, gums and oral mucosa with a pen torch. Note bleeding, ulcerations and colour changes. Check the teeth for any problems which may affect eating, or erosion of enamel (especially on the back teeth) that might suggest bulimia. Assess the tongue, checking for coating, swelling and ulcerations. Note unusual breath odours. (For more detail on examining the mouth and throat, see Chapter 7.)

Check the neck

Assessing the supraclavicular lymph nodes is an important part of your GI examination (see Chapter 10). Pay particular attention to the left side as both sides of the abdomen drain via the thoracic duct into the left subclavian vein. GI disease, especially cancer, may therefore cause left supraclavicular enlargement. But be sure to examine on the right as well for comparison with the left, and also because the upper part of the liver and parts of the upper GI system drain into the right side, so pathology here may cause a right-sided enlargement.

Examining the abdomen

To ensure an accurate assessment:
• Ask the patient to empty their bladder.
• Expose the patient's abdomen from just below the breasts/nipple line to the symphisis pubis.
• If tolerated, place the patient flat with just one pillow.
• Place a pillow under the patient's knees to help relax the abdominal muscles.
• Ask the patient to keep their arms at their sides.
• Keep the room warm. Chilling can cause abdominal muscles to become tense.
• Warm your hands and the stethoscope.
• Ask the patient to point to any areas of pain, and assess painful areas last to help prevent the patient from becoming tense.

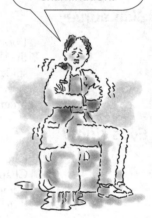

Hold the ice! A cold room can make the abdominal muscles tense, which may affect your examination.

Inspection

Begin by mentally dividing the abdomen into four quadrants and then imagining the organs in each quadrant. (See *Abdominal quadrants*, page 267.)

It's all in the terms

In addition to the quadrants you may also find it helpful to use these three terms to describe organs or findings which sit more centrally:
• epigastric – above the umbilicus and between the costal margins
• umbilical – around the navel
• suprapubic – above the symphysis pubis.

Battle of the bulge

Observe the abdomen for symmetry, checking for bumps, bulges or masses. A bulge may indicate distension or hernia. Shine a good light across the abdomen, as shadows may be cast by uneven contours. Get your eyes level with the patient's abdomen, and look from the foot of the bed/couch as well as the side.

Also note the patient's abdominal shape and contour. The abdomen should be flat to rounded in people of average weight. A protruding abdomen may be caused by obesity, pregnancy, ascites, constipation or abdominal distension with gas. (See *The five Fs*, right.) A slender person may have a slightly concave abdomen.

Innie or outie?

Assess the umbilicus, which should be inverted and located midline. Conditions such as pregnancy, ascites, hernia or an underlying mass can cause the umbilicus to protrude. If the umbilicus protrudes, check whether this is a long-standing or recent change. Ask the patient to put their chin on their chest. This may reveal an umbilical or incisional hernia. If you suspect an inguinal hernia, ask the patient to stand (if feasible) at the end of the examination, and inspect the area. Get them to cough or strain down and inspect again.

Stretched to the limit

The skin of the abdomen should be smooth and uniform in colour. Striae, or stretch marks, can be caused by pregnancy, excessive weight gain or weight loss or ascites. On lighter skin, new striae are pink or blue; old striae are silvery white. In patients with darker skin, striae may be dark brown. Note any dilated or readily visible veins.

See the scars

Note any surgical scars on the abdomen, and pay particular attention to the umbilical area where scars from laprascopic surgery can be easily missed. Also don't mistake these for failed umbilical piercings; ask the patient the reason for any scars which are not explained by the history. Also note any appearance of bruise-like markings either around the umbilicus (Cullen's sign) or on the flanks (Grey–Turner's sign) suggesting haemorrhage or acute pancreatitis.

Riding the peristaltic wave

Note abdominal movements and pulsations. Usually, peristalsis can't be seen. If it can, it will look like slight, wave-like motions, which may indicate bowel obstruction and should be referred urgently. In many patients, even those who are quite obese, pulsation of the aorta is visible in the epigastric area. Pulsation should be slight. Marked pulsations may indicate hypertension, aortic aneurysm or aortic insufficiency. Also look for normal respiratory movement; absence may suggest pain or peritonitis.

Auscultation

To assess bowel sounds, lightly place the stethoscope diaphragm in the right lower quadrant, slightly below and to the right of the

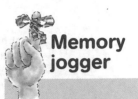

Memory jogger

The five Fs

If the patient has a generalised abdominal distension it is quite likely to be caused by one or more of the five **F**s:

Fat

Flatus

Faeces

Fluid

Foetus.

Visible, rippling waves of peristalsis may signal a bowel obstruction. Be sure to report such a finding immediately.

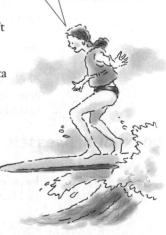

umbilicus. Listen for a minute or so, longer if you think bowel sounds may be absent. (Some texts suggest up to 5 minutes!) Judge their presence or absence, and the approximate number and quality of the sounds.

Bowel sounds are well transmitted through the abdomen, and the amount of sound varies markedly from moment to moment. This means variations between quadrants are of little consequence, and it's usually only necessary to examine one quadrant (Bickley and Szilagyi 2007), moving to another quadrant only if you hear no bowel sounds in the first one.

Silence the suction

Before auscultating the abdomen of a patient with a nasogastric tube (or another abdominal tube) which is connected to suction, briefly clamp the tube or turn off the suction if it is safe to do so. Suction noises can obscure or mimic actual bowel sounds.

Pardon my borborygmus

Normal bowel sounds are high-pitched, gurgling noises caused by air mixing with fluid during peristalsis. The noises vary in frequency, pitch and intensity, and occur irregularly from 5 to 30 times per minute (Jarvis 2008) – although it is often difficult in reality to tell where one sound ends and another begins! They're loudest before mealtimes. Borborygmus is the term for loud, gurgling, 'growling' sounds heard over the intestine as gas passes through it.

Too much activity or not enough?

Bowel sounds are classified as normal, hypoactive or hyperactive. Hyperactive bowel sounds – loud, high-pitched sounds that occur frequently – may be caused by diarrhoea, constipation or laxative use or may signify early small bowel obstruction. Early obstruction may also produce a sound described as 'tinkling bowel sounds'; a bit like the sound of water being poured.

Hypoactive bowel sounds are heard infrequently and indicate diminished peristalsis. These, and absent bowel sounds, are associated with ileus, bowel obstruction and peritonitis. The use of opioid analgesics and other medications can also decrease peristalsis.

Voice of the vessels

Auscultate for vascular sounds with the bell of the stethoscope. (See *Vascular sounds*, page 277.) Listen over the aorta, and the renal, iliac and femoral arteries for bruits, venous hums and friction rubs.

A note of caution

If, as a result of an abnormal pulsation and/or a bruit, you suspect your patient has an abdominal aortic aneurysm, seek help from a more experienced examiner who can palpate the width of the aorta. Lederle and Simel (1999) suggest a width greater than 2.5 cm is a much better predictor of abdominal aortic aneurysm than the force of pulsation. They also dispute the theory that abdominal palpation increases the risk of rupturing an aneurysm, but in view of the seriousness of abdominal aortic aneurysm it is wise to seek advice from an experienced practitioner before proceeding. Also take advice from an expert examiner before proceeding further with the assessment of a patient who has had transplantation of an abdominal organ, again, some authors suggest there is a possible risk of rupture.

Percussion

Percussion is used to detect the size and location of abdominal organs and to detect air or fluid in the stomach or bowel. Begin percussion in the right lower quadrant and proceed clockwise, covering all four quadrants. Be sure to make a few 'hits' in each quadrant, covering the peri-umbilical area as well as the flanks. Some people work in three or four horizontal rows as if they are 'mowing a lawn'. Others work more in a 'star-shaped' pattern, moving in a circular fashion, in and out from the umbilicus.

Hollow or dull?

You normally hear two sounds during percussion of the abdomen: tympany and dullness. When you percuss over hollow air-filled organs, such as an empty stomach or bowel, you hear a clear, hollow sound like a drum beating. It sounds similar to resonance but a bit more 'musical'. The degree of tympany depends on the amount of air and gastric dilation. When you percuss over solid organs, such as the liver, or faeces-filled intestines, the sound changes to dullness. Note the point where the sound changes.

How large is the liver?

Percussion of the liver can help you to estimate its size. (See *Percussing and measuring the liver*, page 278.) Hepatomegaly (liver enlargement) is commonly associated with hepatitis and other liver diseases.

Splenic size?

Because the spleen sits behind the midaxillary line, percussion anterior to the midaxillary line should be tympanic, arising from air

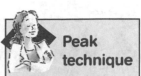

Peak technique

Vascular sounds

Use the bell of your stethoscope to auscultate for vascular sounds at the sites shown in the illustration below.

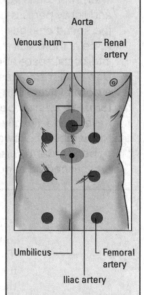

Adapted from Weber, J. and Kelley, J. (2003) *Health Assessment in Nursing.* 2nd edn. Philadelphia, PA: Lippincott Williams & Wilkins.

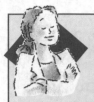

Peak technique

Percussing and measuring the liver

To percuss and measure the liver, follow these steps:

- Identify the upper border of liver dullness. Start in the right midclavicular line in an area of lung resonance, and percuss downward towards the liver. Use a pen to mark the spot where the sound changes to dullness. Note that in adult female patients this may be difficult. If feasible, percuss down from below the breast – but if the sound is already dull, breast tissue may be obscuring the upper liver border.

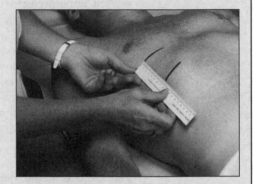

- Then start in the right midclavicular line at a level with the umbilicus, and lightly percuss upwards towards the liver. Mark the spot where the sound changes from tympany to dullness. Note that this is likely to be at the costal margin in a normal liver, so check the lowest intercostal space above the margin to confirm dullness is not due to the bony costal margin.
- Use a ruler to measure the vertical span between the two marked spots, as shown above. In an adult, a normal liver span ranges from 6 to 12 cm (Jarvis 2008). Size is gender, height and age dependent; females, shorter people and those over 80 years old tend to have smaller livers. Note though that infants have proportionally larger livers, usually extending 1 to 2 cm below the cosal margin.
- Remember the lower liver borders may be obscured by the costal margin and difficult to assess, and the upper border by breast tissue. Also, research suggests that liver percussion can be inaccurate (McGee 2007). Any suspected abnormality should therefore be confirmed by ultrasound.

in the colon or stomach. Dullness here suggests an enlarged spleen. To assess for splenic enlargement, percuss along Traubes space. This means percussing along the ninth or 10th intercostal space from the costal margin/midclavicular line to the midaxillary line. (These will be the lowest rib spaces you can feel.) The sound should be tympanic.

Then to further check that the spleen is a normal size, percuss several times in the ninth or 10th intercostal space at the anterior axillary line. As you percuss, ask the patient to take a deep breath in to move the spleen downwards and forwards. Normally tympany should remain. If the sound changes to dull, the enlarged spleen may have been moved under your percussing finger by the deep breath.

If you suspect more severe splenic enlargement (that is, the whole area is dull) percuss diagonally up from the right lower quadrant to the left upper quadrant, noting the point where the note changes from tympany to dullness. Conditions linked with splenic enlargement include glandular fever, trauma, sickle cell anaemia, malaria and some cancers. The spleen frequently enlarges in infancy, even with moderate infections.

Palpation

Abdominal palpation includes light and deep palpation to help determine the size, shape, position and tenderness of major abdominal organs, and to detect masses and fluid accumulation. Palpate all four quadrants, leaving painful and tender areas until last. Always remember to look at the patient's face for signs of pain.

Light touch

Light palpation helps to assess the abdominal musculature for any abnormalities and tenderness. To palpate, put the fingers of one hand close together, depress the skin about 1.5 cm with your fingers and make gentle, rotating movements from the joints between your fingers and hands. Keep your hand flat and avoid short, quick jabs.

What you're feeling for

The abdomen should be soft and non-tender. As you palpate the four quadrants, note any 'lumps or bumps', masses and areas of tenderness or increased resistance. Determine whether resistance is due to the patient being cold, tense or ticklish (guarding) or if it's due to a permanent tensing resulting from peritoneal inflammation (rigidity).

Tickled pink?

Help ticklish or anxious patients, particularly children, to relax by using the hand over hand technique to palpate. (See *Assessing abdominal pain in children*, page 283.)

Pressing the issue

To perform deep palpation, push the abdomen down 5 to 7.5 cm but take care to keep the hand fairly flat. You may find it helps, especially in an obese patient, to put one hand on top of the other, pushing with the upper hand and feeling with the lower. Palpate the entire abdomen in a clockwise direction, checking for tenderness,

> The abdomen should be soft and non-tender when palpated.

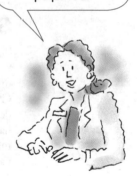

organ enlargement and masses. Don't be discouraged if you can't identify particular organs and structures – it takes lots of practise.

In infants and toddlers the musculature is poorly developed, so you will need to be much more gentle to avoid causing injury. However, this poor musculature does mean the organs are often quite easy to palpate.

Please do not touch

If patient's abdomen is rigid, palpation will be of little use and could be unsafe. An urgent referral based on what you have learned so far is more appropriate. Remember though that a normal but very muscular abdomen can also be difficult to palpate.

Feeling out the situation

Palpate the patient's liver to check for enlargement and tenderness. (See *Palpating the liver*, page 281.) Unless the spleen is enlarged, it isn't palpable. (See *Palpating the spleen*, page 282.) Some authors identify a small risk of rupturing an enlarged spleen on palpation, so if you feel it stop palpating refer the patient for expert assessment.

Special assessment procedures

To check for rebound tenderness or ascites, follow these guidelines.

The rebound tenderness test can help to confirm peritoneal inflammation or localised inflammation (for example, appendicitis). Choose a site away from the painful area, then push down slowly and deeply with your hand at a 90 degree angle. Then withdraw your hand quickly. The underlying structures will rebound suddenly and may elicit a sharp, stabbing pain on the inflamed side. However, this painful test is increasingly viewed as inappropriate, especially for children and those who are confused or anxious. There is growing evidence that normal, gentle palpation may be equally effective. Some authors also suggest there is a small risk of appendix rupture. (See *Assessing abdominal pain in children*, page 283.)

Water logged

Ascites, a large accumulation of fluid in the peritoneal cavity, can be caused by advanced liver disease, heart failure, pancreatitis or cancer. There are tests that you can do which may help you confirm ascites, or monitor changes in the amount of fluid present. (See *Checking for ascites*, page 283.) However, as these tests tend to rely on larger amounts of fluid being present, any suspicion of ascites should be checked with ultrasound.

Peak technique

Palpating the liver

- Place the patient in the supine position. If they can, ask them to bend their knees up to relax the abdomen, and put their arms by their sides.
- Stand at the right side of the patient.
- Place your right hand on the right upper quadrant with your index finger parallel to the costal margin (as shown in the photograph). Make sure that the edge of your index finger lies 2 or 3 cm below the costal margin.

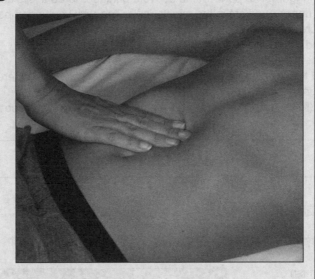

- Place your left hand under their back at the approximate location of the liver.
- Push your fingers 'inwards and upwards' so you can feel under the costal margin. Palpate to see if you can feel a liver edge.
- Now ask the patient to take a deep breath in. As the patient inhales deeply, keep your hand in position and feel again. You may feel the liver move down with the breath to touch or flip over your fingertips. The edge, if felt, should be smooth, firm and somewhat round. A solid, nobbly edge may suggest cirrhosis. Note any tenderness. Remember though that not all patients have a palpable liver edge, and also that the technique takes lots of practice.

Suspected liver enlargement

If the patient's abdomen is dull to percussion in the right upper quadrant below the costal margin, or you have other reason to suspect liver disease, modify your technique. Position your hand as before, but in the right lower quadrant. As the patient takes a deep breath, palpate as before. If you don't feel a liver edge, advance your hand 2 to 3 cm upwards, and repeat until you feel the liver edge or reach the costal margin.

(continued)

Palpating the liver *(continued)*

Variations in technique

Some examiners use their fingertips to perform the above technique. To do this, place your flat hand on the right upper quadrant in the midclavicular line, with you fingertips pointing upwards. Make sure your fingertips lie 2 or 3 cm below the costal margin. Then proceed as described previously, feeling with your fingertips both before and after a deep breath.

It is important to avoid the 'hooking technique' described in some texts, where you hook your curled fingers under the costal margin from above, as there is a suggestion that damage (for example, a ruptured liver cyst) is more likely to occur with this method.

Peak technique

Palpating the spleen

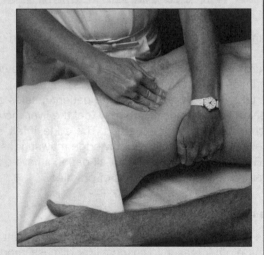

Although a normal spleen isn't palpable, an enlarged spleen is. To palpate the enlarged spleen, stand on the patient's right side. If possible, ask the patient to rotate slightly towards you. Use your left hand to support the posterior left lower rib cage. Position your fingertips so they point towards the left axilla, about 2 to 3 cm below the costal margin. Press inwards and upwards towards the spleen. Feel to see if you can palpate the splenic edge. If not, ask the patient to take a deep breath and feel again.

If the patient's abdomen is dull to percussion in or beyond the left upper quadrant, or you have another reason to suspect marked splenic enlargement (for example, rib trauma), then modify your technique. Position your hand much lower, in the right lower quadrant but again pointing towards the axilla. As the patient takes a deep breath in, palpate to see if you can feel the splenic edge. If you don't feel it, advance your hand 2 to 3 cm and repeat, until you get to the splenic edge or the left costal margin.

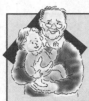

Ages and stages

Assessing abdominal pain in children

There are many conditions which cause abdominal pain in infants and young children. These range from abdominal colic to serious problems such as intussusception (telescoping of the intestine), volvulus (twisting of the intestine) and appendicitis.

Assessing abdominal pain in infants and young children, who can't verbalise how they feel, may be difficult. Be alert for such clues as drawing up of their knees with a reluctance to straighten them, an anguished facial expression, reluctance to let you touch the abdomen or a high-pitched cry. Use a pain scale appropriate to their age to assess the severity of their pain (see Chapter 1).

When attempting to assess symptoms, try techniques that elicit minimal tenderness. For example, if well enough, a child may be happy to hop or jump and tell you if they feel the pain – this is a very gentle way of eliciting rebound tenderness.

When palpating a child's abdomen, if they are finding it too painful, ticklish or frightening, try the 'hand over hand' technique. Tell them that they can be in control, then put your hand over theirs on the abdomen as you palpate. You can feel fairly well through their hand initially, and then slide your fingertips gently over their hand as they relax to feel more precisely.

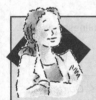

Peak technique

Checking for ascites

There are two tests which you can perform to check for ascites. Remember though that both tests only work if several hundred millilitres (ml) of fluid are present, so always seek an abdominal ultrasound if unsure.

The ballotment test

Ask the patient or an assistant to place the ulnar (little finger) edge of his/her hand firmly on the patient's abdomen at its midline. Then, as you stand facing the patient's head, place the palm of your right hand against the patient's left flank, as shown on the right. Give the right side of the abdomen a firm push with your left hand. If ascites is present, you may feel a 'fluid wave' ripple across the abdomen and hit your right hand. The hand in the midline prevents a 'flesh wave' and a false positive finding.

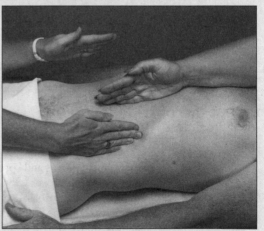

(continued)

Checking for ascites *(continued)*

The shifting dullness test

Standing on the right of the patient, percuss the abdomen in a horizontal line, in 2 to 3 cm steps, from the umbilicus towards the right flank. If the note starts tympanic and changes to dullness, the patient may have ascites. Mark the point where the note changes. Then ask the patient to roll towards you onto their right side and wait 30 seconds. Any ascitic fluid will drain (by gravity) to the right flank. Now percuss again, starting above the umbilicus and percussing horizontally towards the umbilicus and the line you drew. If the note starts tympanic but changes to dullness before you reach the original line, the patient may well have ascites.

This test can also be used to monitor changes in the amount of ascites present in patients with conditions such as cancer.

Supine

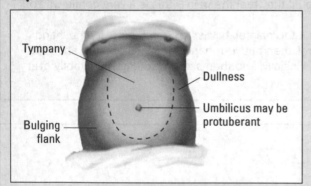

From Bickley, L.S. and Szilagyi, P. (2003) *Bates' Guide to Physical Examination and History Taking*. 8th edn. Philadelphia, PA: Lippincott Williams & Wilkins.

Left lateral position

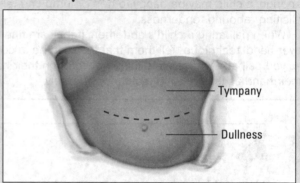

From Bickley, L.S. and Szilagyi, P. (2003) *Bates' Guide to Physical Examination and History Taking*. 8th edn. Philadelphia, PA: Lippincott Williams & Wilkins.

Examining the rectum and anus

Inspect the outside

If indicated (for example, the patient complains of passing fresh blood in their stool, suggesting haemorrhoids fissure), inspect the perianal area. Put on gloves and spread the buttocks to expose the anus and surrounding tissue, checking for fissures, lesions, scars, inflammation, discharge, rectal prolapse and external haemorrhoids. Asking the patient to strain as if having a bowel movement may reveal internal haemorrhoids, polyps or fissures. The skin in the perianal area is normally somewhat darker than that of the surrounding area.

Digital rectal examination

Digital rectal examination is a specialist skill that you should only attempt if indicated by the patient history/examination, and if you have been taught and deemed competent in the technique. Proceed with extreme caution in children, taking advice from senior colleagues, to ensure safeguarding.

To carry out this test, apply a water-soluble lubricant to your gloved index finger. Ask the patient to lie on their left side with their knees drawn up. Ensure only the anal area is exposed. Tell the patient to relax and warn them that they'll feel some pressure. Ask them to bear down. As the sphincter opens, gently insert your finger into the rectum, toward the umbilicus. To palpate as much of the rectal wall as possible, rotate your finger clockwise and then counter-clockwise. The rectal walls should feel soft and smooth, without masses, faecal impaction or tenderness. Inspect the gloved finger for stool, blood and mucous, and test any stool for faecal occult blood. Note that if you don't perform a digital rectal examination it is important to document this in the 'write up' of your GI examination, or it may be assumed that it was done and was normal.

Abnormal findings

GI disorders can affect a patient's ingestion, digestion and elimination. This section describes common abnormalities which you might uncover during a GI assessment.

Nausea and vomiting

Nausea and/or vomiting can be caused by many factors, including viruses, food poisoning, gastric and peritoneal irritation, appendicitis, bowel obstruction, cholecystitis, acute pancreatitis, neurological disturbances, myocardial infarction or by some medications. Be sure to distinguish vomiting from gastro-oesophageal reflux, which tends to be effortless and not accompanied by nausea.

Dysphagia

Dysphagia, or difficulty swallowing, should always be taken seriously, and unless it has an obvious cause (for example, acute sore throat), referral will be needed. It may be accompanied by weight loss. It can be caused by an obstruction, problems with the lower oesophagogastric junction or a neurological disease, such as stroke or Parkinson's disease. Dysphagia can lead to aspiration and pneumonia.

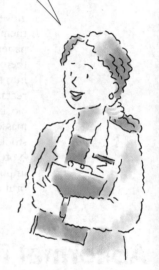

Skin changes, such as Cullen's sign and Grey–Turner's sign, indicate haemorrhage.

Skin colour changes

Dilated, tortuous, visible abdominal veins may indicate inferior vena cava obstruction or portal hypertension. Spider naevi, if there are more than five to six, may signal liver disease. A bruised appearance around the umbilicus (Cullen's sign) or on the flanks (Grey–Turner's sign) suggests pancreatitis or haemorrhage.

Constipation

Constipation, the infrequent passage of hard stool, can be caused by immobility, a sedentary lifestyle, medications (for example, codeine), irritable bowel syndrome or poor fluid intake. The patient may also complain of a dull ache in the abdomen, a full feeling or hyperactive bowel sounds.

Sounds dull!

In constipation, you will probably find left lower quadrant dullness (sometimes even extending to the left upper quadrant) and may palpate a rope-like mass in the left lower quadrant. Constipation occurs more commonly in older patients. Note that a patient with complete intestinal obstruction won't pass flatus or stool and won't have bowel sounds below the obstruction.

Diarrhoea

Diarrhoea may be caused by infection, medications or a GI condition such as Crohn's disease, ulcerative colitis or irritable bowel syndrome. Cramping, abdominal tenderness, anorexia and hyperactive bowel sounds may accompany diarrhoea. Note any accompanying fever which might suggest an infective cause.

Distension

Distension is a generalised term for a protrudent abdomen, and may be caused by any of the five Fs described previously. Localised lumps may be caused by tumours or by herniae; a hernia may protrude more visibly when the patient lifts their head and shoulders whilst lying supine.

Abnormal bowel sounds

Hyperactive, hypoactive and absent bowel sounds have a variety
of causes as noted previously. Importantly, all three are possible
indications of a small bowel obstruction.

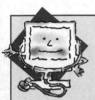

Interpretation station

Abnormal abdominal sounds

The chart below lists abnormal abdominal sounds that you may encounter. The characteristics and location
of a sound can help you determine its possible cause.

Sound and description	Location	Possible cause
Abnormal bowel sounds		
Hyperactive sounds (unrelated to hunger)	Any quadrant	Diarrhoea, laxative use or early intestinal obstruction
Hypoactive, then absent sounds	Any quadrant	Paralytic ileus or peritonitis
High-pitched tinkling sounds	Any quadrant	Intestinal fluid and air under tension in a dilated bowel
High-pitched rushing sounds coinciding with abdominal cramps	Any quadrant	Intestinal obstruction
Systolic bruits		
Vascular blowing sounds resembling cardiac murmurs	Over abdominal aorta	Partial arterial obstruction or turbulent blood flow
	Over renal artery	Renal artery stenosis
	Over iliac artery	Hepatomegaly or partial arterial obstruction
	Over femoral artery	Arterial insufficiency in the legs
Venous hum (rare)		
Continuous, medium-pitched tone created by blood flow in a large, engorged vascular organ such as the liver	Epigastric and umbilical regions	Increased collateral circulation between portal and systemic venous systems, as in cirrhosis
Friction rub (rare)		
Harsh, grating sound like two pieces of sandpaper rubbing together	Over liver and spleen	Inflammation of the peritoneal surface of the liver (as from a tumour) or of the spleen (as from an infarct)

Friction rubs and abdominal bruits

Friction rubs are a grating or 'scratchy' sound over the liver and spleen (these may be heard when listening over the costal margins for the renal arteries). They might indicate splenic infarction or hepatic tumour. Abdominal bruits may be caused by aortic aneurysms or partial arterial obstruction.

Abdominal pain

Abdominal pain may result from a vast number of causes including ulcers, intestinal obstruction, appendicitis, cholecystitis, peritonitis, indigestion, infection or inflammatory disorders. Gastritis, or alternatively a gastric or duodenal ulcer, can cause gnawing, burning abdominal pain in the midepigastrium. Cholecystitis similarly causes severe acute pain, but it is more likely to occur in the right upper quadrant, under the ribs. All of these conditions may be accompanied by nausea and possibly vomiting. Always consider a cardiac cause as an important alternative explanation for any upper abdominal pain, especially if left sided or central. (See *Types of abdominal pain*, below and *Abdominal pain origins*, page 289.)

Tender situation

Rebound tenderness can be caused by peritonitis or appendicitis. Appendicitis may be accompanied by increased abdominal wall

Interpretation station

Types of abdominal pain

If your patient complains of abdominal pain, ask them to describe the pain and ask how and when it started. This chart will help you assess the pain and determine possible causes. Remember that any upper GI pain might also be cardiac in origin.

Type of pain	Possible cause
Burning	Peptic ulcer, duodenal ulcer, gastro-oesophageal reflux disease, gastritis
Cramping	Biliary colic, irritable bowel syndrome, diarrhoea, constipation, diverticulitis, flatulence
Severe cramping	Biliary colic, appendicitis, Crohn's disease, diverticulitis
Stabbing	Appendicitis, pancreatitis, cholecystitis

Interpretation station

Abdominal pain origins

What can you do to figure out which organ might be affected if your patient has abdominal pain? Assess the location of the pain, and then look at this chart to get a quick idea of the possible source of the pain. Pain may be visceral (from the organs), parietal (from the walls of the body cavities) or referred (remote from its origins). Remember that visceral pain may sometimes progress to become parietal pain.

Affected organ	Visceral pain (usually dull)	Parietal pain (usually sharp)	Referred pain
Stomach	Midepigastrium	Midepigastrium and left upper quadrant	Shoulders (more commonly left)
Small intestine	Periumbilical area	Over affected site	Midback (rare)
Appendix	Periumbilical area	Right lower quadrant	Right lower quadrant
Proximal colon	Periumbilical area, and right flank for ascending colon	Over affected site	Right lower quadrant and back (rare)
Distal colon	Hypogastrium, and left flank for descending colon	Over affected site	Left lower quadrant and back (rare)
Gallbladder	Midepigastrium	Right upper quadrant	Right subscapular area, right shoulder and back (rare)
Ureters	Costovertebral angle (middle of back)	Over affected site	Groin; scrotum in men, labia in women (rare)
Pancreas	Midepigastrium and left upper quadrant	Midepigastrium and left upper quadrant	Back and left shoulder
Ovaries, fallopian tubes and uterus	Hypogastrium and groin	Over affected site	Inner thighs

resistance and guarding. Not all patients have the classic right lower quadrant pain initially – appendicitis pain may be generalised in the lower abdomen initially before localising in the right lower quadrant.

Bloody stools

The passage of bloody stools may indicate GI bleeding. As a general rule, the darker the blood, the higher up the GI tract the origin is likely to be. It may result from colorectal cancer, colitis, Crohn's disease, an anal fissure or haemorrhoids.

Redcurrant jelly?

In toddlers and pre-school children the condition intussusception, where the bowel telescopes onto itself, typically causes bloody stools which sometimes appear like redcurrant jelly. Such a finding should be referred urgently.

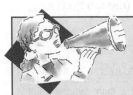

That's a wrap!

Gastrointestinal system review

Functions

- Ingestion and digestion of food
- Elimination of waste products.

Structures

GI tract

- Mouth – responsible for chewing, salivation and swallowing
- Pharynx – allows passage of food from the mouth to the oesophagus
- Epiglottis – closes over larynx when food is swallowed to prevent aspiration into the airway
- Oesophagus – moves food from the pharynx to the stomach
- Stomach – serves as a reservoir for food and secretes gastric juices which aid in digestion
- Small intestine – consists of the duodenum, the jejunum and the ileum; digests carbohydrates, fats and proteins and absorbs end products of digestion into the bloodstream
- Large intestine – consists of the caecum; the ascending, transverse, descending and sigmoid colons; the rectum; and the anus. Responsible for absorbing excess water and electrolytes, storing food residue and eliminating waste products.

Accessory organs

- Liver – metabolises carbohydrates, fats and proteins; detoxifies the blood; converts ammonia to urea; stores glucose as glycogen; and synthesises proteins and essential nutrients
- Gallbladder – stores bile from the liver until it's emptied into the duodenum
- Pancreas – releases insulin and glycogen into the bloodstream; secretes pancreatic enzymes which aid digestion
- Bile ducts – serve as passageways for bile from the liver to the intestines
- Spleen – lymphatic organ which removes damaged red blood cells and platelets, and also stores platelets
- Abdominal aorta – supplies blood to the GI tract.

Health history

Ask the patient about:

- current GI signs or symptoms
- past GI illnesses, surgery and trauma
- any indication of change in bowel habit or blood in the stool
- any signs that might suggest that the pain has a cardiac rather than a GI cause
- medications, including laxative use
- family medical history, especially history of ulcerative colitis, colorectal cancer, gastric or duodenal ulcers and gastric cancer
- diet, exercise patterns and alcohol, caffeine and tobacco use.

Gastrointestinal system review *(continued)*

Assessment

General survey

- Inspect the hands for clubbing, palmer erythaema, Terry's nails and Dupytron's contracture
- Inspect the skin for spider naevi
- Inspect the eyes for anaemia and jaundice
- Inspect the mouth and jaw as well as the inner and outer lips, teeth, gums and oral mucosa.
- Inspect the tongue
- Inspect the neck for left supraclavicular lymph node enlargement.

Abdomen

- Inspect the abdomen for symmetry, shape and contour.
- Note abdominal movements and pulsations.
- Auscultate to assess bowel sounds, and over the abdominal arteries to check for bruits, venous hums and friction rubs.
- Percuss the abdomen, listening for tympany over hollow organs (such as an empty stomach or intestine) and for dullness over solid organs (such as the liver) or faeces-filled intestines.
- Palpate in all four quadrants of the abdomen, leaving painful areas for last.
- Check for rebound tenderness if you suspect peritoneal inflammation; also check for ascites, a large accumulation of fluid in the peritoneal cavity.

Rectum and anus

- Inspect the perianal area if indicated.
- If indicated, palpate the rectum using a water-soluble lubricant on your gloved index finger.

Abnormal findings

- Nausea and vomiting – may be caused by existing illness or by certain medications
- Dysphagia – difficulty swallowing; has various causes; may lead to aspiration and pneumonia
- Skin colour changes – such as Grey–Turner's sign, Cullen's sign, spider naevi, enlarged veins
- Constipation – may occur with a dull abdominal ache, a full feeling and hyperactive bowel sounds
- Diarrhoea – may occur with cramping, abdominal tenderness, anorexia and hyperactive bowel sounds; in children, blood-stained diarrhoea may suggest intussusception
- Abdominal distension – may occur with gas, a tumour or a colon filled with faeces
- Abnormal bowels sounds – may be hyperactive (indicating increased intestinal motility), hypoactive or absent
- Friction rubs – may indicate splenic infarction or hepatic tumour
- Abdominal pain – may result from ulcers, intestinal obstruction, appendicitis, cholecystitis, peritonitis, indigestion, infection or other inflammatory disorders
- Bloody stool – from cancer, colitis, Crohn's disease, haemorrhoids or, in younger children, intussusception.

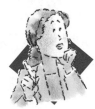

Quick quiz

1. When food is swallowed, the epiglottis:
   - A. opens.
   - B. closes.
   - C. opens or closes, depending on the type of food.
   - D. rotates.

2. A key function of the liver is:
   A. metabolising carbohydrates, fats and proteins.
   B. absorption of water.
   C. synthesising vitamin C.
   D. storage of calcium.

3. Hyperactive bowel sounds may be a sign of:
   A. complete bowel obstruction.
   B. opioid analgesic use.
   C. constipation, diarrhoea, early intestinal obstruction or laxative use.
   D. diminished peristalsis.

4. When you percuss over the liver, you should hear:
   A. dullness.
   B. resonance.
   C. tympany.
   D. hyperresonance.

5. To test a patient for rebound tenderness, position your hand at a:
   A. 30 degree angle to the abdomen.
   B. 45 to 60 degree angle to the abdomen.
   C. 90 degree angle to the abdomen.
   D. 120 degree angle to the abdomen.

For answers see page 401.

12 Genitourinary system

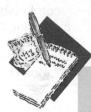

Just the facts

In this chapter, you'll learn:

♦ organs and structures that make up the genitourinary system

♦ methods to obtain a patient history of the genitourinary system

♦ techniques for performing a physical assessment of the genitourinary system

♦ abnormalities of the genitourinary system.

A look at the genitourinary system

The genitourinary (GU) system encompasses the urinary tract and the reproductive organs. Disorders of this system can have wide-ranging effects on other body systems. For example, ovarian dysfunction can alter hormonal balance. Kidney dysfunction can alter blood pressure, disrupt serum electrolytes and affect production of the hormone erythropoietin which regulates the production of red blood cells.

Difficult to discuss

Disorders of the GU system can affect the patient's quality of life, self-esteem and sense of well-being. Reproductive disorders such as infertility can also be extremely distressing. Many patients are reluctant to discuss such problems with a healthcare practitioner, and most patients will understandably find a GU examination embarrassing. Your challenge then, is to perform an assessment that's both skilled and sensitive. If you appear comfortable discussing the patient's problem, they will be encouraged to talk openly too.

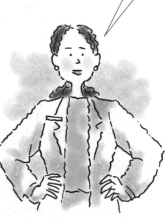

Disorders of the GU system can have wide-ranging effects on other body systems.

Complex questions

There are particular skills in taking a sexual history from some groups of patients. For example, older people, people from certain cultures and teenagers may all have particular sensitivities about the sexual health issues they need to discuss. It's also important to think about young people in particular, in respect of their age, the age of sexual partners, competency to consent, confidentiality and safeguarding (See *Assessing Paediatric Patients*, page 312.) In patients of all ages, you'll need to consider whether you need a chaperone present for the examination which you are going to conduct.

Subtle signs and symptoms

Assessing the GU system can be a challenging task. Many patients with urinary disorders or sexually transmitted diseases don't fully recognise the nature of the problem, because they have only mild signs and symptoms, or no symptoms at all.

To thoroughly and accurately assess your patient's GU system, you'll need to know the organs and structures of the urinary and reproductive systems and how they work.

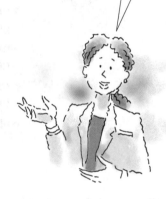

Remember, your patients will take their cues from you. If you're comfortable discussing their problem, they'll be encouraged to talk openly.

Anatomy and physiology of the female GU system

Urinary system

The urinary system helps maintain homeostasis by regulating fluid and electrolyte balance. It consists of the kidneys, ureters, bladder and urethra. (See *Urinary system*, page 295.) Urine output in the average adult varies markedly depending on fluid intake, but probably averages around 1.5 to 2 litres of urine a day.

Kidneys

The two kidneys are highly vascular bean-shaped organs. They are around 10 to 12 cm long, 5 to 7 cm wide and 3cm thick (Tortora 2005). They sit on either side of the lower thoracic vertebrae, under the 11th and 12th ribs. Anteriorly, this equates to a position just below the costal margins. However, they sit retroperitoneally, which places them behind the other abdominal organs, just in front of the muscles attached to the vertebral column. The peritoneal fat layer protects them. Crowded by the liver, the right kidney extends slightly lower

Urinary system

This illustration shows the main structures of the urinary system.

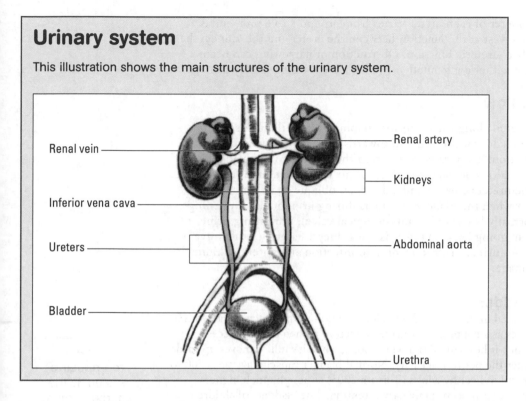

Renal vein

Inferior vena cava

Ureters

Bladder

Renal artery

Kidneys

Abdominal aorta

Urethra

than the left, so is often easier to feel. In infants and younger children the lower pole (section) of the right kidney is usually palpable.

Makin' urine

The main function of the kidneys is to filter out all of the waste products and excess water which the body no longer requires, but to keep the fluid and electrolytes which the body needs, thereby maintaining homeostasis. Closely linked to this is the kidney's role in regulating blood pressure. The functional unit of the kidney is the nephron, about one million in each kidney, which filters the body's entire circulating blood plasma volume about 65 times each day (Tortora 2005). But although this large volume of fluid is filtered out from the bloodstream into the nephrons, most of it (about 99%) is reabsorbed, leaving just the excess fluid and waste products to be passed as urine. Urine gathers in the collecting tubules of the nephrons and drains into the ureters.

Ureters

The adult ureters are around 25 to 30 cm long. The left is slightly longer than the right due to the left kidney's higher position. The diameter of each ureter varies from around 3 to 6 mm, and is narrowest at the junction between the ureter and the kidney; the pelvic–ureteric junction. Obstruction or narrowing can occur here, either congenitally or in later life, causing kidney damage.

The rhythm of the flow

Located along the posterior abdominal wall, the ureters enter the bladder low down and towards the back – the vesico-ureteric junction. They carry urine from the kidneys to the bladder by peristaltic contractions which occur one to five times per minute. The ureters enter the bladder at an oblique angle – meaning that when the bladder contracts during urination, the openings normally 'close off' (a physiological valve), preventing urine from going back up towards the kidneys. Failure of this valve causes urinary reflux, leading to infection and potential kidney damage.

Bladder

Located in the pelvis, the bladder is a hollow, muscular organ which serves as a container for urine collection. When the bladder is empty, it lies behind the pelvic bone; when it's full, it moves upwards under the peritoneal cavity. Normal bladder capacity averages 700 to 800 ml in healthy adults (Tortora 2005) although much higher volumes can occur in urinary retention. The bladders of children and older people have a lower capacity, and women's capacity tends to be lower than men's due to the uterus sitting just above the bladder.

Urethra

The urethra is a small duct which carries urine from the bladder to the outside of the body. A woman's urethra is only about 4 cm long and sits anteriorly to the vaginal opening. In contrast, the male urethra is around 20 cm long because it must pass through the penis.

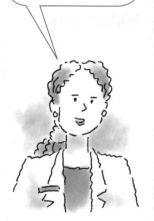

The reproductive system is the source of many health complaints in women.

Female reproductive system

The female reproductive system consists of external and internal genitalia.

External genitalia

The external genitalia, the vulva, consist of the labia majora, labia minora, clitoris, vagina, urethra and Skene's and Bartholin's glands. (See *External female genitalia*, page 297.)

External female genitalia

This illustration shows the main parts of the external female genitalia.

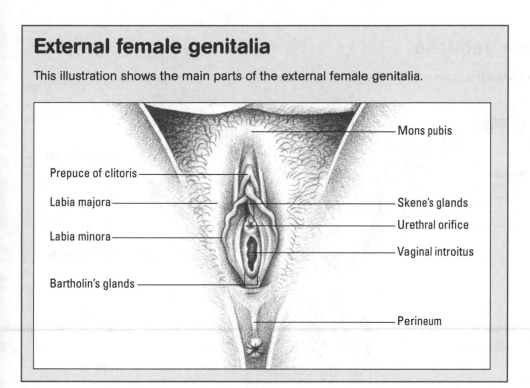

Mons pubis

Prepuce of clitoris

Labia majora

Labia minora

Bartholin's glands

Skene's glands

Urethral orifice

Vaginal introitus

Perineum

Labia majora and minora

The outer vulval lips, or labia majora, are two rounded folds of adipose tissue which extend from the mons pubis to the perineum. The inner vulval lips are the labia minora. Anteriorly they form the prepuce or hood of the clitoris, and posteriorly join to become the fourchette or frenulum. From puberty, the labia majora and the mons pubis above them grow pubic hair.

Clitoris, vestibule and urethral opening

The clitoris, composed of erectile tissue, lies between the labia minora at the top of the vestibule, which also contains the slit-like urethral opening, and the vaginal opening.

Vaginal opening and perineum

The vaginal opening is posterior to the urethral opening. The hymen is a thin fold of mucous membrane (occasionally absent) that partially covers the vaginal opening until it is perforated by sexual or physical activity, making a larger, irregular vaginal opening. The perineum is the area bordered anteriorly by the top of the labial fold and posteriorly by the anus.

Internal female genitalia

The illustration below shows the main internal structures of the female reproductive system.

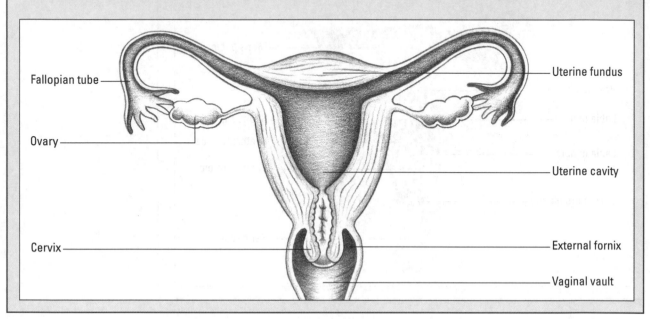

Fallopian tube

Ovary

Cervix

Uterine fundus

Uterine cavity

External fornix

Vaginal vault

Skene's and Bartholin's glands
Skene's and Bartholin's glands produce lubricating fluids important for the reproductive process. They can become infected, leading to abscess formation. Skein's glands are tiny structures just below the urethra, and Bartholin's glands are found posterior to the vaginal opening.

Internal genitalia
The internal genitalia include the vagina, uterus, ovaries and fallopian tubes. (See *Internal female genitalia*, above.)

Vagina
The vagina is a pink, hollow, collapsed passage for intercourse, childbirth and menstruation. It's located between the urethra and rectum, extending from the vulva to the uterus.

Uterus
The uterus is a hollow, pear-shaped, muscular organ which lies between the rectum and bladder. It has an upper fundus and lower cervix, which protrudes into the vagina. The cervix secretes mucous which assists in reproduction and protects the uterus from pathogens. The function of the uterus is to nurture and then expel the foetus during pregnancy.

The cervix's mucous-secreting glands protect the uterus from pathogens.

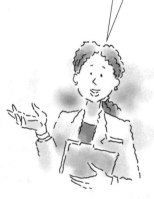

Locations may vary

The position of the uterus in the pelvic cavity may vary, depending on bladder fullness. The uterus may also tilt in different directions.

Ovaries

A pair of oval glands, about 3 cm long, the ovaries are found in the lower abdominal cavity, one each side of the uterus. They produce ova (or eggs) and release the hormones oestrogen and progesterone. The ovaries become fully developed after puberty and shrink after menopause.

Fallopian tubes

Approximately 10 cm long, the two fallopian tubes extend from the ovaries into the upper portion of the uterus. Their funnel-shaped ends help guide the ova to the uterus after expulsion from the ovaries. The fallopian tube is also the usual site of fertilisation of the ova by the sperm.

Male reproductive system

In men, the urethra is also part of the reproductive system because it carries semen as well as urine. The male reproductive system also includes the penis, scrotum, testicles, epididymis, vas deferens, seminal vesicles and prostate gland. (See *Male reproductive system*, page 300.)

Penis

The penile shaft contains three columns of vascular erectile tissue, with the glans, containing the slit-like urethral opening (or meatus), located at its end. The corona is the junction of the glans and the shaft. The prepuce (or foreskin) is the loose skin covering the glans. Its surgical removal is called circumcision. (See *Male circumcision as a religious practice*, page 301.). During sexual activity, sperm and semen are forcefully ejaculated from the urethral meatus.

Scrotum

A loose, wrinkled, deeply pigmented sac, the scrotum is located at the base of the penis. Each of its two compartments contains a testicle, an epididymis and portions of the spermatic cord. The left side of the scrotum is usually lower than the right because the left spermatic cord is longer.

Male reproductive system

This illustration shows the important structures of the male reproductive system.

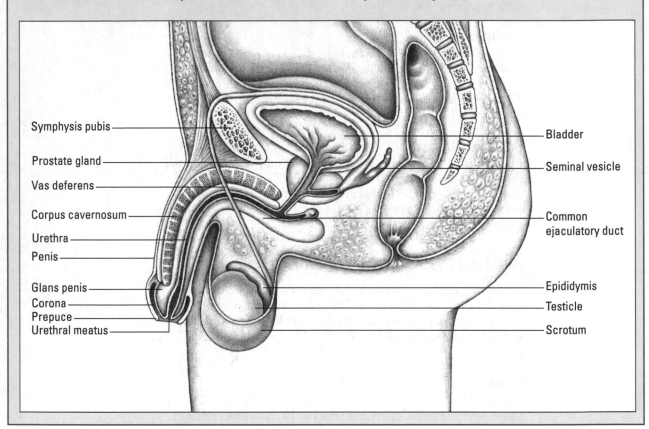

Symphysis pubis

Prostate gland

Vas deferens

Corpus cavernosum

Urethra

Penis

Glans penis

Corona

Prepuce

Urethral meatus

Bladder

Seminal vesicle

Common ejaculatory duct

Epididymis

Testicle

Scrotum

Testicles

The testicles are oval, rubbery structures suspended vertically and slightly forward in the scrotum. They produce testosterone and sperm.

Where it all begins

Testosterone stimulates the changes which occur during puberty, commencing around 9 to 13 years of age. Firstly the testicles enlarge, then pubic hair grows and the penis size increases. Secondary sexual characteristics include facial and body hair, muscle development and voice changes.

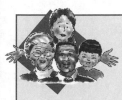

Bridging the gap

Male circumcision as a religious practice

In some religions, such as Judaism and Islam, circumcision is a religious practice. Jewish males are usually circumcised when they're 8 days old by a mohel (a Jew with special training). In the Islamic religion, Islamic boys are often circumcised at around 7-years-old, although there is no fixed age. This circumcision is most likely to be performed in a hospital setting as a day case. Adult males converting to Islam may choose to be circumcised; however, it isn't required.

The practice in both religions, or where practised by parents of other faiths or no faith, who feel it is in their son's best interest, is the subject of ethical debate – with some arguing in its favour and others arguing against it. Currently, though, there are no laws prohibiting male circumcision in the UK. The British Medical Association (BMA) (2006a) states that it is assumed to be lawful if it is:

* performed competently
* believed to be in the child's best interest
* performed with valid consent – this must be from both parents; children who themselves are capable of expressing a view should have their wishes taken into account.

See BMA (2006a) for more information.

Female circumcision

Note you may occasionally come across women who have been circumcised – this usually involves removal of the clitoris. It is a human rights issue now often referred to as genital mutilation. The practice *is* prohibited in the UK (BMA 2006b). However, it is important that women who have been circumcised are cared for sensitively. Health issues such women may experience include problems with menstruation, urination, intercourse, infertility, pregnancy, childbirth and mental health.

Epididymis

The epididymis is a reservoir for maturing sperm. It curves over the posterolateral surface of each testicle, creating a bulge on the surface. Occasionally it's located anteriorly.

Vas deferens

The vas deferens – a storage site and the pathway for sperm – runs from the lower end of the epididymis, up the spermatic cord and through the inguinal canal to the abdominal cavity, where it rests on the fundus of the bladder.

Seminal vesicles

A pair of sac-like glands, the seminal vesicles are found on the lower posterior surface of the bladder in front of the rectum. Secretions from the seminal vesicles help to form seminal fluid.

Prostate gland

About 6 cm long, the prostate surrounds the urethra just below the bladder. It produces a thin, milky, alkaline fluid which mixes with seminal fluid during ejaculation to enhance sperm activity.

Obtaining a health history

Because the urinary and reproductive systems are located so close together, you and your patient may have trouble differentiating signs and symptoms. Use the PQRSTU or OLD CART mnemonic (page 16) to explore the patient's symptoms fully. You will often need to explore both urinary and genital health. (See also *Putting your patient at ease*, below.)

Putting your patient at ease

Here are some tips for helping your patient feel more comfortable during the health history:

- Make sure the room is private and that you won't be interrupted.
- Tell the patient that answers will remain confidential within the healthcare team, and phrase your questions tactfully.
- Start with less sensitive areas and work up to more sensitive areas such as sexual function.
- Don't rush or omit important facts because the patient seems embarrassed.
- Remember that some patients, usually men, may be particularly concerned about discussing sexual problems because it suggests a decrease in sexual prowess.
- Remember that views about sexual practices or reproduction may be influenced by religious or cultural beliefs.
- If the patient uses slang or euphemisms to talk about sexual organs or function, make sure you're both talking about the same thing.

Ease into it

Ask questions about the urinary system first to enable the patient to relax and a rapport to be built, before you ask the more embarrassing genital/sexual health questions.

Asking about the urinary system

The most common complaints of the urinary system include output changes, such as hesitancy, frequency, urgency, burning sensation on micturition (passing urine), nocturia (frequent urination at night), incontinence, urinary colour changes and pain. Patients may also report polyuria (excessive urination), oliguria (reduced urine output) and anuria (passing no urine – an emergency situation).

Make sure 'urine' the know about urination

To explore a urinary problem further, these questions may help.
- Are there any changes in the urine's colour or odour?
- Is there any blood or pus in the urine? Is it clear or cloudy?
- Is there any fever or shivering, indicating infection?
- Is there any pain or burning during urination?
- Have they any problems with incontinence, frequency or poor urinary flow?

Poor urinary flow (hesitancy) may be a particular problem for older male patients, and can be linked to benign or malignant prostatic disease.

Remember that if the patient is passing little or no urine this represents a medical emergency requiring urgent intervention. Less than 0.5 ml/kg/hr in an adult (Resuscitation Council UK 2006), 1 ml/kg/hr in a child or 2 ml/kg/hr in an infant (Mackway-Jones *et al.* 2005) is regarded as a cause for serious concern.

Past medical history

Past illnesses and pre-existing conditions can affect a patient's urinary tract health. For example, has the patient ever had frequent urinary tract infections (UTIs), kidney trauma, kidney stones or surgery on their urinary tract? Kidney stones, surgery or trauma can alter the structure and function of the kidneys and bladder.

Dredging up the past

Be sure to explore whether the patient has, or has had, any other health problems which could affect their urinary system. Patients with diabetes have an increased risk of UTI, whilst cardiovascular disease can alter kidney perfusion.

Has the patient ever had hypertension, or do they have this currently? Remember that the kidneys have a key role in the regulation of blood pressure. Does the patient have any back pain? Do they have any problems with itching? Both symptoms are linked to renal problems.

Discuss drugs and diet

When asking about current medication, note in particular any antihypertensive drugs, any diuretics and any other medication that has side-effects which can affect kidney or bladder function. Some drugs can affect the appearance of urine – for example, rifampicin (used as prophylaxis for tuberculosis) colours the urine a reddish colour. Remember that diet can also affect urine – for example, beetroot causing a red discoloration or asparagus causing an odour.

Familial factors

Also ask about the patient's family history to gather information about the risk of developing kidney failure or kidney disease.

> Remember to ask about what drugs your patient is using. Drugs such as diuretics may cause polyuria or nocturia.

Asking about the reproductive system

The most common concerns about the reproductive system, which affect both genders include pain, discharge, pruritus (itching), infertility and concerns that they have contracted a sexually transmitted disease. If the patient is worried about having caught a sexually transmitted infection (STI), ask if there are any sores, lumps, ulcers or discharge in their genital area. But remember, many sexually transmitted diseases have no symptoms so further screening may be required.

In addition, women may present with menstrual problems such as changes to their cycle or bleeding in between periods. Men may have concerns regarding the scrotum or inguinal area or erectile dysfunction.

To obtain the most complete data about those problems, focus on the patient's current complaints using the PQRSTU or OLD CART mnemonic, and then explore reproductive history, sexual history, social history and family history as appropriate.

> Some of us drugs can affect the appearance of urine or alter GU function. Sorry about that!

Female reproductive history

A woman's menstrual history often provides very valuable information. In older girls find out if menstruation has commenced; it should normally commence by the age of 15. In women over about 45-years-old, ask if she has reached the menopause, and whether there are any problems such as hot flushes, night sweats, mood swings or vaginal dryness. If she is taking hormone replacement therapy find out for how long, as the risks associated with taking it are known to increase with length of use. See NHS Direct (2008b) for more information on this issue.

Menstrual measures

For women who are menstruating, what is her menstrual cycle? Cycles vary greatly from one woman to another. A normal cycle can be anything from 22 to 35 days, whilst normal duration is 7 days or less (Anderson *et al.* 2005). Ask if there have been any interruptions to menstruation other than pregnancies. Also find out if her next period is overdue or if there is any possibility that she might be pregnant currently. In any woman of childbearing age with abdominal pain, always consider ectopic pregnancy as a possible cause.

Go with the flow

Establishing the amount of menstrual flow is difficult – the phrases 'light', 'medium' or 'heavy' may help. If you are concerned, ask about how much sanitary protection a women uses in a typical period or day. Spotting (small amounts of blood loss between periods) may be normal if linked to some oral contraceptives, but can also indicate abnormalities such as infection or cancer. Any unexplained vaginal bleeding should always be investigated urgently.

Smear safety

Ask if your patient is invited for, and attends, regular cervical screening. UK women are invited for regular screening from either the age of 20 (Scotland, Wales, Northern Ireland) or 25 years (England) to age 64 years (60 years in Scotland). Frequency is either 3-yearly or 5-yearly depending on age and country. For full country-specific details, including planned changes for Northern Ireland, see Cancer Backup (2008c).

Also ask teenage girls if they have been immunised against human papilloma virus, the major cause of cervical cancer; a new immunisation programme has recently commenced, and by 2010 all girls 13 to 18-years-old should have been offered immunisation.

Male reproductive history

Ask male patients about any history of genital abnormalities; for example, undescended testicles, testicular torsion or problems with a low sperm count. This is a good time to ask whether he carries out regular testicular self-examination. (See *Testicular self-examination*, page 306.)

Testicular self-examination

Testicular abnormalities which are a cause for concern and should be investigated include:

- A lump
- Swelling
- Tenderness
- A feeling of heaviness or dragging in the scrotum
- A dull ache in the lower abdomen or groin.

During the patient history, ask your male patients whether they perform monthly testicular self-examinations. If not, explain that testicular cancer can be treated successfully when it's detected early. Men should examine their testes once a month. Guidance regarding how to do this, which can be given to male patients, can be found at Cancer Research UK (2005, 2006b).

Circumcised or not?

Ask a male patient with a GU problem whether he's circumcised. If not, can he retract and replace the prepuce (foreskin) easily? An inability to retract the prepuce is called phimosis; an inability to replace it is called paraphimosis. Untreated, these conditions can impair local circulation and lead to infection, oedema and even gangrene.

Scrotal survey

Does the patient have any scrotal swelling, scrotal pain, discomfort or a 'dragging' sensation? These may indicate an inguinal hernia, a haematocele, epididymitis; testicular torsion or a testicular tumour.

The sexual side – men and women

When the patient seems comfortable, consider whether you need to ask about sexual practices. This will depend on whether the presenting problem might have a sexual cause or consequence.

Asking about sexual practices, especially the number and gender of sexual partners, needs to be handled sensitively, with explanation about why this is important. (See also *Don't forget to ask older patients*, page 307.)

Ages and stages

Don't forget to ask older patients

Although sexual performance and drive are likely to be affected by age, don't assume that older people aren't able to have sex or that they aren't interested in sex. Harbouring these beliefs could prevent you from asking older patients about their sexual health. The truth is, your patient may be experiencing a sexual problem that he or she is too embarrassed to bring up on their own – common problems include erectile dysfunction in older men and vaginal dryness in older women. Therefore, be sure not to make assumptions about older patients' sexual health and include it in the history where indicated. Provide advice, support and referral as needed. Also remember that some drugs (for example, some antihypertensives) and some surgeries (for example, prostate surgery) can affect male erectile function. Ensure men are enabled to make informed choices about such healthcare plans which include recognition of these potential side-effects.

Screen for STI

If a patient has an STI, it is vitally important sexual partner(s) are informed and screened themselves. You may also need to ask about the human immunodeficiency virus (HIV) status of the patient and their partner(s); again handle the question sensitively.

Contraception concerns?

Asking about contraception and 'safe sex' may well also be relevant. Exploring these issues offers the opportunity for health promotion as well as links with possible presenting symptoms. Pain during intercourse (dyspareunia), most often reported by women, should be followed-up to exclude underlying physical causes.

Past pregnancy?

Asking women about previous pregnancies may well be important – or asking both partners if the problem is infertility. Remember though that incidence of miscarriage and infertility is high, or a woman may have had a termination, so again ask the questions sensitively and appropriately.

Assessing the GU system

To perform a physical assessment of the GU system, you'll use the techniques of inspection, percussion and palpation.

Examining the urinary system, urine and serum electrolytes

In practice, the examination of the urinary system is typically combined with examination of the gastrointestinal system to form an integrated abdominal examination. Whether you are conducting a combined examination or a specific urinary system examination, remember that several aspects of the general survey will be relevant.

Vital values

Evaluate your patient's vital signs and weight. Vital signs might reveal hypertension, which can cause renal dysfunction if it's uncontrolled. Pyrexia suggests infection, such as UTI. Weight changes provide information about fluid status, and are important for patients with urinary disorders or renal failure, especially those receiving dialysis. The appearance of the skin, eyes and mouth may convey pallor associated with anaemia, or indications of dehydration.

Telltale behaviour

Assessing mental status can offer clues in your assessment. Renal dysfunction can cause tiredness, lethargy, confusion or disorientation. Advanced renal disease can cause coma or seizures.

Inspection

Inspect the abdomen as described in Chapter 11. Look for differences in the contours of the abdomen which suggest swelling of the kidneys or bladder. Signs of ascites may be suggestive of a renal problem such as nephrotic syndrome.

Percussion

Percuss the abdomen in all four quadrants as described in Chapter 11. Ascitis or gross enlargement of the kidneys may cause dullness – although because the kidneys lie behind the intestines, you might still hear tympany, despite a severely enlarged kidney lying behind it.

A thud from behind

A specialised form of kidney percussion can be performed from the back – this is the test for costovertebral angle tenderness which occurs with kidney inflammation. (See *Performing fist percussion*, page 309.)

Peak technique

Performing first percussion

To perform this test, ask the patent sit up so you can access his/her back, and stand behind them. Place the ball of the palm of your non-dominant hand on the back at the level of the 12th rib. Make a fist with the other hand, and use its ulnar surface to strike the first hand just below the knuckles. Use just enough force to cause a perceptible thud. This should be painless, and is abnormal if marked tenderness is felt.

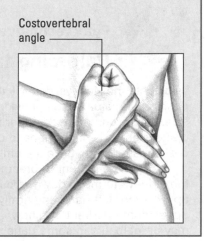

Costovertebral angle

The bladder matters

To percuss the bladder, first ask the patient to empty it if they can. Then ask them to lie supine. Start at the umbilicus and percuss down towards the symphisis pubis until the note changes from tympany to dullness. Note the level of the change. A normally full bladder is indicated by dullness a few cm above the symphisis pubis, but tympany should remain until you reach the symphisis pubis if the bladder is empty. Dullness above the symphisis pubis after voiding, or associated with an inability to void, suggests retention. Note that a markedly distended bladder can reach close to the level of the umbilicus.

Palpation

Because the kidneys lie behind other organs and are protected by muscle, they normally aren't palpable unless they're enlarged. However, in very thin patients, in babies/young children and in older patients, you may be able to feel the lower pole of the right kidney as a smooth round mass in the right upper quadrant. (For technique see *Palpating the kidneys*, page 310.)

If the kidneys feel enlarged, the patient may have hydronephrosis, a cyst or a tumour.

If the bladder is full, you'll feel it

You won't be able to palpate the bladder unless it's distended. With the patient supine, use the fingers of one hand to palpate the lower abdomen in a light dipping motion. A distended bladder will feel firm and relatively smooth, extending above the symphysis pubis. If a female patient is 12 or more weeks pregnant, you may feel the fundus of the uterus.

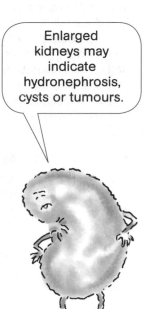

Enlarged kidneys may indicate hydronephrosis, cysts or tumours.

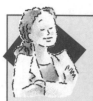

Peak technique

Palpating the kidneys

To palpate the kidneys, first ask the patient to lie in a supine position. To palpate the right kidney, stand on the patient's right side. Place your left hand under the back just below the level of the liver, and your right hand on the abdomen just below the costal margin and above the umbilicus.

Instruct the patient to breathe in deeply, as this helps the kidneys to move downwards. As the patient inhales, press up with your left hand and firmly down with your right in the upper right quadrant, as shown. The lower pole of the kidney may be palpable in some patients, and the kidney should be palpable if enlarged. If felt, it should feel like a firm, smooth, rounded mass. The procedure is sometimes described as a 'duck bill' procedure, describing the two hands as operating in a duck bill fashion.

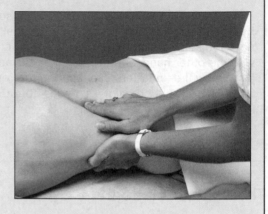

To palpate the left kidney, reach across the patient's abdomen, placing your left hand behind the left flank. Place your right hand over the area of the left kidney – that is, below the costal margin and above the umbilicus. Alternatively, walk around the bed or couch and proceed as for the right kidney. Ask the patient to inhale deeply again. As they do so, pull up with your left hand and press down with your right. The left kidney is less likely to be palpable in a normal patient.

Auscultation

Auscultate the renal arteries by listening with the bell of the stethoscope at the costal margins, as described in Chapter 11. Bruits in this area may indicate renal artery stenosis, and are particularly important to consider in patients with severe hypertension.

Urinalysis

A 'clean catch' urine specimen can be examined for its colour, debris and odour. It can also be assessed for its specific gravity (which measures concentration) and via a 'dipstick' urine test for its pH, and the presence of blood leukocytes, nitrates, protein, ketones, bilirubin or glucose. Common findings include glucose which may suggest diabetes, or protein, leukocytes and/or blood which may suggest infection (although negative dipstick testing doesn't exclude abnormality). More detailed analysis, including bacterial culture of infected urine, is achieved through laboratory testing. For further detail of these tests see Hastings (2008). (See also *Assessing urine appearance*, page 311.)

Assessing urine appearance

How your patient's urine looks can provide clues about general health and the source of a GU problem. During the health history, ask whether there has been any change in colour. If there has, or when you inspect a urine sample, use this list of possible causes to help you interpret the changes:

- Pale and diluted – diabetes insipidus, diuretic therapy, excessive fluid intake
- Dark yellow or amber and concentrated – acute febrile disease, inadequate fluid intake, severe diarrhoea or vomiting
- Blue–green – methylene blue ingestion
- Green–brown – bile duct obstruction
- Dark brown or black – acute glomerulonephritis, intake of such drugs as chlorpromazine
- Orange, red, brown or a combination – obstructive jaundice, urobilinuria, intake of drugs such as rifampin or phenazopyridine
- Red or red–brown – haemorrhage, porphyria, intake of drugs such as rifampicin or phenazopyridine.

Blood testing for kidney function

Laboratory testing of blood levels of urea and electrolytes is commonly used to investigate renal function. High levels of urea and/or creatinine may indicate renal disease. Abnormal levels of sodium, potassium, chloride and bicarbonate may also suggest renal disease, although all such findings have many other causes.

Examining the reproductive system

Some assessment techniques in the field of sexual health require specialist techniques. This includes bimanual vaginal examination and cervical cytology, which are taught on specialist certificated courses. Testicular palpation and prostatic examination are also specialised skills, and like breast examination should be used with caution as there are risks of false reassurance; palpation by a non-expert cannot confirm the absence of a tumour. Suggestions of testicular or prostatic disease from the history therefore require further assessment by an expert. It is for this reason that these skills are not covered in this text.

Inspecting male and female external genitalia is, however, an important skill to learn. If the patient is a child be cautious and follow guidelines carefully. (See *Assessing paediatric patients*, page 312.)

Inspecting the female external genitalia

Before the examination, ask the patient if she would like to pass urine. Ensure her privacy by offering a gown, and using a drape or sheet to cover her on the bed or couch until you are ready, and to keep exposure to a minimum. Ensure the door is locked, or that people know not to enter the area.

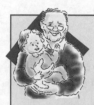

Ages and stages
Assessing paediatric patients

Routine testicular examination should only be undertaken once during childhood, on infants at their 6 to 8 week check, to make sure that both testes have descended into the scrotum. If not, referral for further assessment by a paediatrician is required. Thereafter, testicular examination is only performed if clinically indicated – for example, the parent has noticed a swelling in the testes.

Before palpating a boy's scrotum for a testicular examination, explain what you'll be doing and why. A younger child will probably want his parent present for comfort; however, an older boy is likely to want privacy. Make sure he's comfortably warm and as relaxed as possible. Cold and anxiety may cause his testicles to retract so that you can't palpate them.

Hernia and hydroceles

If a parent is concerned about scrotal swelling, suspect a scrotal extension of an inguinal hernia, a hydrocele or both. Hydroceles are common in children under about 2 years of age, although can occur in older children. To differentiate between the two, remember that hydroceles transilluminate (that is, you can shine a light through the scrotum which will show through the tissue surrounding the testicle) and are unlikely to be tender.

Ages and stages
Pubic hair development

Pubic hair changes in density, colour and texture throughout a person's life. Before adolescence, the pubic area is covered only with normal body hair. In adolescence, this body hair grows thicker, darker, coarser and curlier. In full maturity, it spreads over the symphysis pubis, and also the labia and inner thighs in women. In later years, the hair grows thin, grey, and brittle. Pubic in women. hair development before puberty may suggest hormonal imbalance and should be investigated.

Then ask the patient to draw her heels up towards her bottom and allow her legs to fall apart sideways. An older or disabled patient, or one who has had a hip replacement, may need help with this, or may need to lie in a different position, such as on her side with her legs drawn up.

First, look to identify the structures described in *External female genitalia*, page 297. Note the presence of any discharge (a possible sign of urethral or vaginal infection) or ulcerations (a possible sign of a sexually transmitted disease). Notice any piercings, or any lesions or other abnormalities.

A look at the labia

Put on gloves before spreading the labia to locate the urethral meatus. It should be a pink, irregular, slit-like opening at the midline, just above the vagina. Look again for signs of discharge. The labia minora should be pink, moist and free from lesions, as should the areas around Bartholin's or Skein's glands.

Don't forget discharge

You may see a normal vaginal discharge outside menstruation. This varies from clear and stretchy before ovulation, to white and opaque after ovulation. A curdy discharge, an odour or a different colour would be abnormal. Swab any abnormal looking discharge or exudate from a lesion. Palpate any lump or lesion with your fingers to detect tenderness, consistency and mobility.

Inspecting the male genitalia

Depending on the history, inspection may be required of one or more parts of the male genitalia. Note both penile and especially scrotal skin tends to be darker than the patient's normal skin tone.

Penis

Penile skin should be slightly wrinkled. Check for lesions, nodules, redness, inflammations and swelling, asking the patient to lift the penis so you can see underneath. Use a gloved hand to palpate any lumps. Ask the patient to retract the foreskin if there are problems in that area. Check the meatus which should be at the tip, and take a swab of any discharge if required.

Scrotum and testicles

To inspect the scrotum, ask the patient to hold his penis out of the way so you can observe for swelling, nodules, redness, ulceration and distended veins. If a patient describes a scrotal change such as a lump, pain, tenderness, numbness, feeling of heaviness or unexplained groin pain, it is important to seek prompt assessment by an expert. Testicular cancer is the most common cancer in boys and men aged 15 to 44 (Cancer Research UK 2008c), but younger boys and older men are at risk too. Prompt diagnosis means an excellent chance of successful treatment.

It might be perfectly normal!

Men sometimes worried that one testicle is lower than the other, but this is usually normal. Sebaceous cysts – firm, white to yellow, non-tender skin lesions – can be normal, but check with an experienced examiner until you are confident at distinguishing them.

Assessing the inguinal and femoral areas – men and women

If the patient reports lower abdominal/inguinal pain, or has seen a lump in their groin, assess for an inguinal hernia as described in Chapter 11. Also remember to check other important structures in this area, including the femoral pulse, femoral arteries and inguinal lymph nodes.

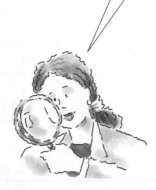

Inspect the inguinal and femoral areas for hernias.

Notice the nodes

The inguinal lymph nodes comprise two chains. The horizontal chain lies along the line of the groin where the abdomen joins the leg, and drains the superficial abdomen, the buttock and the external genitalia including the scrotum or vagina. However, it doesn't drain the testes or the cervix – so will not offer clues to tumours in these areas. The vertical group lies down the inner thigh and drains parts of the leg. Both chains should be palpated if the history suggests possible infection or malignancy in the areas of drainage.

Abnormal findings

This section discusses common abnormalities of the GU system.

Urinary abnormalities

Common abnormal findings in the urinary system include polyuria; haematuria; urinary frequency, urgency and hesitancy; nocturia; urinary incontinence and dysuria.

Polyuria

A fairly common finding, polyuria is the production and excretion of an excessive quantity of urine, typically more than 2500 ml daily. It most commonly results from diabetes insipidus, diabetes mellitus or diuretic use, although there are several possible causes. Patients with polyuria are at risk of dehydration.

Haematuria

Haematuria, the presence of blood in the urine, may cause brown or bright red urine, or flecks/streaks of blood in the urine if the volume is smaller. It requires further investigation. There are numerous potential causes including trauma, infection, renal calculi, kidney disease and cancer. Remember, urine may be contaminated with blood from the vagina or GI tract.

Urinary frequency, urgency and hesitancy

Urinary frequency (that is, abnormally frequent urination) commonly results from decreased bladder capacity. It is a common symptom of a UTI. It also occurs with urethral stricture, neurological disorders, pregnancy, uterine tumours, prostatic disease, diabetes, diuretic use and stress.

It's a pain

In many cases the sudden urge to urinate (urgency) is accompanied by bladder pain, which may suggest a UTI. Urgency without pain may be a symptom of an upper motor neurone lesion which affects bladder control.

Trouble starting up

Difficulty starting a urine stream, or urinary hesitancy, can occur with a UTI, a partial obstruction of the lower urinary tract, neuromuscular disorders, prostatic disease or the use of certain drugs.

Nocturia

Excessive urination at night, or nocturia, is a common sign of kidney or lower urinary tract disorders. Prostatic disease is another common cause. It may also be caused by cardiovascular, endocrine or metabolic disorders and is a common adverse effect of diuretics or excess caffeine intake. Getting up to urinate a couple of times a night can be a normal finding in older people.

Urinary incontinence

Urinary incontinence is a common complaint which may be temporary or permanent. The amount of urine released may be small or large. Urge incontinence is when the urgent need to urinate can't be overcome, and stress incontinence is when leakage occurs as a result of coughing, sneezing or laughing. Possible causes include a UTI, tumour, renal calculi, uterine prolapse and neurological disorders. Again it can be a problem associated with ageing, but it is important to assess for a possible underlying cause, whatever the age of the patient.

Dysuria

Dysuria, or pain during urination, signals a possible UTI. Other causes include bladder irritation or distension, prostatic enlargement, bladder outlet obstruction, bladder spasm and pylonephrosis. In babies and small children, symptoms of UTIs tend to be vague; for example, nausea, vomiting or fever. So always carry out routine urinalysis in such cases.

Sexually transmitted infections

STIs are amongst the most common diseases in the world, with a steady rise in incidence in recent years. Always consider the possibility of STI in patients with a vaginal or penile discharge, or with skin changes in the genital area. (See *Sexually transmitted infections*, page 316.) Remember many STIs can be asymptomatic, so sexual history is an important part of your care. Also remember that sexual partner(s) of a patient with STI need screening too. Handle this sensitively but stress the importance.

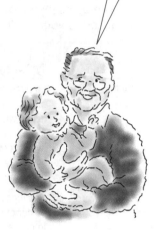

Thanks to my enlarged prostate, we have opposite problems – he goes all the time, and I can't go at all!

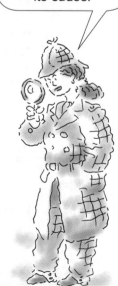

The onset of dysuria is a clue to its cause.

Interpretation station

Sexually transmitted infections

STIs are one of the most common diseases in the world. The likelihood of coming across these conditions is therefore high. It takes considerable experience to diagnose these conditions, and swabs should always be taken where there is any discharge or exudate in order to help confirm the diagnosis. However, the following chart may help you to think about the different clinical signs and symptoms to look for, and will also help you to describe your findings when you refer your patient to a GU medicine clinic or other specialist.

Condition	Typical symptoms	Typical presentation in female patients	Typical presentation in male patients
Syphilis	Papules that become a syphilitic chancre, a red, painless, eroding lesion with a raised border. If internal, may be missed. Regional lymphadenopathy. Secondary syphilis presents with fever and a maculopapular rash.	Lesions typically appear inside the vagina, on the cervix, on the external genitalia or in the rectum.	The lesion typically appears on the penis or in the rectum.
Genital warts	Small painless warts. Typically the colour of the flesh. Occur singly or in clusters. May enlarge to form cauliflower-like masses.	Appear on the vulva or anus. Often begin around the fourchette. Vagina and cervix may be affected.	Appear on the penis (especially penile shaft) or anus.
Genital herpes	Small, often red vesicles, lesions or crusts. Regional lymph node inflammation and fever may be present. Patients often experience recurrent attacks.	Occur on external genitalia, buttocks and thighs, also internally in the vagina and cervix.	Occur on external genitalia, buttocks and thighs.
Chlamydia	Often has minimal or no symptoms, especially in women. If seen, discharge is the most likely symptom.	Mucopurulent cervical discharge, cystitis, lower abdominal pain, post-coital or intramenstrual bleeding. Up to 80% of women are asymptomatic.	Penile discharge and irritation around the urethra (although this often resolves spontaneously leaving the infection still present). May lead to epdidymitis. Asymptomatic in up to 50% of men.
Gonorrhoea	Discharge and dysuria. Can be asymptomatic, especially in women.	Watery or purulent discharge (often green/yellow), cystitis, pain on urination, pelvic pain. Around 50% of women are asymptomatic.	Most likely to be painful urination and penile discharge. 10% of men are asymptomatic.
Trichomoniasis	Purulent discharge.	Offensive yellowy/green discharge and local irritation. Red strawberry-like papules on cervix and/or vaginal wall. Very occasionally asymptomatic.	Penile discharge, irritation and urinary frequency. Much more likely to be asymptomatic than women.

Adapted from NHS Direct (2008c), Seidel *et al.* (2003), and Kumar and Clarke (2002).

Abnormalities affecting women

Common female genital/menstrual abnormalities include cervical changes, vaginal infection, vaginal and uterine prolapse, retrocele and menstrual problems.

Cervical changes

Many women will report previously diagnosed cervical abnormalities in their history. Although sometimes these will be cervical cancer, they will more commonly be a cervical intra-epithelial neoplasm. These are abnormal cellular 'precancerous' changes in the outer layer of the cervix which are graded and treated according to depth. Treatments range from 'watch and wait' (more frequent screening but no immediate treatment) to colposcopy (a more detailed cervical examination) or a cone biopsy to remove part of the cervix.

Vaginal inflammation and discharge

Vaginitis is caused by a variety of organisms, and can lead to redness, itching, dyspareunia (painful intercourse), dysuria or a malodorous discharge. Common causes are bacterial infection and candidiasis. Antibiotics and pregnancy increase the risk of candidiasis infection.

Vaginal and uterine prolapse

Also called cystocele, vaginal prolapse occurs when the anterior vaginal wall and bladder prolapse into the vagina. It may even be visible outside the body.

Rectocele

Rectocele is the herniation of the rectum through the posterior vaginal wall. On vaginal examination, it will be seen as a pouch or bulging on the posterior wall as the patient bears down.

Dysmenorrhoea

Dysmenorrhoea – painful menstruation – is a very common and at times disabling problem for menstruating women. It's usually characterised by mild to severe cramping or colicky pain in the pelvis or lower abdomen which may radiate to the thighs and lower sacrum. It is worst at the beginning of menstruation and gradually subsides as bleeding tapers off.

What a pain! Dysmenorrhoea affects more than 50% of menstruating women.

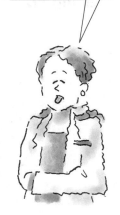

Amenorrhoea

The absence of menstrual flow, amenorrhoea, can be primary (no onset of menstruation by the age of 16) or secondary (absence of menstruation for 3 or more months). Other than the normal causes (pregnancy, lactation or menopause), amenorrhoea may result from imperforate hymen, cervical stenosis, intrauterine adhesions, medication, hormonal treatments or anorexia nervosa.

Abnormalities affecting men

A number of male reproductive system problems may occur, including those discussed below.

Penile lesions

Lesions on the penis can vary in appearance. In addition to STIs, consider other causes. A hard, non-tender nodule, especially in the glans or inner lip of the prepuce, may indicate penile cancer.

Zip up slowly

Trouser zip injury is a common cause of penile trauma. Patients will typically be embarrassed and may present on a hot summer's day wearing an overcoat! Injuries are seldom serious.

Paraphimosis

In paraphimosis, the prepuce is so tight that, when retracted, it gets caught behind the glans and can't be replaced. Oedema can result and more severe damage can occur if left untreated.

Cleaning up

Instruct uncircumcised men to retract the prepuce each time they clean the glans and then to replace it afterward. This prevents excessive tightness.

Displacement of the urethral meatus

Hypospadias means a urethral meatus is located on the underside of the penis. This can occur anywhere on the length of the shaft. It is commonly treated in early childhood, but if untreated can lead to infertility and also teasing if a child needs to sit down to urinate. Epispadias, the opening on top of the penis, is rarer, and the whole penis may be congenitally malformed.

Testicular tumour or torsion

A lump or other symptoms such as pain, tenderness, numbness, heaviness or unexplained groin pain in the testes may be a testicular tumour, and should always be further investigated. Testicular pain and swelling of sudden onset may indicate testicular torsion (interruption of testicular blood supply). These symptoms require immediate referral.

Hydrocele

Scrotal swelling commonly results from a hydrocele, a collection of fluid in the testicle. It may indicate cirrhosis, heart failure and testicular tumour, but can occur spontaneously, especially in children. A hydrocele can be transilluminated – that is, you can shine a light through it.

Hernia

An inguinal or a femoral hernia (femoral hernias also affect women) is a loop of bowel which comes through a muscle wall in the groin. On palpation it feels like a bulging mass of tissue under your fingers. It can descend into the scrotum. Suspected inguinal or femoral hernias should be referred urgently if the lump is permanently visible (doesn't disappear and reappear), and immediately if there are other signs or symptoms of intestinal obstruction. They are particularly common in premature babies and older men.

Prostate gland enlargement

Prostatic enlargement may indicate benign or malignant changes, most commonly occurring after 50 years of age. Symptoms may include nocturia, hesitancy, frequency and recurring UTIs. In acute prostatitis, or if the patient has a UTI, a fever will also be common.

Erectile dysfunction

Erectile dysfunction is the inability to achieve and maintain penile erection sufficient to complete satisfactory sexual intercourse; it may also affect ejaculation. It may occur occasionally or be a continual problem. Causes can be psychological, vascular, neurological or hormonal, or the side-effect of some medications. Erectile dysfunction can be an initial symptom of other problems, including cardiovascular, metabolic or neurological disease.

Priapism

Priapism, a persistent, painful erection unrelated to sexual excitation, is an emergency situation. It can last several hours or days, accompanied by severe, constant, dull aching in the penis. Patients may be embarrassed to seek help, but lack of prompt treatment can cause penile ischaemia and thrombosis. Causes include sickle cell anaemia, neoplasm, trauma and medication.

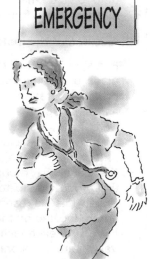

Priapism is a urologic emergency!

EMERGENCY

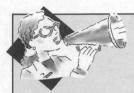

That's a wrap!

Genitourinary system review

Structures of the urinary system

- Kidneys – form urine, maintain homeostasis, contain nephrons
- Ureters – carry urine from the kidneys to the bladder
- Bladder – container for urine collection
- Urethra – carries urine from the bladder to outside of the body.

Structures of the female genitalia

- Vagina – route of passage for childbirth and menstruation
- Uterus – nurtures and then expels the foetus during pregnancy; divided into the fundus and cervix
- Ovaries – produce ova and release the hormones oestrogen and progesterone
- Fallopian tubes – the usual site of fertilisation of the ova by the sperm; help to guide the ova to the uterus after expulsion from the ovaries.

Structures of the male genitalia

- Penis – consists of the shaft, glans, urethral meatus, corona and prepuce (foreskin); discharges urine as well as sperm
- Scrotum – loose, wrinkled sac that contains the testicles, epididymides and portions of the spermatic cords
- Testicles – oval, rubbery structures that produce testosterone and sperm
- Epididymis – a reservoir for mature sperm located on the posterolateral surface of each testicle
- Vas deferens – storage site and pathway for sperm

- Seminal vesicles – sac-like glands found on the lower posterior surface of the bladder, whose secretions help form seminal fluid
- Prostate gland – produces a thin, milky fluid which mixes with seminal fluid to enhance sperm activity.

Health history

Ask about:

- Presenting urinary problems, such as urinary tract infections, kidney disease, kidney stones and past medical history of urinary problems
- Any changes to the urine
- Presenting genital problems, such as discharge, menstrual abnormalities, lesions, erectile problems, infertility and pain
- Medication history
- Potentially associated health factors, such as cardiovascular disease or hypertension
- Other symptoms such as back pain, fever, itching
- Menstruation (onset and last menstrual period), pregnancy, cervical screening and menopause in women
- Sexual health.

Assessment

Urinary system

- Inspect the areas over the kidneys and bladder.
- Percuss the kidneys (to check for costovertebral angle tenderness) and bladder.

Genitourinary system review *(continued)*

- Attempt to palpate the kidneys and bladder, although they aren't normally palpable unless the kidneys are enlarged or the bladder is distended.
- Palpate the bladder, and be aware of the areas where percussion dullness might occur in marked kidney enlargement.
- Auscultate the renal arteries.

Reproductive system

- Inspect the external genitalia to assess for any abnormalities in appearance, including lumps, lesions, discharge, swelling and discoloration.
- Discuss cytology screening with women, and testicular self-examination in men.
- Assess the groin for possible inguinal or femoral hernia; assess femoral arteries and inguinal lymph nodes.

Abnormal findings

Urinary system

- Polyuria – overproduction of urine
- Haematuria – blood in the urine, causing urine to turn brown or bright red
- Urinary frequency – abnormally frequent urination
- Urinary urgency – sudden urge to urinate
- Urinary hesitancy – difficulty starting urine stream
- Nocturia – excessive urination at night
- Urinary incontinence – involuntary release of urine
- Dysuria – painful urination.

Reproductive system

Both genders

- Sexually transmitted diseases – note chlamydia and gonorrhoea especially are often asymptomatic
- Hernia – protrusion of an organ through a muscle wall.

Women

- Cervical polyps – bright, red, soft and fragile lesions
- Vaginal and uterine prolapse – anterior vaginal wall and bladder prolapse into the vagina
- Rectocele – herniation of the rectum through the posterior vaginal wall
- Dysmenorrhoea – painful menstruation
- Amenorrhoea – the absence of menstrual flow.

Men

- Paraphimosis – tight prepuce that, when retracted, gets caught behind the glans and can't be replaced
- Hypospadias – urethral meatus located on the underside of the penis
- Epispadias – urethral meatus located on top of the penis
- Hydrocele – collection of fluid in the testicle
- Testicular tumour – neoplasm, or torsion – acute interruption to blood supply
- Erectile dysfunction – inability to achieve and maintain penile erection sufficient to complete satisfactory sexual intercourse
- Priapism – persistent, painful erection unrelated to sexual excitation.

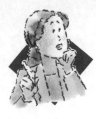

Quick quiz

1. Testicular self-examinations should be performed every:
    A. day.
    B. week.
    C. month.
    D. 6 months.

2. Your patient complains of lower abdominal discomfort, and you note a firm mass that is dull to percussion extending above the symphysis pubis. The patient has attempted to empty their bladder. You suspect:
    A. a distended bladder.
    B. an enlarged kidney.
    C. a hydrocele.
    D. an inflamed ovary.

3. An inguinal hernia is best palpated with the patient:
    A. sitting.
    B. in a supine position.
    C. standing.
    D. lying on their right side.

4. Your patient reports a 32-day menstrual cycle. You know this cycle is probably:
    A. a normal variation.
    B. a sign of hormonal imbalance.
    C. a precursor to uterine cancer.
    D. a precursor to menopause.

5. Your patient complains of a thick, white, vaginal curd-like discharge and vaginal itch. You suspect:
    A. gonorrhoea.
    B. Candida albicans.
    C. bacterial vaginosis.
    D. trichomoniasis.

6. Although the male and female urinary system functions in the same way, there's a difference in the length of the:
    A. bladder neck.
    B. ureters.
    C. kidneys.
    D. urethra.

For answers see page 401.

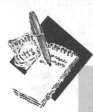

13 Musculoskeletal system

Just the facts

In this chapter, you'll learn:

♦ structures of the musculoskeletal system
♦ questions to ask during a health history
♦ techniques to assess the musculoskeletal system
♦ ways to identify abnormal findings and understand their significance.

A look at the musculoskeletal system

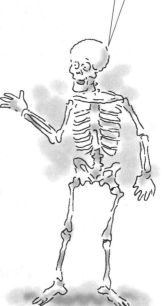

Besides giving the body its shape, my 206 bones serve as storage sites for minerals and my bone marrow produces blood cells.

During a musculoskeletal assessment, you'll use sight, hearing and touch to determine the health of the patient's muscles, bones, joints, tendons and ligaments. These structures give the human body its shape and ability to move. Your assessment skills will help to uncover musculoskeletal abnormalities and evaluate the patient's ability to perform normal activities.

The three main parts of the musculoskeletal system are the bones, joints and muscles.

Bones

The 206 bones of the skeleton form the body's framework, supporting and protecting organs and tissues (Tortora 2005). The bones also serve as storage sites for minerals and contain bone marrow, the main site of blood cell production. (See *A close look at the skeletal system*, page 324.)

Bones come in a variety of types:
- Long bones – such as the tibia or femur
- Short bones – cube-like bones such as the carpal bones of the hand
- Flat bones – such as those that make up the skull, or the scapula
- Irregular bones – such as the vertebrae
- Sesamoid bones – small bones held in place by tendons in positions of high friction, such as the kneecap.

A close look at the skeletal system

Of the 206 bones in the human skeletal system, 80 form the axial skeleton (skull, facial bones, vertebrae, ribs, sternum and hyoid bone) and 126 form the appendicular skeleton (arms, legs, shoulders and pelvis). Shown below are the body's major bones.

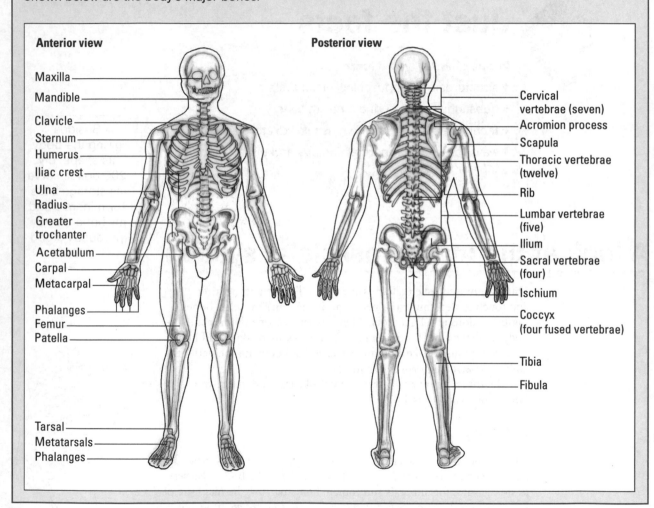

Anterior view

Maxilla
Mandible
Clavicle
Sternum
Humerus
Iliac crest
Ulna
Radius
Greater trochanter
Acetabulum
Carpal
Metacarpal
Phalanges
Femur
Patella
Tarsal
Metatarsals
Phalanges

Posterior view

Cervical vertebrae (seven)
Acromion process
Scapula
Thoracic vertebrae (twelve)
Rib
Lumbar vertebrae (five)
Ilium
Sacral vertebrae (four)
Ischium
Coccyx (four fused vertebrae)
Tibia
Fibula

Joints

The junction of two or more bones is called a joint. Joints stabilise the bones and allow a specific type of movement. The two types of joints are non-synovial and synovial.

Non-synovial

In non-synovial joints, the bones are connected by fibrous tissue, or cartilage. The bones may be immovable, like the sutures in the skull (usually joined by fibres), or slightly movable, like the vertebrae, usually joined by cartilage.

Synovial

Synovial joints move freely; the bones are separate from each other and meet in a cavity filled with synovial fluid, which is a lubricant. (See *Synovial joint*, right.) In synovial joints, a layer of resilient cartilage covers the surfaces of opposing bones. This cartilage cushions the bones and allows full joint movement, by making the surfaces of the bones smooth. (See *Types of joint motion*, page 326.) These joints are surrounded by a fibrous capsule which stabilises the joint structures and contains the synovial fluid.

Linked by ligaments

The capsule also surrounds the joint's ligaments – the tough, fibrous bands which join one bone to another. Ligaments are largely responsible for holding the bones close together in a synovial joint.

Six synovials

Synovial joints come in various types, such as ball-and-socket joints and hinge joints. Ball-and-socket joints – the shoulders and hips being the only examples of this type – allow for the fullest range of movement (ROM). These movements include flexion, extension, adduction, abduction and circumduction, as well as internal and external rotation. Hinge joints, such as the knees, elbows, fingers and toes, typically move in flexion and extension only. The knees and elbows have a slightly different design to the other hinge joints. Pairs of condyles – specialised bone endings that are either concave (hollow) or convex (rounded) – articulate against each other in the joint.

The four other kinds of synovial joint are:
• saddle joints (for example, joint between carpal and metacarpal in the thumb)
• pivot (for example, the atlanto-axial joint at the top of spine)
• gliding (for example, joints between the carpal bones in the hands)
• rotational (for example, wrist).

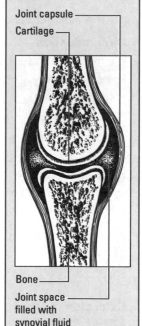

Synovial joint

Normally, bones fit together. Cartilage – a smooth, fibrous tissue – cushions the end of each bone, and synovial fluid fills the joint space. This fluid lubricates the joint and eases movement, in much the same way as the brake fluid functions in a car.

Joint capsule

Cartilage

Bone

Joint space filled with synovial fluid

Types of joint motion

Joint movement

Joints produce many different types of motion which can be assessed.

- Circumduction – moving in a circular manner (for example, shoulder)
- Flexion – bending, decreasing the joint angle (for example, elbow and knee)
- Extension – straightening, increasing the joint angle (for example, elbow and knee)
- Abduction – moving away from midline (for example, shoulder and hip)
- Adduction – moving toward midline (for example, shoulder and hip)
- Retraction and protraction – moving backward and forward (for example, jaw)
- Pronation – turning downward (for example, forearm)
- Supination – turning upward (for example, forearm)
- Internal rotation – rotating toward midline (for example, shoulder and hip)
- External rotation – rotating away from midline (for example, shoulder and hip)
- Inversion – turning inward (for example, foot)
- Eversion – turning outward (for example, foot).

The illustrations below show some examples of these movements.

Circumduction

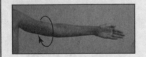

Abduction

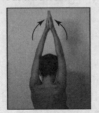

Supination

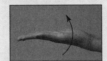

Flexion

Adduction

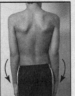

Internal rotation

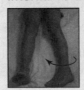

Extension

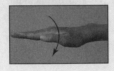

Pronation

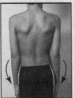

External rotation

Muscles

Muscles are groups of contractile cells or fibres which effect movement of a part of the body, or in some cases an organ (for example, the heart). Skeletal muscles, which are the focus of this chapter, contract and produce skeletal movement when they receive a stimulus from the central nervous system. The central nervous system is responsible for both involuntary and voluntary muscle function.

Tenacious tendons

Tendons are tough fibrous portions of muscle which attach the muscles to the periosteum, the outer covering of the bone. They are made of connective tissue.

Bursae

Bursae are superficial sacs filled with friction-reducing synovial fluid; they're located in areas of high friction such as the knee, elbow, shoulder and hip. Bursae cushion the movement of muscles and tendons, allowing them to glide smoothly over the underlying bones, and each other, during movement. They can become inflamed due to injury or infection, causing bursitis.

Obtaining a health history

The patient's reason for seeking care is important because it can determine the focus of your examination. Patients with joint injuries usually complain of pain, swelling, stiffness and/or noticeable deformities. Deformity can also occur with a bone fracture, which causes sharp pain especially when the patient moves the affected area. Muscular injury is commonly accompanied by pain, swelling, stiffness and weakness.

Size up for severity

When assessing musculoskeletal injuries, it is important to exclude serious injury (for example, a neck injury) first, and if suspected, to intervene immediately to protect the patient from further harm. Consider whether the patient needs pain relief before you carry out the assessment.

When, how and what?

To explore the presenting problem use the PQRSTU or OLD CART mnemonic (page 16) to help you gain a clear picture. Or, depending on the presenting problem, a simplified 'when, how and what' formula can be helpful. It is also important not to overlook other symptoms which might appear unrelated. For example, back pain associated with a change to bladder and bowel function signifies a combination of symptoms which requires urgent intervention; shoulder pain may have many other causes such as a cardiac or gastrointestinal problem.

Asking about current and past health

As you explore the presenting problem there are some particular questions you may want to ask.
• Has the patient noticed any redness, heat, pain or swelling in the affected area, particularly if this is now resolved and thus not apparent to you on examination?
• Has the patient noticed any restriction in ROM, or any grating or other unusual sounds when moving the affected body part, or other parts of the body?
• Has the patient felt any numbness, tingling or other altered sensation which could suggest nerve involvement? For example, a patient with back pain may have an associated numbness or tingling sensation running down their buttock and leg, suggestive of possible sciatica.

Long standing?

If the condition is long standing (for example, arthritis), does the condition affect the patient's normal daily activities? Is pain perhaps the main reason for seeking care? Do they use a walking stick or walking frame? This information will help you assess the priorities in terms of management.

Ancient history

As you explore the past medical history, find out whether the patient has ever had, or currently has, gout, arthritis or tuberculosis. If the patient has a past or present history of cancer, you will need to consider bony metastases as a possible source of bone pain. Has the patient had a number of fractures in the past, or ever been diagnosed with osteoporosis? (See *Biocultural variations in bone density*, page 329.)

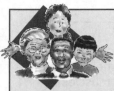

Bridging the gap

Biocultural variations in bone density

Studies of bone density have shown that Afro–Caribbean men have the densest bones, hence their relatively low incidence of osteoporosis, a bone disorder characterised by a decrease in bone mass that leaves bones porous, brittle and prone to being fractured. Caucasian people have lower bone density than Afro–Caribbean people, but higher than Chinese, Japanese and Inuit people, all of whom are at particular risk of osteoporosis (Overfield 1995).

Another key risk factor for women is being postmenopausal, as hormonal changes lead to a loss of bone density. Other risk factors in both genders include poor diet, obesity, smoking, lack of exercise and corticosteroid use.

Asking about medications

Question the patient about the medications he/she takes regularly. Many drugs can affect the musculoskeletal system. Corticosteroids, for example, can cause muscle weakness, myopathy, osteoporosis and pathological fractures, as well as avascular necrosis of the heads of the femur and humerus. Potassium-depleting diuretics can cause muscle cramping and weakness. Some antibiotics can cause tendon weakness. Anticoagulants such as warfarin can affect the joints.

Asking about lifestyle

Ask the patient about lifestyle issues, particularly their employment and hobbies. For example, frequent computer use or use of power tools can cause repetitive strain injury in the wrist/arms, but so can knitting or playing tennis. Regularly carrying a heavy bag or toddler can cause musculoskeletal damage to the back and neck.

Assessing the musculoskeletal system

Because the neurological and the musculoskeletal systems are interrelated, you will frequently need to assess them together, and will thus need to work closely between the guidance given in this chapter and the next as you refine your skills. You will also need to think about the peripheral vascular system and the blood supply to the injured part. To assess the musculoskeletal system, use the techniques of inspection and palpation to test all the major bones, joints and muscles.

Complete or focused examination?

Perform a complete examination if the patient has generalised symptoms such as aching in several joints. You can perform a focused examination if they have a presenting complaint in only one body area, but always ensure you consider the wider context. As a minimum, examine the joints above and below the one where the problem is, and make a comparison between the affected side and the unaffected side. So in a shoulder injury, for example, you will look at the elbow, the neck and the other shoulder.

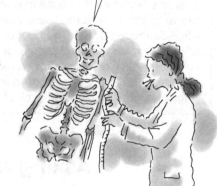

I'm really much larger when I have my muscles on.

Going head to toe

Before starting your assessment, or at an appropriate time, make sure the body part in question is fully exposed. Use a gown if required. If possible, make sure the room is warm. Explain each procedure as you perform it. The only special equipment you might need is a tape measure.

. . . from the top

Begin your examination with a general observation of the patient. If you are undertaking a full musculoskeletal examination, work from head to toe (departing from the usual practice of starting with the hands, because the neck should be assessed first for safety) and from proximal (nearest the chest/abdomen) to distal (furthest from the chest/abdomen) structures. Because muscles and joints are interdependent, interpret these findings together.

Look, feel move

As you work your way down the body, follow the key three-stage principle of 'look, feel, move':
• Look – inspect the size and shape of joint, limb, body region and skin

- Feel – palpate the skin and tissues around the joint, limb and body region
- Move – assess the movement of the joint. This will include assessing the approximate angle of the movement and whether it is normal.

Get moving

There are three distinct types of movement that you are likely to want to assess:
- Active – by the patient
- Passive – by you, the examiner
- Resisted – where you push or pull against the patient to assess power/strength.

Get active

Ask the patient to perform an active ROM of the joint, if possible. Active ROM assesses whether the patient can perform all the relevant joint movements of the body part without assistance.

Passive patients

If the patient struggles to perform an active ROM, or you need to gain additional information, perform a passive ROM examination. This doesn't require any effort by the patient, as all the movement is done by the examiner. Support the joint, and move it gently though its ROM to avoid causing pain or spasm. Never force movement.

Can you resist me?

Consider whether you also need to perform resisted movement (movement where you and the patient work in opposition, pulling or pushing in different directions) to test muscle strength. This is particularly relevant where there might be a muscular or neurological cause to the problem.

Walk the walk

Whenever possible, (but not if you suspect an acute neck or back injury) observe how the patient stands and moves. Watch them as they walk into the room or, if they are already in the room and their condition allows, ask them to walk to the door, turn around and walk back towards you. The torso should sway only slightly, the

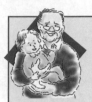

Ages and stages

Identifying congenital abnormalities

Congenitally dislocated hip

Unilateral or bilateral congenitally dislocated hip is a congenital condition where the head of the femur (ball) is either intermittently or permanently displaced outside the acetabulum (socket). This common abnormality is routinely screened for after birth and during postnatal checks. Some infants respond to conservative treatment with a harness that holds the hips in abduction for a number of weeks. More severe cases need corrective surgery. A missed congenitally dislocated hip may be spotted in the infant or toddler due to difficulty walking, typically with a wide, waddling gait; unequal leg length; or noting asymmetry of the leg creases and/or position of the knees. Such children should be referred promptly for assessment to maximise the chances of successful treatment.

Talipes equinovarus (club foot)

Club foot is a congenital abnormality where the foot is not in correct alignment; most commonly it is inverted and pointing downwards. Mild cases may respond to strapping and physiotherapy in the first few weeks of life; other children will require corrective surgery during the second 6 months of life. Any seemingly missed club feet should be referred promptly.

arms should swing naturally at the sides, the gait should be even and the posture should be erect. As the patient walks, each foot should flatten and bear the weight completely, and the toes should flex as the patient pushes off with their foot. In midswing, the foot should clear the floor and pass the other leg.

Learning to walk?

In young children you may see a range of abnormal gaits linked to congenital anomalies. For example, a waddling 'duck-like' gait which is suggestive of musculodystrophy or a missed congenital hip dislocation. Toe walking due to a tight Achilles tendon is a relatively common finding in toddlers. You may also see abnormal gait linked to talipes equinovarus ('club foot' deformity). (See *Identifying congenital abnormalities*, above.)

Assessing the bones and joints

As you assess the bones and joints, remember the systematic approach of 'look, feel, move'.

Safety first

If the history or your inspection suggests further examination would be unsafe (for example, a problem affecting the neck), stop and seek immediate advice rather than continuing with other stages of the examination – immobilising the affected area, or some other form of intervention, may be the priority. In any limb where trauma has occurred or swelling is evident, check the pulses distal to the problem. If pulses are absent, and/or the distal limb is pale and cool, immediate referral is needed. (See *The 5 Ps of musculoskeletal injury*, below.)

As you examine, ask the patient to tell you whether they experience any pain or discomfort. Watch facial expression for signs of pain. Also judge the approximate angle of the joint to assess whether there is a full ROM – normal angles are given for each joint, taken from Jarvis (2008). Remember a full circle is 360 degrees, and a quarter or right angle is 90 degrees.

The 5 Ps of musculoskeletal injury

To swiftly assess a musculoskeletal injury, remember the 5 Ps: **p**ain, **p**aresthesia, **p**aralysis, **p**allor and **p**ulse.

Pain

Ask the patient whether they feel pain. If they do, assess the location, severity and quality of the pain.

Paresthesia

Ask the patient about loss of sensation, and if indicated undertake sensory tests as described in Chapter 14. Abnormal sensation or loss of sensation suggests neurological involvement.

Paralysis

Assess whether the patient can move the affected area. If they can't, they might have nerve or tendon damage.

Pallor

Paleness, discoloration and coolness on the injured side may indicate neurovascular compromise, and should be investigated immediately.

Pulse

Check all pulses distal to the injury site. If a pulse is decreased or absent, blood supply to the area is reduced. Again this needs immediate investigation.

The neck

Inspect the patient's face and neck for swelling, symmetry and evidence of trauma. The mandible should be in the midline, not shifted to the right or left, and the neck should be straight. Note that in any incidence of trauma to the neck, great caution is needed. This invariably includes immobilisation with a collar to avoid risk to the cervical spine, and an X-ray examination. *Do not* attempt palpation and ROM assessment. Seek expert advice in such situations and be aware of local protocols for dealing with neck injuries.

Hmm . . . Your neck is going to be a little challenging to palpate.

Check the neck

Inspect the front, back and sides of the patient's neck, noting muscle asymmetry or masses, or any deformity of the cervical spine (the first seven vertebrae down from the base of the skull) – for example, 'step deformity' where the vertebrae sit out of line. If and when you are happy that inspection is normal, palpate the spinous processes of the cervical vertebrae for tenderness, misalignment, swelling or lumps. Also palpate down either side of the vertebrae (the paravertebral muscles). You may find placing your other hand on the forehead helps you to press more firmly.

Side to side

Now, if all is well, check ROM in the neck. First, carefully assess rotation. Ask the patient to turn their head to each side without moving the trunk; the chin should be almost parallel with the shoulders (rotation of around 70 degrees either side). Putting your hands on their shoulders may help the patient to just move their neck and not their body.

Chin up

Next, ask the patient to touch their chin to their chest, and then to point their chin towards the ceiling. The neck should flex forward 45 degrees (the chin should be able to touch the chest) and extend backwards 55 degrees (assuming straight is 0 degrees). Note that on leaning back the patient can feel dizzy, so this test may be more safely performed whilst sitting. Ensure that the patient does not stay in this position for more than a second or so.

Ear, ear!

Now to assess lateral rotation, ask the patient to try touching their right ear to their right shoulder and left ear to left shoulder. Hold your hands on the shoulders so they move only their neck. The usual ROM is 40 degrees on each side.

Head circles

Ask the patient to move their head in a circle to test all the movements linked together, and note whether movement is fluent, symmetrical and pain free.

Crack or crepitus?

As the patient moves the neck in different positions, listen for crepitus. Crepitus is an abnormal grating sound.

The jaw

Next, evaluate the temporomandibular joint. First, inspect for any abnormality or asymmetry. Then place the tips of your first two or three fingers in front of the ears and palpate the joint.

Is the temporomandibular joint OK?

Now, if there is no history of jaw dislocation, keep palpating as you assess the ROM of the jaw. Firstly, ask the patient to open and close their mouth, then ask them to move the jaw from side to side, and lastly forwards and backwards (protraction and retraction). The patient should be able to perform all six movements easily, without pain or tenderness.

Clock the click

Hearing or feeling a 'click' as the patient moves their jaw is a common finding that may suggest the jaw isn't properly aligned. However, you are unlikely to refer this finding in the absence of any other symptoms. Temporomandibular joint dysfunction may also lead to swelling of the area, crepitus or pain. Remember jaw pain might suggest injury, arthritis or even a myocardial infarction.

The spine

To examine the spine, it should be fully exposed. First, check the patient's spinal curvature from the side as they stand in profile (assuming the nature of the problem allows this, otherwise examine with the patient prone). In this position, the spine has a double reverse 'S' shape. (See *Scoliosis, kyphosis and lordosis*, page 336.)

Scoliosis, kyphosis and lordosis

The spine normally has a double 'S'-shaped curve – a cervical lordosis (concave curvature), a thoracic kyphosis (convex curvature), a lumbar lordosis and a sacral kyphosis.

If the curvature is exaggerated, this is abnormal. These abnormalities are concerning because they decrease lung capacity and may lead to respiratory problems in later life.

These illustrations show the difference between scoliosis, kyphosis and lordosis.

Scoliosis

If the patient has pronounced scoliosis, a lateral deviation of the spine is present and the patient leans to the side. Hip height, shoulder height and waistline are likely to be uneven.

Kyphosis

If the patient has pronounced kyphosis, the thoracic curve is abnormally rounded, as shown below. Note kyphosis and scoliosis are often combined – known as kyphoscoliosis.

Lordosis

If the patient has pronounced lordosis, the lumbar spine is abnormally concave. Lordosis (as well as a waddling gait) is normal in pregnant women and young children.

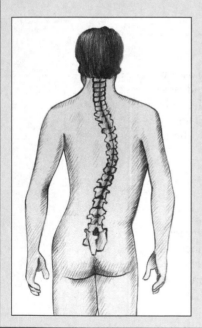 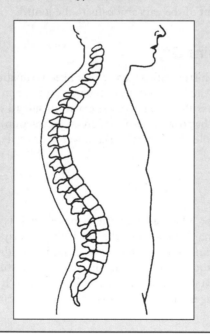 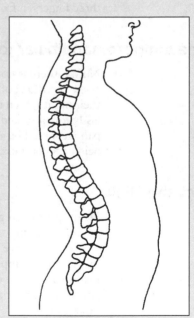

Back to back!

Next, observe the spine posteriorly. It should be in the midline position, without deviation to either side. Lateral deviation suggests scoliosis; it often combines with a kyphosis to form a 'lateral-outwards' deformity – kyphoscoliosis. You may also notice that one shoulder is lower than the other. To assess further for scoliosis, ask the patient

Peak technique

Testing for scoliosis

When testing for scoliosis, ask the patient to remove their shirt and stand as straight as possible with their back to you. Look for:

* uneven shoulder height and shoulder blade prominence
* unequal distance between the arms and the body
* asymmetrical waistline
* uneven hip height
* sideways lean
* uneven creases or skin folds.

Bent over

Then ask the patient to bend forwards, keeping head down and palms together. Look at the back during bending and also as they straighten up for:

* asymmetrical thoracic spine or prominent rib cage (rib hump) on either side
* asymmetrical waistline.

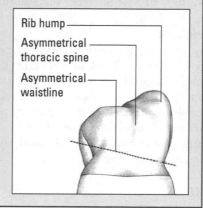

Rib hump
Asymmetrical thoracic spine
Asymmetrical waistline

to bend forwards at the waist if they are able to, and stand behind them. As you look across the back, and again as they straighten up, the deformity may become more apparent. Normally, the spine remains in the midline. (See *Testing for scoliosis*, above.)

Spine-tingling procedure

Next palpate the spinal processes and the paravertebral muscles lateral to the spine firmly with your fingertips. This can be done standing but may be easier with the patient lying prone. Note tenderness, swelling, spasm or deformity.

Bend and stretch

Now assess the ROM of the spine. If the patient seems able, ask them to try and touch their toes. They may well not quite reach their toes, but normal flexion at the waist should be about 90 degrees and the back should be concave. Then test extension by asking the patient to lean backwards from the waist, but take care to assess appropriateness first. If done, ensure

How do I measure up? Nice spine, wouldn't you say?

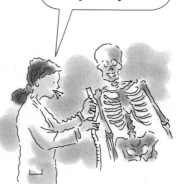

safety by positioning the patient with their back close to the bed/couch, and having your hands close to the shoulders as they bend back. Normal ROM is about 30 degrees.

To the left and the right

Now assess rotation by asking the patient to sit on the edge of the bed/couch (to stabilise the pelvis), and then ask them to rotate their upper body to face one side and then the other. Normal rotation is 30 degrees from the waist. Finally, assess lateral bending by asking the patient to stand, and then ask them to run their hand down their leg towards their knee on either side – normal is about 35 degrees.

Shoulders

Start by observing the patient's shoulders, noting asymmetry, muscle atrophy or deformity. Look from different directions – the back, the front, each side and from above (with the patient sitting). Remember to compare sides. Look for any signs of swelling or loss of the normal rounded shape. Remember, if the patient's reason for seeking care is shoulder pain, the pain could be referred – neck pain, cardiac pain, pancreatic pain or even lower abdominal pain can radiate to the shoulder, so explore carefully.

Feel those landmarks

Next palpate the shoulders with the fingertips to locate bony landmarks; noting tenderness or swelling. Palpate the following:
• the sternoclavicular joint (just to the left and right of the sternal notch)
• the clavicle
• the acromioclavicular joint (the joint between the clavicle and the acromion – which is the 'tick-shaped' forward projection from the scapula)
• the greater tuberosity (top of the humerus)
• the coracoid process (a small beak-like projection from the scapula which can be felt just below the clavicle lateral to the midclavicular line).

Assess for tenderness, swelling or deformity. Then using your entire hand, palpate the shoulder muscles for firmness and symmetry.

Feelin' groovy?

Palpate the bicipital groove by asking the patient to brace their upper arm to the body, and placing your fingertips lengthways on the top of the arm where it sits adjacent to the torso. Ask the patient to rotate their lower arm outwards and inwards without the upper arm moving away from the side of the body. Palpate the tendon in the bicipital groove under your fingers. Movement should be smooth and painless.

Lift and rotate

If the patient's shoulders don't appear to be dislocated, assess ROM. (See *Types of joint motion*, page 326 for diagrams.) Although you are going to start with active movement, remember you might need to use passive and/or resisted movement to complete your examination. Start with the patient's arm straight at the side – the neutral position.

Flex and extend

Firstly assess flexion and extension. To assess flexion, ask the patient to move the straight arms forward in an arc, as if doing a 'Mexican wave'. Full flexion is 180 degrees, with the arms pointing to the ceiling. To assess extension, ask them to move their straight arms from the neutral position posteriorly back as far as possible. Normal extension is up to 50 degrees. Do assess both arms together where possible to compare sides.

Swing into position

To assess abduction, ask the patient to move their arms from the neutral position laterally as far as possible in an arc. The arms should remain straight throughout. Normal ROM is 180 degrees – the hands should be able to touch or clap above the head. In some shoulder injuries the patient may get 'stuck' at 90 degrees, but with a little help from you be able to continue to 180 degrees. To assess adduction, ask the patient to move the arm down from the abducted position back to the neutral position, and then together and across the front of their body as far as possible. Normal ROM is 50 degrees. To help you remember which is which, see *Memory Jogger*, right.

Internal or external?

To assess external rotation, ask the patient to place both hands behind their head, with their elbows fully flexed. Then for internal rotation, ask them to reach up behind their back with elbows flexed, getting the hands as high as possible towards the scapulae. Look carefully at the back of the patient as they perform each manoeuvre – are both hands level and is the shoulder rotation around 90 degrees? If you can't remember which is which, remember internal rotation is nearer the intestines!

Memory jogger

Here's an easy way to remember the difference between adduction and abduction.

Adduction is moving a limb toward the body's midline; think of it as adding two things together.

Abduction is moving a limb away from the body's midline; think of it as taking something away, like abducting or kidnapping.

Big circles

Finally, assess circumduction which uses all the movements. Ask the patient to make big circles with their arms (elbows can be bent or straight). As they do so, feel for crepitus by placing your hands on their shoulders. Don't confuse it with the occasional 'crack' that can be heard from synovial joints. Full ROM should be possible and the same on both sides.

Elbows

Next inspect the elbows for any sign of redness or swelling. Then palpate the elbow. The most prominent point, the olecranon, is the tip of the ulna, and the other two prominent points are the medial and lateral epicondyles at the base of the humerus. These three promontories form a visual triangle when the elbow is flexed. The ulna and humerus form the hinge joint that flexes and extends the elbow. Palpate around the joint for any loss of the normal concavities, indicating joint swelling or bursitis of the olecranon bursae.

Hurts at the head

Palpate the lateral area just below the joint to feel the radial head; this is normally slightly tender but will be very tender in a fracture. The joint between the radial head and the humerus allows supination and pronation of the forearm. Also palpate the medial side of the inner arm just above the joint to check for epitrochlear node enlargement.

He's up to his elbows

Next, assess the elbows for flexion and extension. Ask the patient to rest their arms at their sides. Ask them to flex their elbows from this position and then extend them. Normal flexion is about 160 degrees; extension, 0 degrees.

Flip the forearm

To assess supination and pronation of the elbow, ask the patient to place the ulnar side of their hand and lower arm on a flat surface with the thumb on top. Ask them to rotate their palm down toward the table for pronation and then rotate the back of their hand onto the table for supination. The normal angle of elbow rotation is 90 degrees in each direction. The patient must move from the elbows not the shoulders. If no table is to hand you can do this passively by holding the arm above the elbow to isolate the lower arm, and then holding the hand in a handshake position and rotating it both ways.

Wrists and hands

Inspect the wrists and hands for contours, and compare them for symmetry. Also check for nodules, redness, swelling, deformities or any other abnormalities. Pay particular attention to the finger joints (distal and proximal interphalangeal joints) and the knuckles (metacarpal–phalangeal joints) as these are common sites for arthritic changes. (See *Heberden's and Bouchard's nodes*, page 352.)

Knuckle down

Note any swelling or fixed flexion of the knuckles, suggestive of rheumatoid arthritis. Inspect both the backs of the hands and the palms. Note any redness of the palms (which may suggest rheumatoid arthritis) or muscle atrophy. Look at the nails. Pitting may indicate psoriasis, which is sometimes linked with a type of arthritis. Note any pulling in (contracture) of the ring and little finger, suggesting Dupytron's contracture.

All fingers and thumbs

Use your thumb and index finger to palpate down each finger, paying attention to the interphalangeal joints. To assess the metacarpal–phalangeal joints, flex the knuckles to about 90 degrees with the fingers straight, and palpate with your finger and thumb, or both thumbs, just below the knuckle to feel the joint space. Then palpate the hands and wrists, noting any hardness or thickening of the tendons. Note any tenderness, nodules or bogginess. To avoid causing pain, be especially gentle with older patients and those with arthritis.

Snuff anyone?

Assess the 'anatomical snuff box' by asking the patient to hold the hand in a handshake position with their thumb raised. Palpate in the hollow area at the base of the thumb. It may feel slightly tender; if the patient has injured the area, significant tenderness may indicate a scaphoid fracture. Finally do Tinel's test. (See *Testing for carpal tunnel syndrome*, page 342.)

Lift a finger; make a fist

To assess movement, start with extension and flexion of the fingers. Ask the patient to make a fist, and then straighten their fingers out and back as far as possible. Normal extension of the metacarpal–phalangeal

Peak technique

Testing for carpal tunnel syndrome

Two simple tests – Tinel's sign and Phalen's test – can help to confirm carpal tunnel syndrome.

Tinel's sign

Lightly percuss the transverse carpal ligament, which sits over the median nerve. To do this, percuss at the point where the patient's palm and wrist meet. If this action produces discomfort, such as numbness and tingling shooting into the palm and fingers, the patient has Tinel's sign and may have carpal tunnel syndrome.

Phalen's test

If flexing the patient's wrist for about 30 seconds causes tingling or numbness in the hand or fingers, they have a positive Phalen's sign. The more severe the carpal tunnel syndrome, the more rapidly the symptoms develop.

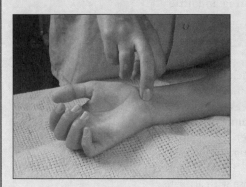

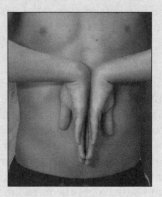

joints is 30 degrees; normal flexion, 90 degrees. Then ask them to spread their fingers apart to demonstrate abduction and draw them back together to demonstrate adduction.

Thumb's up

To assess flexion and extension of the thumb, ask the patient to place the palms uppermost and bring the thumb as far as possible across the palm (flexion) and as far out as possible so the whole hand is flat (extension). Now ask them to bring their thumb up at right angles to the palm (abduction) and return it to lie in line with the fingers (adduction). Finally, ask the patient to touch the tip of each finger in turn on the same hand with their thumb (opposition).

Wristy business

To assess extension of the wrists, ask the patient to adopt a 'praying position', getting their fingers as close to each other as possible, and their wrists as close to 90 degrees as possible. There should be no gaps between the fingers; gaps may indicate previous injury or arthritis. Then to test flexion ask them to put the backs of the hands together, with wrists flexed. Again the angle should be close to 90 degrees. Leave this for 30 seconds to perform Phalen's test. (See *Testing for carpal tunnel syndrome*, page 342.)

Side to side

Finally, to assess radial and ulnar movement, hold the patient's hands at the wrists (placing them palm down on a table may be helpful) and ask the patient to move the hands left and right as far as they can. Normal movement is 20 degrees either way.

Hips

Inspect the hip area for contour and symmetry. An externally rotated hip may suggest femoral fracture. Note that three pairs of bursae protect the hip joint – the greater trochanteric bursae sits over the top of the femur (trochanteric bursitis is a common hip problem); the iliopectineal bursae sits in the groin; and the ischial bursae sits on the inschium (posterior base) of the pelvis (this may be more easily inspected with the leg fully flexed, or with the patient prone).

How do you like that for great hip flexion and rotation?!

Hip, hip, hooray!

Palpate each hip over the iliac crest (anterior superior bony prominence in the hip) and trochanteric area for tenderness or instability and over the bursae for swelling.

Hip and happening!

Assess ROM in the hip with the patient in a supine position; if the patient has had a hip replacement seek expert advice before performing any of these tests to assess the risk of dislocation. To assess hip flexion, ask the patient to bend one knee and pull it toward the abdomen and chest as far as possible. As the patient flexes the knee, the opposite hip and thigh should remain flat on the bed. Repeat on the opposite side.

Be passive

You will need to assess hip abduction and adduction passively to isolate the joints. Stand alongside the patient and press down on the superior iliac spine of the opposite hip with one hand to stabilise the pelvis. With your other hand, hold the patient's leg by the ankle and gently abduct the hip until you feel the iliac spine move. This movement indicates the limit of hip abduction. Then, while still stabilising the pelvis, move the ankle medially across the patient's body to assess hip adduction. Repeat on the other side (you will probably need to walk around the bed/couch or reposition the patient).

Normal ROM is about 45 degrees for abduction and 30 degrees for adduction. To assess hip extension, ask the patient to lie prone (facedown), and gently extend the thigh upwards. Repeat on the other thigh. ROM is normally about 15 degrees.

As the hip turns

To assess internal and external rotation of the hip, ask the patient to bend their knee. Rock the knee medially and then laterally until you feel resistance. Normal ROM for internal rotation is 40 degrees; for external rotation, 45 degrees.

The knee

Inspect the position of the knees, noting any loss of concavities either side of the patella (indicating swelling) and whether they are symmetrical, as hip damage can lead to leg shortening and asymmetric knee positions may give this away. Note whether the patient is bowlegged (varus), with knees that point out, or knock-kneed, (valgus) with knees that turn in. Check the back of the knees for any lumps or swelling – such as popliteal lymph nodes or cystic (fluid-filled) sacs.

Knees up

Palpate around both knees with the knee straight, and again with it bent at 90 degrees. Note any sign of swelling, tenderness or lumps. They should feel smooth, and the tissues should feel solid. Undertake specific tests for effusion. (See *Tests for excess fluid in the knee*, page 345.)

On bended knees

To assess ROM in the knee, ask the patient to bend the knee as far as it will go so the heel touches the buttocks. Alternatively, ask the patient to draw the knee up to the chest. The calf should touch the thigh. Normal ROM for flexion is 120 degrees. Knee extension returns the knee to a neutral position of 0 degrees. If the patient can't extend the leg fully or if the knee pops audibly and painfully, consider the response abnormal. Other abnormalities include pronounced crepitus, which may signal a degenerative disease of the knee, and sudden buckling, which may indicate a ligament injury. (See *Assessing the ligaments of the knee*, page 346.)

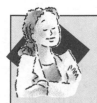

Peak technique

Tests for excess fluid in the knee

Bulge sign

The bulge sign indicates excess fluid in the knee joint. To assess the patient for this sign, elevate the knee on a bed or stool so the leg is straight. Then give the medial side of the knee two to four firm strokes, as shown, to displace excess fluid. Then palpate the lateral aspect of the knee to check for fluid displacement. You may then be able to push or tap the fluid back across to the medial aspect.

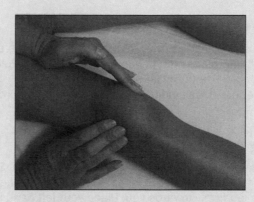

Balloon sign

The balloon sign also assesses for excess fluid in the knee joint. Use the curve between your thumb and index finger to milk down the thigh three or four times, pushing any fluid towards the knee. Now compress the same part of your hand firmly above the patella, and feel the medial and lateral aspects either side of the patella for swelling.

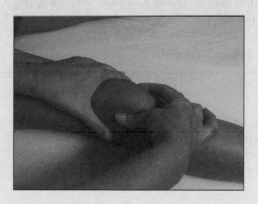

Patella tap

Keep your hand in the same position, and percuss on the patella with three or four finger strokes. If there is fluid you may feel the patella move up and down against the underlying bottom end of the femur.

Ankles and feet

Inspect the ankles and feet for swelling, redness, nodules and other deformities. Remember to look at the soles of the feet, and note any areas of callosities; suggesting that the patient is transferring their weight abnormally or asymmetrically. Check the arch of the foot and look for toe deformities. Also note oedema, bunions, corns, ingrown toenails, plantar warts, ulceration or unusual pigmentation.

Assessing the ligaments of the knee

Four ligaments support the knee – the medial and lateral ligaments down either side, and the anterior and posterior cruciate ligaments that cross over behind the patella. Testing these takes a lot of practice, so work with an experienced examiner until you are confident. Remember, in an acute injury the patient may not be able to tolerate these tests. Increasingly, magnetic resonance imaging scanning is being used to detect such injuries.

Anterior and posterior draw test

To assess the anterior cruciate ligaments have the patient lying on the bed/couch, with their knee flexed to 90 degrees. Sit on the foot, and place both hands behind the knee. Pull it towards you – the 'anterior draw test'. The joint should be stable – note any laxity or pain.

Now to assess the posterior cruciate adjust your hands so you can push the bent knee away from you – the 'posterior draw test'.

Medial and lateral ligaments

To assess the medial and lateral ligaments, ask the patient to lie back. Start with the right leg. Hold the leg above the ankle with the knee flexed to about 20 to 30 degrees, resting the elevated lower leg against your body and pulling the lower leg firmly towards you. Place your left hand just above the knee on the lateral side and push to try and open the joint on the medial side – note any pain or laxity. Now adjust your hands so that you can push against the medial side of the knee and try to open up the lateral side. To examine the left leg you will need to move round the bed or couch and reverse the movement.

Adapted from Bickley and Szilagyi (2007).

Feel the feet

Use your fingertips to palpate the bony and muscular structures of the ankles and feet. Palpate each toe joint by compressing it with your thumb and fingers. Start with the ankle joint and work your way down the foot towards the toes.

The ankle angle

Then examine ROM of the ankle and foot. Have the patient sitting, or on the couch. To assess plantar flexion, ask the patient to point their toes towards the floor. Then test dorsiflexion by asking them to point their toes towards the ceiling. Normal ROM for plantar flexion is about 45 degrees; for dorsiflexion, 20 degrees.

In and out

Next, ask the patient to demonstrate inversion by turning the feet so the soles face inwards, and eversion by turning the feet outwards. Normal ROM for inversion is 30 degrees; for eversion, 20 degrees.

To test flexibility in the foot itself, hold the heel firmly and then passively invert and evert the foot with the ankle stabilised. Ask the patient to wiggle their toes, and then flex and straighten them.

The long and short of it

If you suspect that one leg is longer than the other, take measurements. Put one end of the tape on the bony point of the iliac crest on the pelvis, and run the tape over the medial side of the knee to the medial malleolus. Make sure the foot is dorsiflexed. Now compare with the other side. A difference of more than 1 to 2 cm is abnormal.

Assessing the muscles

Assessment of the muscle strength and tone will be relevant to most skeletal examinations depending on the nature of the problem. It will also be relevant in many neurological examinations. Where the cause of a presenting problem is unknown, or where both musculoskeletal and neurological damage are suspected, you will need to conduct bony, muscular and neurological assessment on the affected joint or limb and the corresponding uninjured side. (See Chapter 14 for more information.)

Muscling in

You will need to assess muscles for bulk, tone, strength and symmetry. If a muscle appears atrophied or hypertrophied, compare it with the muscles on the other side. Comparisons of circumference can be measured with a tape measure, but accuracy and reliability are often low so if you do this, check that the positions are perfectly matched, and the tape straight and flat. Other abnormalities of muscle appearance include contracture and abnormal movements, such as spasms, tics, tremors and fasciculation (a fine muscular twitching under the skin).

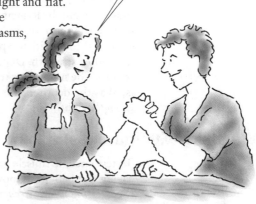

This really isn't necessary to prove that you have good arm muscle tone.

Muscle tone

Muscle tone describes muscular resistance to passive stretching. Muscles are normally held in a state of partial tone or tension – like a piece of elastic – firm but not yet stretched. If tone is increased the muscles are tight, like the elastic being stretched. If tone is decreased the muscles are floppy, like elastic which has been around the washing machine too many times!

Abnormal findings include muscle rigidity and flaccidity. Rigidity is a resistance to passive movement, indicating increased muscle tone, possibly caused by an upper motor neurone lesion such as a stroke or cerebral palsy. Flaccidity, characterised by floppiness, may result from a lower motor neurone lesion. (See Chapter 14 for explanation of upper and motor neurone lesions.)

Tuning in to arm tone

To test the patient's arm muscle tone, passively circumduct the shoulder, then passively flex and extend the elbow and passively circle the wrist/forearm. You should feel a slight resistance. Then let the arm drop. It should fall easily but not heavily to the patient's side.

Leg roll

Test leg muscle tone with the patient on the bed/couch. Start by rolling the upper leg under your outstretched hands (like rolling out a piece of plasticine). Watch the foot. If tone is normal it will lag slightly behind the leg. If tone is increased the leg and foot will move together, and if tone is decreased the foot will flop from side to side.

Knee flip

Now lift the patient's knee off the bed – if tone is normal the heel should stay on the bed; tone is increased if the foot comes off the bed too. A flaccid leg will feel very heavy. Finally, rotate the ankle as you did the wrist, feeling for slight resistance.

Muscle strength

Observe the patient's gait and movements to form an idea of general muscle strength. Remember that muscular or neurological problems may be the cause of abnormal findings. Grade muscle strength on a scale of 0 to 5, with 0 representing no strength and 5 representing maximum strength. Document the results like a fraction, with the score as the numerator (top number) and maximum strength (that is, 5) as the denominator (bottom number). (See *Grading muscle strength*, right.)

Wrestling with muscle strength

To test specific muscle groups, use resisted movement. This means asking the patient to move the muscles while you apply resistance. (See *Testing muscle strength*, page 349.) Part of the skill is ensuring

---

Grading muscle strength

Grade muscle strength on a scale of 0 to 5, as follows:

- 5/5 – Normal power.
- 4/5 – Movement against resistance but weaker than normal.
- 3/5 – Movement against gravity but not against resistance.
- 2/5 – Movement with gravity eliminated.
- 1/5 – Flicker of contraction but no movement.
- 0/5 – No movement or contraction visible.

Medical Research Council scale for grading muscle power, cited by Pentland et al. (2005).

that neither of you have a mechanical advantage. For example, test strength in the opposed little finger and thumb with *your* little finger and thumb, not your index finger and thumb.

Shouldering the load

Test the strength of the patient's shoulder girdle by asking them to hold their arms out in front of them and cross their forearms on top of each other. Now press down on the elbows, asking the patient to stop you from pushing the arms down, and then push up from below, asking the patient to stop you pushing their arms upwards. Note that the pronator drift test for coordination (see Chapter 14) also assesses shoulder girdle strength among other things.

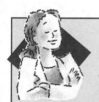

Peak technique

Testing muscle strength

To test the muscle strength of your patient's arm, leg and ankle muscles, use the techniques shown here.

Biceps strength

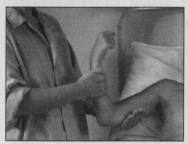

Leg strength: knee flexion

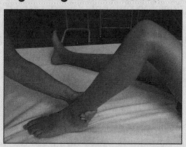

Ankle strength: plantar flexion

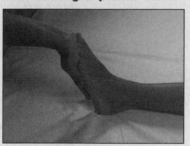

Triceps strength

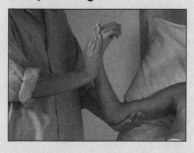

Leg strength: knee extension

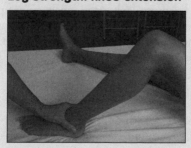

Ankle strength: dorsiflexion

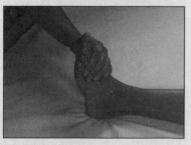

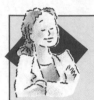

Peak technique

Testing hand strength

When testing handgrip strength, face the patient, hold out the first and second fingers of each your hands, and ask them to grasp your fingers and squeeze as hard as possible. Don't extend fingers with rings on them; a strong handgrip on those fingers can be painful.

Remember that grip is a primitive reflex, so it may be possible even in muscle weakness. If you are unsure whether your handgrip strength test is reliable, try the abduction test. Ask the patient to hold out their hand flat, with fingers together. Place your thumb on one side, and your index and middle fingers on the other. Ask the patient to spread their fingers against your resistance.

To test finger strength further, ask the patient to touch their little finger to their thumb. Link your touching little finger and thumb through theirs and try to break the chain. You can repeat this for any fingers whose strength you want to test.

Testing the bi's and tri's

Next, ask the patient to hold their arms in front of them, with the elbow bent to 90 degrees and their palm facing inwards. To test bicep strength, pull down on the inner (flexor) aspect of the forearm as they pull against you. Support under the upper arm with your other hand if need be. To test tricep strength, ask the patient to try and straighten their flexed forearm as you push against the outer (extensor) surface of the forearm or hand.

Forcing the hand

Assess the strength of the patient's wrist flexion by holding just above the wrist with one hand (so they don't use the whole arm), and asking them to bend their wrist and push their clenched fist down into your palm as you push upwards. To test extension, ask the patient to bend the wrist back as you push your cupped hand downwards over their clenched fist. Make sure they bend from the wrist and not the elbow. Test the strength of finger abduction, thumb opposition and handgrip in a similar way. (See *Testing hand strength*, above.)

Hip strength

To test hip strength, ask the patient to lie in a supine or sitting position on the bed/couch, and ask them to raise one leg at a time whilst you push down on their anterior thigh.

Leg it

Then, ask the patient to flex one knee at a time to 90 degrees with the foot flat on the bed. Assess leg strength by asking the patient to pull their heel towards their bottom whilst you oppose the movement with your hand held around the back of the heel. Then, ask them to straighten their knee as you push against the front of the ankle. Finally, assess ankle strength by asking the patient to straighten their legs on the bed/couch. Ask them to push their feet down against your hands, and then ask them to pull their feet upwards as you try to hold them down.

Abnormal findings

Abnormalities in the musculoskeletal system occur for many reasons. Some general abnormalities have already been discussed; more specific abnormalities are described below.

Arm pain

Arm pain (pain anywhere from the hand to the shoulder) usually results from musculoskeletal disorders, but it can also stem from neurovascular or cardiovascular disorders. In some cases, it may be referred pain from another area, such as the chest, neck or abdomen.

Crepitus

Crepitus is an abnormal crunching or grating you can hear and feel when a joint with roughened articular surfaces moves. It occurs in patients with rheumatoid arthritis or osteoarthritis, or when broken pieces of bone rub together. However, it is extremely common in many patients, and as an isolated finding probably needs noting rather than referral.

Footdrop

Footdrop – plantar flexion of the foot with the toes bent towards the instep – results from weakness or paralysis of the dorsiflexor muscles of the foot and ankle. A characteristic and important sign of certain peripheral nerve or motor neurone disorders, footdrop may also stem from prolonged immobility when inadequate support, improper positioning or infrequent passive exercise produces shortening of the Achilles tendon.

Heberden's and Bouchard's nodes

Heberden's and Bouchard's nodes are hard nodes which develop on the distal and proximal joints of the fingers in patients with osteoarthritis. (See *Heberden's and Bouchard's nodes*, below.) Patients with osteoarthritis may also experience joint swelling, pain, crepitus, limited movement and contracture. Gait may be affected if knees and hips are involved.

Leg pain

Although leg pain commonly indicates a musculoskeletal disorder, it can also result from more serious vascular or neurologic disorders. The pain may occur suddenly or gradually and may be localised or affect the entire leg. Constant or intermittent, it may feel dull, burning, sharp, shooting or tingling.

Muscle atrophy

Muscle atrophy, or muscle wasting, results from denervation or prolonged muscle disuse. When deprived of regular exercise, muscle fibres lose both bulk and length, which produces a visible loss of muscle size and contour, and apparent emaciation or deformity in the affected area.

Heberden's and Bouchard's nodes

Heberden's and Bouchard's nodes are typically seen in patients with osteoarthritis.

Heberden's nodes

Heberden's nodes appear on the distal interphalangeal joints. Usually hard and painless, these bony and cartilaginous enlargements typically occur in middle-aged and elderly patients with osteoarthritis.

Bouchard's nodes

Bouchard's nodes are similar but less common and appear on the proximal interphalangeal joints.

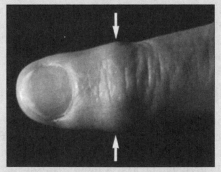

From Bickley, L.S. and Szilagyi, P. (2003) Bates' *Guide to Physical Examination and History Taking*. 8th edn. Philadelphia, PA: Lippincott Williams & Wilkins.

Wasting away

Wasting usually results from neuromuscular disease or injury but may also stem from metabolic and endocrine disorders and prolonged immobility. Some muscle atrophy also occurs with ageing. It will also be seen in a limb which has been immobilised for a period of time – for example, when plaster of Paris is removed.

Muscle spasm

Muscle spasms, or cramps, are strong, painful contractions. They can occur in virtually any muscle but are most common in the calf and foot. Muscle spasms typically occur from simple muscle fatigue, after exercise, and during pregnancy. However, they may also develop in electrolyte imbalances and neuromuscular disorders, or as the result of certain drugs.

Muscle weakness

Muscle weakness may be reported to you by the patient, or you may detect it by observing and measuring the strength of an individual muscle or muscle group. It can result from a malfunction in the cerebral hemispheres, brain stem, spinal cord, nerve roots, peripheral nerves or myoneural junctions, as well as problems with the muscle itself. For more detail regarding muscle weakness in relation to nervous system function see Chapter 14.

Trauma

Most musculoskeletal emergencies result from trauma. Specific traumatic injuries include fractures, dislocations, amputations, crush injuries and serious lacerations. If the patient is alert they will be able to describe how the injury occurred, but if their level of consciousness is reduced or deteriorates you will need to get the history from others, such as the relatives or paramedics. Causes of reduced level of consciousness include head injury, shock, drugs, alcohol or illness that preceded the injury (for example, heart attack preceding the fall). Remember in such cases not to focus on the most obvious injury, but on an ABCDE assessment. (See also The 5 Ps of musculoskeletal injury, page 333.)

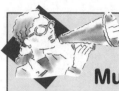

That's a wrap!

Musculoskeletal system review

Structures

Bones

- Support and protect organs and tissues
- Serve as storage sites for minerals
- Produce blood cells in bone marrow
- Five types – long, short, flat, irregular and sesamoid.

Joints

- Defined as the junction of two or more bones
- Consist of two types:
  - Non-synovial – immovable or slightly movable bones connected by fibrous tissue or cartilage (such as the skull and vertebrae)
  - Synovial – freely movable bones which meet in a cavity filled with synovial fluid (a lubricant); include ball-and-socket, hinge, saddle, gliding, rotational and pivot joints
- Perform different types of motion.

Related structures

- Muscles consist of groups of contractile cells or fibres
- Ligaments attach bone to bone
- Tendons attach to bone to muscle
- Bursae are fluid-filled sacs over joints which reduce friction.

The health history

- Determine the patient's reason for seeking care, such as pain, swelling, stiffness and obvious deformities.
- Ask about current health, such as affects on normal activity, and the use of ice, heat or other remedies to treat the problem.
- Ask about past health, including arthritis, cancer, osteoporosis and trauma, and inquire about the patient's use of a walking frame or stick.

- Ask about medications, especially those that may affect the musculoskeletal system (such as corticosteroids and potassium-depleting diuretics).
- Ask about lifestyle, including the patient's job and hobbies.

Assessing the musculoskeletal system – principles

- Work from head to toe and from proximal to distal.
- Note the size and shape of joints, limbs and body regions.
- Inspect and palpate around joints, limbs and body regions.
- Ask the patient to perform active ROM exercises; if not possible, or to gather additional information, perform passive ROM exercises. Never force any movement!
- Observe the patient's posture and gait whenever possible.
- Perform resisted movement where indicated.

The 5 Ps of musculoskeletal injury

- Pain
- Paresthesia
- Paralysis
- Pallor
- Pulse.

Assessing bones and joints

Head, jaw and neck

Caution – report any history of neck trauma immediately. Do not palpate or assess ROM.

- Inspect the front, back and sides of the patient's neck.
- If safe, palpate the cervical vertebrae and the neck area. Listen for crepitus as the patient moves their neck.
- If safe, assess ROM in the neck.

Musculoskeletal system review *(continued)*

- Inspect the patient's face.
- Evaluate ROM in the temporomandibular joint.

Spine

- Inspect the patient's spine posteriorly and as they stand in profile.
- Palpate the spinal processes and areas lateral to the spine.
- Assess for scoliosis by asking the patient to bend at the waist.
- Assess the range of spinal movement.

Shoulders

- Inspect and palpate the shoulders.
- Assess internal and external rotation, flexion and extension, abduction and adduction and circumduction of the shoulders.

Elbows

- Inspect and palpate the elbows.
- Assess flexion and extension and supination and pronation of the forearm.

Wrists and hands

- Inspect and palpate the wrists and hands. Also inspect and palpate each finger joint.
- Assess ROM in the wrist: rotation, flexion and extension. Assess for carpal tunnel syndrome if any history of pain, tingling or numbness.
- Assess flexion, extension, abduction and adduction of the fingers and thumbs.

Hips

- Inspect the hip area.
- Palpate the hips.
- Assess hip flexion, extension, abduction and adduction as well as internal and external hip rotation.

Knees

- Inspect the knees.
- Palpate the knees.

- Perform tests to assess for excess fluid in the knee joint.
- Perform additional tests on the ligaments where indicated.
- Assess flexion and extension in the knee.

Ankles and feet

- Inspect and palpate the ankles and feet.
- Assess dorsiflexion, plantar flexion, inversion and eversion of the ankles.
- Assess flexibility of the foot.
- Assess the metatarsophalangeal joints by having the patient flex and extend the toes.
- Measure both legs if you suspect one is longer than the other.

Assessment of the muscles

- Assess muscle tone as you move each limb through passive ROM exercises.
- Assess shoulder, arm, wrist and hand strength.
- Assess leg strength.

Abnormal musculoskeletal findings

- Arm pain
- Crepitus – abnormal crunching or grating which may be heard or felt when a joint with roughened articular surfaces moves
- Footdrop – plantar flexion of the foot with the toes bent toward the instep
- Leg pain
- Heberden's nodes and Bouchard's nodes – hard nodes on the interphalangeal joints in patients with osteoarthritis
- Muscle atrophy
- Muscle spasms – muscle cramps; strong, painful muscle contractions
- Muscle weakness
- Trauma.

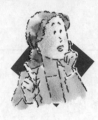

Quick quiz

1. Crepitus is only found in which of the following joint types?
   A. Synovial
   B. Non-synovial
   C. Fixed
   D. Slightly movable

2. If your patient feels tingling in the hand when you percuss on the inner aspect of the wrist, this is most likely due to:
   A. carpal tunnel syndrome.
   B. broken metacarpal bones.
   C. wrist dislocation.
   D. rheumatoid arthritis.

3. A patient with kyphosis has an:
   A. exaggerated lateral spinal curvature.
   B. unusually rounded thoracic curve.
   C. abnormally concave lumbar spine.
   D. inability to bend forward at the waist.

4. Your patient can't move his right arm outwards away from his side in a lateral arc, so you document this as impaired:
   A. supination.
   B. abduction.
   C. adduction.
   D. eversion.

5. To assess a swollen knee:
   A. perform the bulge sign test.
   B. perform Tinel's test.
   C. palpate for Heberden's nodes.
   D. palpate the trochanteric bursa.

For answers see page 402.

14 Neurological system

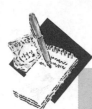

Just the facts

In this chapter, you'll learn:

♦ characteristics of the organs and structures of the neurological system

♦ methods to obtain a patient history of neurological function

♦ techniques to conduct a physical assessment of the neurological system

♦ ways to recognise neurological abnormalities.

A look at the neurological system

The neurological system controls body function and is related to every other body system. Consequently, patients who suffer from diseases of other body systems can develop neurological impairments related to the disease. For example, a patient who has heart surgery may then suffer a stroke.

Help!

Because the neurological system is quite complex, evaluating it can seem overwhelming at first. But although tests for neurological assessment are extensive, they're also straightforward. In fact, you may well find you already routinely include some of these tests in your care delivery.

Just talking with a patient helps you assess orientation, level of consciousness and ability to formulate and produce speech. Simple tasks such as walking allow you to evaluate motor ability. Your knowledge of neurological assessment techniques will enhance your patient care and may save some patients from irreversible neurological damage.

Because the neurological system is related to every other body system, patients who suffer from diseases of other systems can develop neurological impairments.

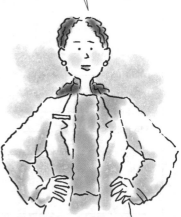

Divvy it up

The neurological system is divided into the central nervous system (CNS), the peripheral nervous system and the autonomic nervous system. Through complex and coordinated interactions, these three parts integrate all physical, intellectual and emotional activities. Understanding how each part works is essential to conducting an accurate neurological assessment.

Central nervous system

The CNS comprises the brain and spinal cord. These two structures collect and interpret voluntary and involuntary motor and sensory stimuli. (See *A close look at the CNS*, below.)

A close look at the CNS

This illustration shows a cross-section of the brain and spinal cord, which together make up the CNS. The brain joins the spinal cord at the base of the skull and ends near the second lumbar vertebrae. Note the butterfly-shaped grey matter in the spinal cord.

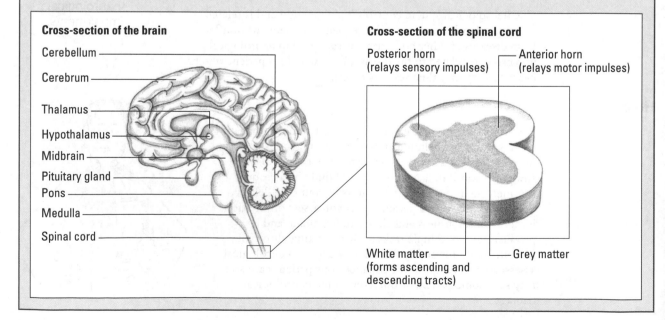

Cross-section of the brain

- Cerebellum
- Cerebrum
- Thalamus
- Hypothalamus
- Midbrain
- Pituitary gland
- Pons
- Medulla
- Spinal cord

Cross-section of the spinal cord

- Posterior horn (relays sensory impulses)
- Anterior horn (relays motor impulses)
- White matter (forms ascending and descending tracts)
- Grey matter

Brain

The brain consists of the cerebrum (or cerebral cortex), the brain stem and the cerebellum. It collects, integrates and interprets all stimuli, and initiates and monitors voluntary and involuntary motor activity.

The reasons for your cerebrum

The cerebrum gives us the ability to think and reason. It's encased by the skull and enclosed by three membrane layers (outer dura mater, middle arachnoid mater and inner pia mater) called meninges. The space between the arachnoid mater and pia mater (called the subarachnoid space) contains cerebrospinal fluid. If blood or fluid accumulates between these layers, pressure builds inside the skull and compromises brain function.

Four lobes are better than one

The cerebrum is divided into four lobes and two hemispheres. The right hemisphere largely controls the left side of the body, and the left hemisphere largely controls the right side of the body. Each lobe controls different functions. Two key areas within the cerebrum are the sensory area at the front of the parietal lobe, and the motor area at the back of the frontal lobe. The sensory area receives and interprets sensory information from the body, and the motor area initiates voluntary and involuntary movement. (See *A close look at the cerebrum and its functions*, page 360.) Cranial nerves I and II originate in the cerebrum.

Meet the muses – Thala, Hypothala and Epithala

The diencephalon, a division of the cerebrum, contains the thalamus, hypothalamus and epithalamus. The thalamus is a relay station for sensory impulses travelling from the body to the brain. The hypothalamus has many regulatory functions, including temperature control, sleep, pituitary hormone production, water balance and thirst/hunger. The epithalamus – the pineal gland – is the body's biological clock.

Quite the sy-stem!

The brain stem lies below the diencephalon and is divided into three parts, with the midbrain sitting uppermost, and then the pons and the medulla. The brain stem contains cranial nerves III to XII, and is a major route for sensory and motor impulses running to and from the cerebral cortex.

All in an inch!

The medulla extends only to about 3 cm of the brain stem (just over an inch) (Tortora 2005) yet is the part of the brain stem

A close look at the cerebrum and its functions

The cerebrum is divided into four lobes, based on anatomic landmarks and functional differences. The lobes – parietal, occipital, temporal and frontal – are named for the cranial bones that lie over them.

   This illustration shows the locations of the cerebral lobes and explains their functions. It also shows the location of the cerebellum.

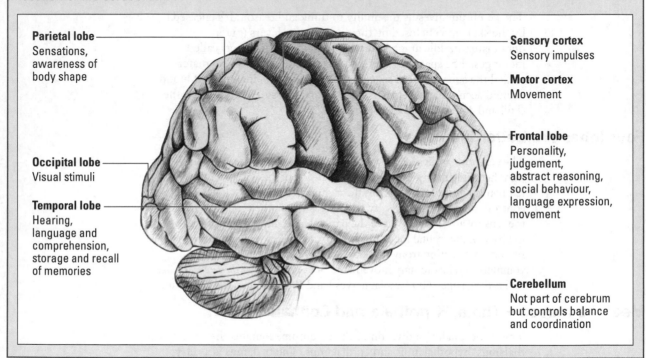

Parietal lobe
Sensations, awareness of body shape

Occipital lobe
Visual stimuli

Temporal lobe
Hearing, language and comprehension, storage and recall of memories

Sensory cortex
Sensory impulses

Motor cortex
Movement

Frontal lobe
Personality, judgement, abstract reasoning, social behaviour, language expression, movement

Cerebellum
Not part of cerebrum but controls balance and coordination

where crucial functions essential to life are located – automatic body functions such as heart rate, breathing, vascular circulation, swallowing and coughing.

Go to the back of the brain

The cerebellum, at the base of the brain, is a leaf-shaped structure containing branches of the major motor and sensory pathways. It is sometimes described as the body's 'autopilot'. It facilitates smooth, coordinated muscle movement, awareness of the body in space (proprioception) and balance.

Spinal cord

The spinal cord is the primary pathway for messages travelling between the peripheral areas of the body and the brain. It also mediates the sensory-to-motor transmission pathway known as the reflex arc. Messages which pass through the reflex arc (such as the message to move your hand away from a flame) enter and exit the spinal cord at the same level, thus initiating movement without involving the need for messages to travel to and from the brain, although the brain is 'told' afterwards that it's happened. (See *Reflex arc*, below.)

So long spine

The spinal cord extends from the upper border of the first cervical vertebrae at the top of the neck, to the lower border of the first lumbar

Reflex arc

Spinal nerves, which have sensory and motor portions, control deep tendon and superficial reflexes. A simple reflex arc requires a sensory (or afferent) neurone and a motor (or efferent) neurone. The knee-jerk, or patella reflex, illustrates the sequence of events in a normal reflex arc.

First, a sensory receptor detects the mechanical stimulus, produced by the reflex hammer striking the patellar tendon. Then the sensory neurone carries the impulse along its axon by way of the spinal nerve to the dorsal root, where it enters the spinal column.

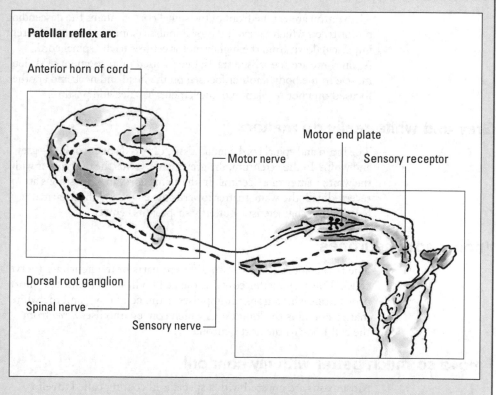

Patellar reflex arc

Anterior horn of cord

Motor end plate

Motor nerve

Sensory receptor

Dorsal root ganglion

Spinal nerve

Sensory nerve

Next, in the anterior horn of the spinal cord, the sensory neurone joins with a motor neurone, which carries the impulse along its axon by way of a spinal nerve to the muscle. The motor neurone transmits the impulse to the muscle fibres through stimulation of the motor end plate. This impulse triggers the muscle to contract and the leg to extend. *Don't stand directly in front of a patient when testing this reflex!*

vertebrae in the middle of the back. It's encased by a continuation of the meninges and cerebrospinal fluid which surrounds and protects the brain, and is also protected by the bony vertebrae of the spine.

Getting your back up . . .

The ascending tracts carry sensory (sometimes called afferent) impulses from the peripheral nervous system to the brain. They enter the spinal cord at the back (dorsal area). Different areas of the cord contain bundles of nerves called tracts (or pathways) which have particular functions – such as feeling 'crude touch', feeling 'pain and temperature' or feeling 'fine touch, vibration and position sense'. Partial damage to part of the spine might therefore leave a person with touch sensation but no pain sensation, for example, in a particular area of the body.

. . . and all down your front

The ventral area at the front of the spinal cord contains the descending motor tracts which transmit motor impulses (sometimes called efferent impulses) down from the higher motor centres to the spinal cord. Again there are specialised tracts; one focused on movement of skeletal muscle in the body, another focused on the head and neck and another focused on finer regulation of movement, balance and posture.

Grey and white really do matter

The brain and spinal cord contain tissue of two distinct colours – grey and white. In the cerebrum, the grey matter forms the outer layer with the white matter more central. In the spinal cord, these positions are reversed with the white matter towards the edges and the grey matter forming the characteristic butterfly shape at its centre.

Know about neurones

The two colours relate to two different parts of the neurones (nerve cells). The grey matter contains the cell bodies and dendrites (short projections which transmit impulses *to* the cell body), and the white matter contains the long axons which convey impulses *away* from the cell body to the next neurone.

I move so much better with my coat on!

Most axons are covered with a specialised coating called myelin which speeds up transmission of impulses. This coating is not fully formed at birth. Historically this may have influenced the incorrect assumption that infants didn't feel pain, but in fact recent evidence suggests they actually experience pain hypersensitivity.

Peripheral nervous system

The peripheral nervous system includes the 12 pairs of cranial nerves, which have specific names and functions. (See *Identifying cranial nerves*, below.) The 31 pairs of spinal nerves are labelled according to the position at which they exit the spinal cord (for example, C3, T1, L2). Peripheral sensory nerves transmit stimuli from sensory receptors located in the skin, muscles, sensory organs and viscera to the posterior horn of the spinal cord. Motor nerves transmit information from the anterior horn cells to different muscles, in order to initiate movement.

Identifying cranial nerves

The cranial nerves have either just a sensory function, a predominant motor function or both sensory and motor functions. They are assigned Roman numerals – for example, cranial nerve I, cranial nerve IV, cranial nerve X. This illustration lists the function of each cranial nerve.

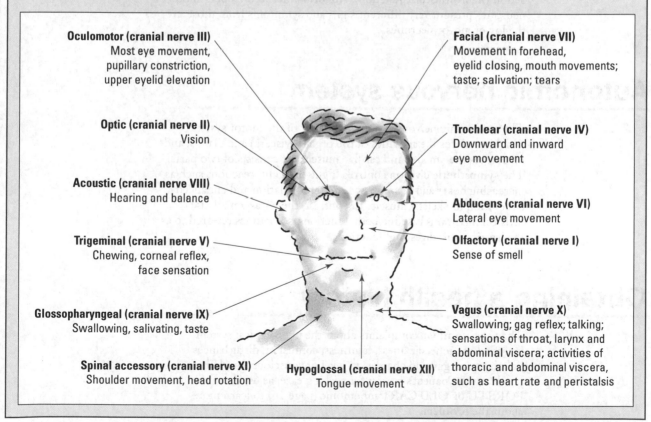

Oculomotor (cranial nerve III)
Most eye movement, pupillary constriction, upper eyelid elevation

Optic (cranial nerve II)
Vision

Acoustic (cranial nerve VIII)
Hearing and balance

Trigeminal (cranial nerve V)
Chewing, corneal reflex, face sensation

Glossopharyngeal (cranial nerve IX)
Swallowing, salivating, taste

Spinal accessory (cranial nerve XI)
Shoulder movement, head rotation

Hypoglossal (cranial nerve XII)
Tongue movement

Facial (cranial nerve VII)
Movement in forehead, eyelid closing, mouth movements; taste; salivation; tears

Trochlear (cranial nerve IV)
Downward and inward eye movement

Abducens (cranial nerve VI)
Lateral eye movement

Olfactory (cranial nerve I)
Sense of smell

Vagus (cranial nerve X)
Swallowing; gag reflex; talking; sensations of throat, larynx and abdominal viscera; activities of thoracic and abdominal viscera, such as heart rate and peristalsis

Sensory body mapping

For the purpose of documenting sensory function, the body is divided into dermatomes. Each dermatome represents an area which transmits sensory nerve impulses via sensory fibres to a particular spinal root – either cervical, thoracic, lumbar or sacral. For example, C5 to C8 transmit sensory impulses from the arms, and T4 from the nipple line. This body map is used when testing sensation and describing the location of a finding. (See *Dermatomes*, page 365.)

Is your motor upper or lower?

The distinction between the parts of the motor system is also important. Upper motor neurones are central neurones running from the brain to the anterior horn cells of the spinal cord. Lower motor neurones are peripheral neurones running from the anterior horn cells to the point where the nerve meets the muscle to initiate action (neuromuscular junction). Abnormalities in the upper motor neurones present very different signs and symptoms from those in the lower motor neurones.

Autonomic nervous system

The autonomic nervous system is the part of the motor system which regulates the activities of the organs (viscera) and glands, and innervates the smooth and cardiac muscles. It consists of two parts. The sympathetic division controls 'fight-or-flight' reactions such as increasing heart and respiratory rate, pupil dilation and enhanced circulation to skeletal muscle. In contrast, the parasympathetic division maintains baseline body functions, sometimes referred to as the 'resting and digesting' functions.

Obtaining a health history

The most common complaints about the neurological system include headache, dizziness, faintness, confusion, disturbances in balance or gait and changes in level of consciousness. When you learn the patient's reason for seeking care, as usual use the PQRSTU or OLD CART mnemonic (page 16) to learn more about the problem.

Dermatomes

The following diagram shows the distribution of the sensory dermatomes both anteriorly and posteriorly.

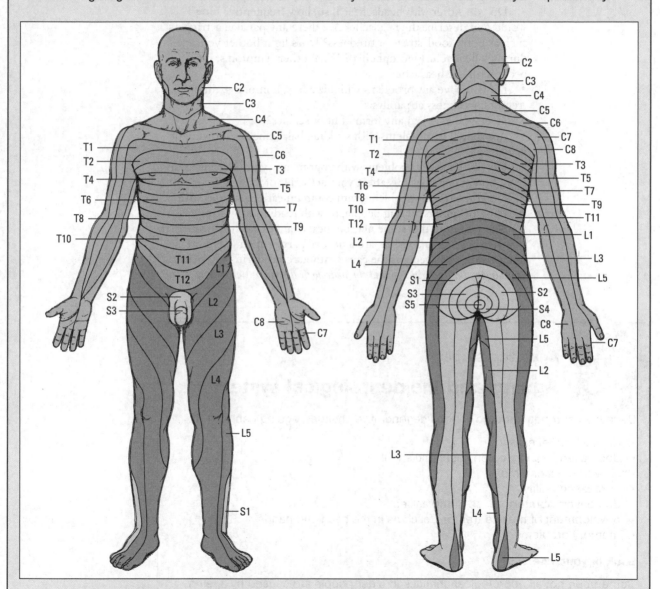

From *Stedman's Medical Dictionary* (2000) 27th edn. Baltimore, MD: Lippincott Williams & Wilkins.

Asking about current health

It is important to consider a range of issues when assessing the neurological system. Consider asking the following questions.

• Do you suffer with headaches? If so, how frequently? How would you describe the headache? Are there any particular triggers such as light, food, stress or tiredness? Does light bother your eyes during a headache (photophobia)? What other symptoms, if any, occur with the headache?

• Do you have any problems with dizziness, numbness, tingling, tremors, weakness or paralysis?

• Have you ever had any form of fit or seizure?

• Are there any problems with walking, balancing, swallowing or urinating?

• Do you have any problems with your memory or concentration? If so, how much does this affect your activities of living?

• Do you have any problems with communication, such as with speaking or understanding people, or with reading or writing?

Keep in mind that some neurological changes, such as decreased reflexes, hearing and vision, are a normal part of ageing, but do not assume that ageing is the cause without considering alternative explanations. (See *Ageing and the neurological system*, below.)

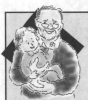

Ages and stages

Ageing and the neurological system

Because neurones undergo various degenerative changes, ageing can lead to:

• diminished reflexes
• decreased hearing, vision, taste and smell
• slowed reaction time
• decreased agility
• decreased vibratory sense in the ankles
• development of muscle tremors, such as in the head and hands
• memory problems.

Look beyond age

Remember, not all neurological changes in older people are caused by ageing. Some drugs and conditions can cause them as well. See whether the changes are asymmetric, indicating a pathological condition, or whether they link to other abnormalities or factors in the history which need further investigation.

Asking about past health

Because many chronic diseases can affect the neurological system, ask the patient about past health or chronic illnesses. Those which might be particularly relevant include epilepsy, migraine, cerebral vascular accident (stroke), diabetes (where neuropathy is a complication) or a previous head injury. When asking about medication, remember that many medications can affect the neurological system.

Asking about family history

As you ask about family history, again pay particular attention to neurological conditions A number of neurological conditions have a genetic risk factor, including epilepsy and multiple sclerosis (Pentland *et al.* 2005)

Assessing the neurological system

A complete neurological examination is so long and detailed that you will rarely if ever perform one in its entirety. Often you will perform an examination of a particular body area, comparing problems on one side with the normal 'opposite side'. However, if your initial screening examination suggests a more complex neurological problem, you may want to perform a detailed assessment. Whist the order of the examination will vary somewhat depending on the patient's problem, always examine the patient's neurological system in a systematic fashion.

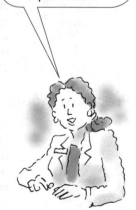

When assessing mental status, be sure to ask more than just 'yes or no' questions.

Assessing consciousness and intracranial pressure

Your assessment often begins when you talk to the patient during the health history. How they respond to your questions gives clues to orientation and memory, and guides you during your physical assessment. Be sure to ask questions that require more than 'yes' or 'no' answers. Otherwise, confusion or disorientation may not be immediately apparent.

ABCDE

Begin the examination by considering ABCDE, and use AVPU (see Chapter 2) to initially assess the patient's level of consciousness. If they are alert or responsive to voice, are they orientated to time ('do you know what time it is?'), place ('do you know where you are?') and person ('can you tell me your name?').

Glasgow Coma Scale

If you have any doubt about the patient's level of consciousness, or the history suggests a risk of deterioration in consciousness (for example, a head injury), you should perform a full set of neurological observations using the Glasgow Coma Scale. This internationally recognised scoring system considers eye opening, verbal response and motor response, and offers an objective way to assess the patient's level of consciousness. This test is not always performed as well as it might be, so even if you feel it is familiar take time to revise the techniques. (See *Glasgow Coma Scale*, page 369.) Note that paediatric adaptations exist and should be used with babies and younger children. For further guidance see NICE (2007d) and Hastings (2008).

Very vital signs

Assessment of vital signs is also crucially important when examining a patient suffering from an acute neurological presentation, particularly if you suspect raised intracranial pressure (ICP). Full details on vital signs monitoring is covered in Chapter 2. Most charts for monitoring the Glasgow Coma Scale incorporate a recording of vital signs on the same chart, so that the two data sets can be viewed alongside each other. Pupil equality and reaction to light is also recorded, with unilateral or bilateral pupil dilation which is not responsive to light a serious finding requiring urgent review. These are typically collectively referred to as neurological observations.

Pressure monitor?

As ICP rises, cerebral blood flow is significantly reduced. This affects the medulla oblongata which is situated at the base of the skull, causing a rise in blood pressure, bradycardia and a reduced respiratory rate. However, do not overly rely on this traditional picture of raised ICP; it is a relatively late sign and consciousness will already have begun to deteriorate before these signs are observed. Temperature may also be altered as a result of damage to the hypothalamus.

(See also *Detecting increased ICP*, page 387 and further guidance on neurological observations by Dougherty and Lister (2004b) and Blows (2007).)

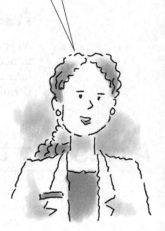

A patient's orientation to time is usually disrupted first, and orientation to person is disrupted last.

Glasgow Coma Scale

The Glasgow Coma Scale provides an easy way to describe the patient's level of consciousness, and helps to detect and interpret changes from baseline findings. To use the Glasgow Coma Scale, test the patient's ability to respond to verbal, motor and sensory stimulation, and grade your findings according to the scale.

If a patient is alert, can follow simple commands and is orientated to time, place and person, their score will total 15 points. Scores should be recorded out of the maximum of 15 (for example, 15/15).

Each element should also be separately recorded; eye opening (E4), motor response (M6) and verbal response (V5) is the maximum score possible (NICE 2007d).

A decreased score in one or more categories signals neurological concern. A total score of 7 or less indicates very severe neurologic damage.

Test	Score	Patient's response
Eye-opening response (E)		
Spontaneously	4	Opens eyes spontaneously
To speech	3	Opens eyes when told to
To pain	2	Opens eyes only on painful stimulus
None	1	Doesn't open eyes in response to stimulus
Motor response (M)		
Obeys	6	For example, shows two fingers when asked
Localises to pain	5	For example, reaches towards painful stimulus on nail bed and tries to remove it
Withdraws from pain	4	For example, moves away from painful stimulus on nail bed
Abnormal flexion response to pain	3	Abnormal flexion – a decorticate posture (shown below)
Abnormal extension response to pain	2	Abnormal extension – a decerebrate posture (shown below)
No response to pain	1	No response; just lies flaccid – an ominous sign
Verbal response (V)		
Orientated	5	Orientated to time, place and person
Confused	4	Responds in conversational manner. Answers are logical but incorrect; suggests disorientation or confusion
Inappropriate words	3	Replies randomly if at all. Not conversational. Illogical answers, words or comments
Incomprehensible	2	Moans or screams
None	1	No response
Total score		

Assessing mental health and cognitive functioning

As you assess the patient, observe appearance, mood, speech and behaviour for clues which might suggest self-neglect. Such changes can suggest an emergent health problem, often neurological in nature. Also consider your patient's cognitive functioning. If you are uncertain use the Mini Mental Examination (Patient UK 2007b). For more information regarding assessing mental health and cognitive function see Chapter 3.

Assessing cranial nerve function

There are 12 pairs of cranial nerves. (See *Remembering the cranial nerves*, below and *Cranial nerve functions*, page 371.) These nerves transmit sensory and motor messages, primarily between the brain and brain stem, and the head and neck. Some carry sensory functions, some predominantly motor functions and some both.

Memory jogger

Remembering the cranial nerves

Remembering the names of the cranial nerves can be challenging. Various mnemonics exist to help you.

One to try is:

On	**O**lfactory
Old	**O**ptic
Olympus'	**O**culomotor
Towering	**T**rochlear
Tops	**T**rigeminal
A	**A**bducens
Fin	**F**acial
And	**A**coustic
German	**G**lossopharyngeal
Viewed	**V**agus
Some	**S**pinal accessory
Hops	**H**ypoglossal

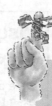

Memory jogger

Cranial nerve functions

Some cranial nerves have just sensory functions (I, II and VIII), some have both functions (V, VII, IX and X) and some have primarily motor functions (III, IV, VI, XI and XII) – these also have a small sensory component allowing awareness of the body part in space, known as proprioception.

How will you ever remember which does what?

Use the following mnemonic to help you remember which cranial nerves have sensory functions (S), motor functions (M) or both (B).

I:	**S**ome
II:	**S**ay
III:	**M**arry
IV:	**M**oney
V:	**B**ut
VI:	**M**y
VII:	**B**rother
VIII:	**S**ays
IX:	**B**ad
X:	**B**usiness
XI:	**M**arries
XII:	**M**oney.

Cranial nerve I

Cranial nerve I – *the olfactory nerve* – is often not routinely assessed in a standard cranial nerve assessment. This is because it requires specialist equipment and because reliability can be questionable. If you need to assess cranial nerve I, see Chapter 7 'Name that smell . . .', page 165.

Cranial nerve II

Next, assess cranial nerve II – the *optic nerve*. This process comprises three components – testing visual acuity using the Snellen chart, testing peripheral vision (fields by confrontation) and examining the optic disc with an ophthalmoscope. Blurring, swelling or bulging of the optic disc may indicate increased ICP. All three tests are fully described in Chapter 6.

Headline check

If you need to test visual acuity for near vision quickly and informally, ask the patient to read a newspaper, starting with large headlines and moving to small print. Let them use reading glasses if normally worn; you are checking differences to what is normal for the patient. Test one eye at a time. For a quick test of distance vision ask the patient to read a poster on the wall, again one eye at a time, and with vision corrected with glasses or contact lenses if that is normal for the patient.

Seeing eye to eye

Precise testing of peripheral vision is covered in Chapter 6. A quick test of peripheral vision can be performed by putting your index fingers over the patients head, about 20 to 30 cm apart, and then wiggling them and moving them forward. The patient should look straight ahead. Ask them to tell you when they see the fingers, and if they see one or both; they should see them a few centimetres after they move in front of the forehead. Repeat, moving into the visual fields from either side of the jaw line, and from behind the ears (in this instance, fingers should be seen when you are level with the eyes). (See *Visual field defects*, right.)

Cranial nerves III, IV and VI

The *oculomotor nerve* (cranial nerve III), the *trochlear nerve* (cranial nerve IV) and the *abducens nerve* (cranial nerve VI) all control eye movement, so they are tested together.

Three real lookers

Remember, as explained in Chapter 6, that downwards–inwards movement is controlled by cranial nerve IV, lateral movement by cranial nerve VI and all other movements by cranial nerve III, which is also responsible for elevation of the eyelids and pupillary constriction. Remember that abnormalities include ptosis, lid retraction, lid lag and pupil inequality. To assess these nerves follow the guidance as described in Chapter 6 for assessing:
- Appearance of the eyes and eyelids
- Direct and consensual pupil reaction
- Light reflection

Visual field defects

Here are some examples of visual field defects. The black areas represent visual loss.

Left	**Right**

A: Blindness of right eye

B: Bitemporal hemianopsia, or loss of half the visual field

C: Left homonymous hemianopsia

D: Left homonymous hemianopsia, superior quadrant

- Accommodation (near–far response)
- Six cardinal positions of gaze
- Nystagmus.

Cranial nerve V

The *trigeminal nerve* (cranial nerve V) is tested from both a sensory and a motor perspective. It supplies sensation to the corneas, facial skin and nasal/oral mucosa. It also supplies motor function for the jaw and all chewing muscles. Corneal testing is not done routinely, but if indicated see Chapter 6 for the technique.

Feeling in the face

To assess the sensory component, check the patient's ability to feel crude touch on the face. Ask them to close their eyes; then touch the face with a wisp of cotton wool on either side of the forehead, cheek and jaw. This will separately test the three branches of the trigeminal nerve. Try to stay fairly close to the midline of the face; if you drift too far out towards the ears, the three separate branches are less distinct.

Does that hurt?

Next, test pain perception by touching the face in the same areas with a 'neuro tip' or similar tool (that is, a special assessment tool with a sharp end and a blunt end). Remember, all such equipment is single use and should be disposed of as 'sharp'. Make sure you use the sharp end in all six areas, and blunt end in some or all areas as a control. Ask the patient to tell you if the sensation is sharp or dull.

'Tri' chewing without this nerve

To test the motor component of cranial nerve V, which innervates the temporal and masseter muscles, ask the patient to clench their teeth or mimic chewing while you palpate above the ears (temporal) and on the cheeks (masseter).

Cranial nerve VII

The *facial nerve* (cranial nerve VII) also has a sensory and a motor component. The motor component is responsible for the facial muscles including closing the eyelids. Assess it by looking for symmetry and normal movement in the following:
- inspecting the patient's face at rest
- asking the patient to smile
- asking the patient to frown
- asking the patient to raise their eyebrows

- asking the patient to screw their eyes tight shut whilst you try to open them, to assess eyelid closure
- asking the patient to puff out their cheeks and hold the air in, whilst you try to 'pop' the cheeks with a finger pressing on either side simultaneously.

A tale of two halves

If a weakness caused by a stroke or other condition damages the cerebral cortex, the patient will normally be able to raise their eyebrows and close their eyes, but will not be able to smile, frown or cheek puff. This is because each half of the upper face is controlled by nerves from both sides of the cerebrum, but the lower face only by nerves from the opposite side of the cerebrum. If the weakness is due to an interruption of the facial nerve or other peripheral nerve involvement – for example, a Bell's palsy – the entire side of the face will be immobile.

Taking the taste test

The sensory component of cranial nerve VII controls taste perception on the anterior two-thirds part of the tongue. This tends not to be routinely tested, as accuracy is difficult. If need be you can assess taste by placing items with various tastes on the patient's tongue – for example, sugar (sweet), salt, lemon juice (sour) and tonic water (bitter). Ask the patient to wash away each taste with a sip of water before moving on.

Cranial nerve VIII

The *acoustic nerve* (cranial nerve VIII – sometimes called vestibulocochlear, which perhaps better describes both functions) is responsible for hearing and balance. The cochlear division controls hearing, and the vestibular division controls balance.

Let's hear it for the acoustic nerve!

To test hearing, use the whisper test, Weber Test and Rinne test as described in Chapter 7. To test the vestibular portion of this nerve, ask the patient if they have any problem with their sense of balance, or test using the coordination tests (particularly normal gait, heel-to-toe walking and Romberg test) described later in this chapter.

Cranial nerves IX and X

The *glossopharyngeal nerve* (cranial nerve IX) and the *vagus nerve* (cranial nerve X) are tested together because their innervation overlaps in the pharynx. The glossopharyngeal nerve is responsible for swallowing, salivation, phonation (speech production) and taste perception on the posterior one-third of the tongue. The vagus nerve controls swallowing and is also responsible for voice quality, as well as providing nerve supply to the major organs and controlling vital functions such as heart rate and peristalsis.

Say aah!

Throughout the assessment you will hopefully have been listening to the patient's voice. Assess the throat as described in Chapter 7, noting in particular the symmetrical position of the uvula and symmetrical rising of the soft palate when the patient says 'Aah'.

Not so hard to swallow

Also test swallowing, but use a dry swallow if you have any doubt regarding risk of aspiration. If indicated (but not routinely as it is very unpleasant), check the gag reflex by touching the tip of a tongue blade against the posterior pharynx.

Cranial nerve XI

The *spinal accessory nerve* (cranial nerve XI) controls the sternomastoid muscles and the upper portion of the trapezius muscle in the neck. To assess this nerve, test the strength of both muscles.

A very important accessory

First, inspect the muscles for any sign of atrophy. Then, to assess the sternomastoid, place your palm against the patient's cheek and ask them to turn their head against your resistance. Repeat on the other side. Then test the trapezius muscle by placing your hands on the patient's shoulders and asking them to shrug their shoulders against your resistance. Do both sides together so you can compare muscle strength.

Cranial nerve XII

The *hypoglossal nerve* (cranial nerve XII) controls tongue movement involved in swallowing and speech. At rest (inspect the open mouth) and when 'stuck out', the tongue should be midline, without sign of atrophy, tremors or fasciculations.

Speaking about the tongue

Test tongue strength by asking the patient to push their tongue against their cheek as you apply resistance with the tip of your finger. Test both sides. Finally, ask the patient to say 'light, tight, dynamite'. (Try saying it yourself without moving your tongue and you will understand the purpose of this test!)

Assessing the spinal nerves

Assessing the spinal nerves involves testing in five broad areas:
- Tone
- Muscle strength
- Sensation
- Coordination
- Reflexes.

Although these tests focus on different aspects of neurological functioning, there is a great deal of overlap between the different tests and the aspects of the nervous system they assess. For example, tests of tone and reflexes both help you to decide whether a problem is affecting the upper motor neurones or the lower motor neurones.

It might be your nerves – or it might be your muscles

There is also considerable overlap between the nervous system and the musculoskeletal system; many of the tests, especially of tone and muscle strength, require both systems to be intact for a normal finding. It is for this reason that testing of tone and muscle strength has already been covered in the musculoskeletal chapter. (See Chapter 13 for an explanation of these tests.)

Assessment of the sensory system

Sensory system evaluation involves checking a number of key aspects of sensation.

Crude touch

To test for the sense of crude touch, ask the patient to close their eyes; then assess all the relevant dermatomes with a wisp of cotton wool. (See *Dermatomes*, page 365.) Ask the patient to say 'now' when they feel the touch. If the patient is not able to understand or say 'now', watch to see if they try to brush the cotton wool away.

Getting in touch

Lightly touch the patient's skin – don't sweep the cotton wool, because you might miss an area of lost sensation. If the patient has major deficits, reassess the area in small steps, starting in the area with poor sensation and moving towards the area with normal sensation, to help you determine the level or boundaries of sensory deficit.

Pain

To test the patient for pain sensation, again assess all the relevant dermatomes using a 'neuro tip' (as described earlier for testing pain sensation in the face). Be sure to test sharp in all areas and use dull as the control. You don't have to assess dull in all areas.

This may hurt a bit

Ask the patient to tell you whether the stimulus is sharp or dull. Compare your findings with the findings for crude touch – a patient with a peripheral neuropathy might retain sensation for crude touch but have lost pain sensation. Avoid this test in children unless its absolutely essential. A non-verbal patient may withdraw from a pain sensation. (See *Glasgow Coma Scale*, page 369.)

Temperature

Temperature sensation sits in the same nerve pathways as pain sensation, so it is often not necessary to test both. If pain sensation is abnormal, testing temperature sensation is a good idea. You need two test tubes containing hot and cold water (but be sure the hot is not too hot – test on your own forearm first). Place them on different dermatomes to assess if the patient can tell hot from cold.

Vibration sense

Use a long, low-pitched (128 Hertz) tuning fork over certain bony prominences to test vibration sense. (See *Evaluating vibratory sense*, page 378.)

Position sense

To test position sense, ask the patient to close their eyes. Then grasp the sides of the big toe (not the pad – it gives away your movement), and move the toe up or down. Ask whether the movement is up or down. Make sure you don't just alternate the movement, and gradually make the movements finer; the patient should be able to detect quite subtle movement. Repeat on the other foot.

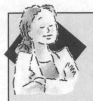

Peak technique

Evaluating vibratory sense

To evaluate vibratory sense, apply the base of a vibrating 128-Hertz tuning fork to the base of the patient's big toe, as shown below. Ask the patient to close their eyes, and then tell you if they feel vibration; and if they do, ask them to tell you when it stops. Then, after an interval, deaden the vibration by grasping the tines of the tuning fork. The patient telling you they feel the vibration stop helps you to be sure they are feeling vibration and not just the fork touching the skin (that is, crude touch).

   If the patient doesn't feel the vibration at the toe, try the medial malleolus. Then continue moving proximally up the bony prominences until sensation is felt. Once vibration is felt, there is no need to carry on up as everything above that level will be intact. Repeat the process on the other leg. Then test vibration sense in both thumbs, moving to the wrist and elbow if need be.

Vibratory sense – toe

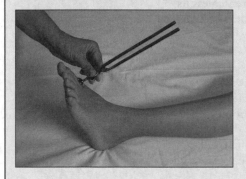

Vibratory sense – thumb

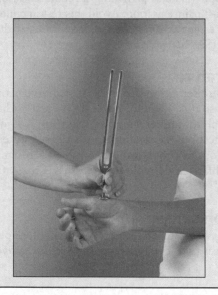

Fingers on the move

To perform the same test on the patient's upper extremities, grasp the sides of the thumb and move it back and forth in the same way. Repeat on the other thumb. To demonstrate position sense, the patient needs intact vestibular and cerebellar function.

Discrimination testing

Discrimination testing assesses the ability of the cerebral cortex to interpret and integrate sensory information.

I have to hand it to you

Stereognosis is the ability to discriminate the shape, size, weight, texture and form of an object by touching and manipulating it. To test this, ask the patient to close their eyes and open their hand. Then place a common object, such as a key, coin or ring in their hand, and ask them to identify it. Repeat with the other hand and a different object.

On its own – number 9!

Graphesthesia is an additional or alternative test. This may be easier for a patient with poor finger movement (for example, arthritis), and can also be done on the foot. Ask the patient to keep their eyes closed and hold out their palm or foot while you draw a large number on it. Ask them to identify the number. Be aware though that findings can be less reliable than stereognosis.

Point localisation and extinction

To test point localisation, ask the patient to close their eyes. Then touch a body part with your finger, and ask them to touch where you touched. Do this in various areas. Touch sometimes in two contralateral (that is, matched) areas at once – for example, both thighs – and sometimes just one area.

Can you touch where I touch?

An abnormal finding is where the patient doesn't feel your finger so makes no attempt to touch the area, or where the patient's finger is placed a long way from the area you pointed to. If the patient only touches one area when you touch two, this is called extinction, and suggests damage to the sensory cortex.

Diabetic patients – special considerations

A special kind of sensory testing instrument – a monofilament – is used with diabetic patients. The fine flexible plastic filament should be pressed 'end on' in different positions on the big toe and across the ball of the foot, with enough force to make it bend, for about 1.5 seconds. The patient should respond 'yes' when they feel the filament. Failure to feel it suggests peripheral diabetic neuropathy.

Assessment of coordination

Cerebellar testing looks at the patient's coordination and general balance. Sensory or motor problems will also affect coordination.

Romberg's test

Firstly perform Romberg's test. (See *Romberg's test*, below.) Take great care with patient safety during this test.

Pronator drift and arm tap

Then test pronator drift. Ask the patient to stand with feet slightly apart to ensure balance, and extend their arms with palms facing up (supine). The patient should then close their eyes and maintain this position for 30 seconds, without pronation of the hands or downwards drift of the arms.

Maintaining the arm-y

Then test further by pushing down on the outstretched arms and seeing if the oustretched position can be maintained.

Romberg's test

Before performing the Romberg test think of patient safety. If in any doubt ask a second person to help you. Position the patient with their back to (but not touching) the bed or couch, and hold your arms out on either side to protect them if they sway. Observe the patient's balance whilst they are standing with their eyes open, feet together and arms at their sides. Then, if they are stable with their eyes open, ask them to close their eyes. They should be able to maintain the position for 60 seconds (McGee 2007). A slight wobble is normal (Romberg negative), but if the patient cannot stand without swaying notably, the result is Romberg positive. Stop the test as soon as you recognise that the finding is positive. This will be almost immediately in some patients.

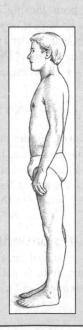

Gait

Can the patient sit and stand without support? If so, observe them as they walk across the room, turn and walk back. Note imbalances or abnormalities of gait. (See *Identifying gait abnormalities*, page 392.) With cerebellar dysfunction, the patient may well have a wide-based, unsteady gait. Deviation to one side may indicate a cerebellar lesion on that side.

Walking the tightrope

Now, if it seems safe to do so, ask the patient to walk heel to toe, like you would walk on a tightrope, and observe balance. Stay close to the patient throughout. Fitter patients can also be assessed by asking them to stand on one leg and then the other, walk on their heels and walk on tip toe.

Point to point

Test extremity coordination by asking the patient to alternately touch their nose and your outstretched finger as you move your finger into different positions on both sides of the patient's face. Hold your finger about 40 to 50 cm away. Be sure to get the patient to repeat the test with both hands. Movements should be accurate and smooth.

Heel to shin

Ask the patient to place the heel of one leg just under the patella on the other leg, and run it down their shin. Inability to place the heel, or the heel running off the side of the shin, is an abnormal finding. Repeat with the other leg. If the patient has rough skin on the heel and/or fragile skin on the shin, make sure that the leg is covered with clothing.

Rapid alternating movement

Other tests of cerebellar function assess rapid alternating movements. In these tests, the patient's movements should be accurate and smooth.

All fingers and thumbs

First, ask the patient to touch the thumb of their right hand to their right index finger and then to each of their remaining fingers. Get them to repeat, more quickly. Observe the movements for accuracy and smoothness.

Thigh slapping

Next, ask them to place their palms on their thighs and turn the palms up and down, gradually increasing speed.

Sole tapping

If you want to do a similar coordination test on the lower extremities, ask the patient to lie on the bed or couch. Then hold your palms near the soles of the feet. Ask the patient to alternately tap the sole of the right foot and the sole of the left foot against your palms. Get them to increase speed as you observe coordination.

Testing young children and patients who are unable to understand instructions

Many of these tests require the patient to have sufficient cognitive function to understand the instructions and respond to them. If the specific tests are not possible, much can be learned from observing the patient – for example, a young child playing or an older person feeding themselves. Are movements purposeful and successful, or do they frequently 'miss' their intended target?

Assessing reflexes

Evaluating reflexes involves testing deep tendon and superficial reflexes, and observing for primitive reflexes. The more times you try to elicit the same reflex, the less of a response you'll get. So observe carefully the first time you stimulate.

Deep tendon reflexes

The key to testing deep tendon reflexes is to make sure the patient is relaxed and the joint is flexed appropriately, placing a partial stretch through the tendons. First, distract the patient by asking them to focus on a point across the room or shut their eyes. Always test deep tendon reflexes by moving from head to toe and comparing side to side. (See *Assessing deep tendon reflexes*, page 383.) Remember, a common mistake is not swinging the hammer hard enough (or occasionally too hard!), and not allowing it to hit the point of impact as a dead weight. Practise on yourself to refine your technique – your own patella reflex is ideal.

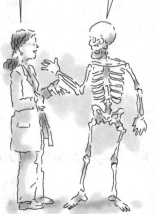

I'm supposed to assess your deep tendon reflexes.

You may find this hard to believe, but I used to have great tendons.

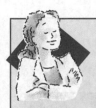

Peak technique

Assessing deep tendon reflexes

During a neurological examination, you'll assess the patient's deep tendon reflexes. Test the biceps, triceps, brachioradialis, patella and tendon Achilles reflexes. Tendons will respond best when they are partly stretched, so the positions described are important to ensure reliable findings. In addition to the specific limb movements described below, you should also see muscle contraction.

Brachioradialis reflex

Ask the patient to rest the ulnar (little finger) edge of their hand on their abdomen or lap with their elbow partially flexed. Place your finger on radial edge, in line with the thumb, at the dip in the wrist (about where the watchstrap would go). Strike your finger with the hammer, or strike the radial area directly. Watch for supination of the hand and/or flexion of the fingers.

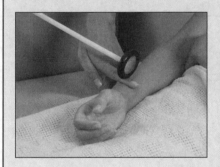

Biceps reflex

Position the patient's arm so the elbow is flexed at a 45-degree angle and the arm is relaxed. Place your thumb or index finger over the biceps tendon, which sits near the medial side of the inner elbow. You should feel it under your thumb/finger as the patient moves their arm inwards to 90 degrees. Press firmly with your thumb/finger, and strike the base of it with the hammer. Watch and feel for the contraction of the biceps muscle and flexion and/or supination of the forearm.

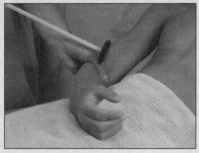

Triceps reflex

If the patient is able, sit them upright and ask them to put their arm out sideways, and then to flex the elbow to 90 degrees, so that it hangs downwards in an upside-down L shape. Strike the triceps tendon about 5 cm above the olecranon process on the extensor surface of the upper arm. Watch for contraction of the triceps muscle and extension (outward swing) of the forearm. Or, if this is not possible, ask the patient to adduct their arm and place their forearm across their chest. Hold it lightly and strike the tendon as described above.

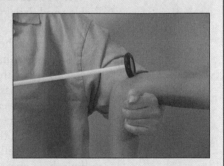

(continued)

Assessing deep tendon reflexes (continued)

Patella reflex

If possible, ask the patient to sit with legs dangling freely. If they need to remain in bed, flex the knee at a 45-degree angle and place your non-dominant hand behind it for support. Strike the patella tendon just below the patella, and look for contraction of the quadriceps muscle in the thigh with extension of the lower leg.

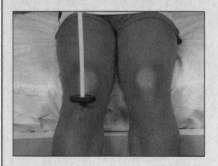

Tendon Achilles reflex

Ask the patient to bend and externally rotate their knee, crossing the foot and ankle over the other leg so that the tendon is easily accessible (avoid this position if the patient has had a hip replacement). Ask the patient to relax their foot. Then support the plantar surface of the foot, passively bending it up to 90 degrees to partially stretch the tendon. Strike the Achilles tendon, and watch for plantar flexion of the foot at the ankle. Alternatively, the test can be performed with patient lying prone with feet over the end of the bed or couch, or with the patient kneeling on a chair (but ensure that the patient is safely supported if you try this method). Always passively flex the foot to about 90 degrees with your other hand.

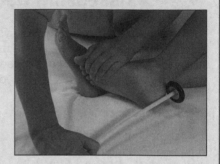

Grade deep tendon reflexes using the following scale – based on Bickley and Szilagyi (2007):
- 0 – absent reflexes, no response
- +1 – diminished, low normal
- +2 – normal impulses
- +3 – brisker than average (may be normal)
- +4 – very brisk reflexes, indicative of disease.

If a reflex is weak or absent, try reinforcement. This distracts the patient and may help elicit the reflex. For upper reflexes, ask the patient to clench their teeth when you say 'now' (just before you hit). For lower reflexes, ask them to interlock their fingertips and try pulling them apart.

Superficial reflexes

Stimulating the skin is a method of testing superficial reflexes.

Tickling the feet

To elicit the plantar reflex, use a tongue depressor to draw a line up the lateral side of the patient's sole from the heel up to the toe, curving across the ball of the foot to end at the base of the big toe. The normal response in an adult or child is downwards (plantar) flexion of the toes. Upwards movement of the toes and fanning of the toes – called Babinski's reflex – is abnormal except in infants/ toddlers. (See *Babinski's reflex in infants*, right.)

For men only

The cremasteric reflex is tested in men by using a tongue depressor to stimulate the inner thigh. Normal reaction is contraction of the cremaster muscle and elevation of the testicle on the side of the stimulus.

Tickling the tummy

Abdominal reflexes can be tested with the patient in a supine position, with their arms at their sides and knees slightly flexed. Briskly stroke both sides of the abdomen with a finger or tongue depressor above and below the umbilicus, moving from the periphery towards the midline. Movement of the umbilicus towards the stimulus is normal.

Primitive reflexes

Primitive reflexes are abnormal in an adult but normal in an infant, whose CNS is immature. As the neurological system matures, these reflexes disappear. But the reflexes can return abnormally in neurological disease. The primitive reflexes you can assess for are the grasp, snout, sucking and glabella reflexes. Note Babinski is also a primitive reflex.

Just get a grip

Assess abnormal grip reflex by applying gentle pressure to the patient's palm with your fingers. If they grasp your fingers, suspect cortical or premotor cortex damage.

Read my lip

The snout reflex is assessed by lightly tapping on the patient's upper lip. Pursing of the lip is a positive snout reflex that may indicate frontal lobe damage.

Ages and stages

Babinski's reflex in infants

The Babinski reflex is a normal finding in infants and toddlers. It is commonly seen in newborns. The age at which the normal plantar reflex emerges varies considerably and can occur at any point between 6 months and 2 years.

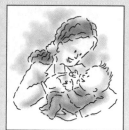

The urge to suck

Observe the patient while they are eating, or if they have an oral airway or endotracheal tube in place. If you see a sucking motion, this suggests cortical damage. This reflex is commonly seen in patients with advanced dementia.

Tap, tap, blink, blink

The glabella response is elicited by repeatedly tapping the bridge of the patient's nose. The abnormal response is persistent blinking, which suggests diffuse cortical dysfunction.

Abnormal findings

During your assessment, you may detect a number of different abnormalities caused by neurological dysfunction.

Altered level of consciousness

Consciousness may be impaired by any one of several disorders which can affect the cerebral hemisphere of the brain stem. Consciousness is the most sensitive indicator of neurological dysfunction. (See *Detecting increased ICP*, page 387.)

Consciousness-altering disorders

Disorders which affect consciousness include toxic encephalopathy, haemorrhage and extensive, generalised cortical atrophy. Compression of brain stem structures by tumour or haemorrhage can also affect consciousness, by depressing the reticular activating system which maintains wakefulness. In addition, sedatives and opioids can depress consciousness.

Cranial nerve impairment

Damage to the cranial nerves causes many abnormalities, including olfactory, visual, auditory and muscle problems. Vertigo and dysphagia can also indicate cranial nerve damage.

Olfactory impairment

If the patient can't detect odours with both nostrils, they may have a dysfunction in cranial nerve I. This dysfunction can result from any disease which affects the olfactory tract, such as a tumour, haemorrhage or facial bone fracture. Loss of sense of smell has also been linked to Alzheimer's disease.

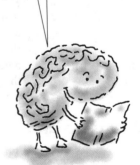

Compression of brain-stem structures can affect consciousness. Oof. That doesn't sound good.

Detecting increased ICP

The earlier you can recognise the signs of increased ICP, the more quickly you can intervene, and the better the patient's chance of recovery. By the time late signs appear, interventions may be useless.

These early signs should be considered alongside use of the Glasgow Coma Scale. If you observe any of the early signs, but are not undertaking full neurological observation, take this as a cue to conduct a full set of neurological observations, and request urgent review of the patient. Observation of a late sign constitutes a medical emergency and need for immediate intervention.

	Possible early signs	Late signs
Level of consciousness	• Requires increased stimulation • Subtle orientation loss • Restlessness and anxiety • Sudden quietness	Unrousable
Pupils	• Pupil changes on side of lesion • One pupil constricts but then dilates (unilateral hippus) • Sluggish reaction of both pupils • Unequal pupils	Pupils fixed and dilated or 'blown'
Muscle weakness	• Muscle weakness evident – may be quite sudden • Positive pronator drift; with palms up, one hand pronates	Profound weakness
Vital signs	• Intermittent increases in blood pressure	Increased systolic pressure, profound bradycardia, abnormal respirations (Cushing's triad)

Visual impairment
Visual problems include visual field defects, pupillary changes and eye muscle impairment.

Far afield

Visual fields are affected by tumours or infarcts of the optic nerve head, optic chiasma (point where the optic nerves cross over) or optic tracts.

Peer at the pupils

If the patient's pupillary response to light is affected, they may have damage to the optic nerve and/or oculomotor nerve. Pupils are sensitive indicators of neurological dysfunction. Raised ICP typically causes dilation of the pupil ipsilateral (on the same side) to the cause; without treatment, both pupils can become fixed and dilated. (See *Recognising pupillary changes*, page 389.) Pinpoint pupils may well suggest narcotic overdose, overdose of other recreational drugs or poisoning. Remember that a minor (less than 0.5 mm) difference can be normal in some people.

Don't move a muscle!

Weakness or paralysis of the eye muscles can result from cranial nerve damage. Increased ICP and intracranial lesions can affect the motor nuclei of the oculomotor, trochlear and abducens nerves.

The drifters

Damage to the peripheral labyrinth, brain stem or cerebellum can cause nystagmus. The eyes drift slowly in one direction and then jerk back to the other.

Feeling droopy

Drooping of the eyelid, or ptosis, can result from a defect in the oculomotor nerve.

Facing the pain

If the patient responds inadequately to sensory stimulation of the skin or cornea, the trigeminal nerve may be affected. Trigeminal neuralgia causes severe piercing or stabbing pain over one or more of the facial dermatomes.

Auditory impairment

Sensorineural hearing loss can result from lesions of the cochlear branch of the acoustic nerve or from lesions/ damage in any part of the nerve's pathway to the brain stem. A patient with this type of hearing loss may have trouble hearing high-pitched sounds, or may have a total loss of hearing in the affected ear.

Which end is up?

Vertigo is the illusion of movement and can result from a disturbance of the vestibular centres. If the patient reports vertigo it might be caused by a peripheral or central lesion.

Vertigo is the illusion of movement that can result from a disturbance of the vestibular centres.

Recognising pupillary changes

Several different pupil abnormalities may be observed. Observe pupil size in relation to what might be expected based on the lighting conditions, and in relation to each other. Also note whether either or both reacts to light. There are numerous neurological causes for pupil abnormalities. Use this chart as a guide to pupillary changes.

Pupillary change

Unilateral, dilated. Causes include trauma, glaucoma, parasympathetic nerve damage, occulomotor nerve damage and raised ICP.

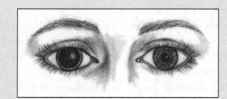

Bilateral, dilated. Normal in a dark room if reactive to light. Abnormal if fixed or seen in a bright light. Abnormal causes include damage to the sympathetic nervous system, sympathomimetic drugs, use of dilating drops and cardiopulmonary arrest.

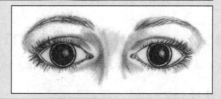

Bilateral, midsize/moderately dilated. Normal in dull light if reactive. Abnormal if fixed/non-reactive to light; associated with lesions or haemorrhage in the midbrain – 'midbrain pupils'.

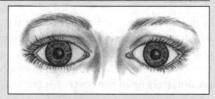

Bilateral, pinpoint. Pupils will normally appear small in a bright light. Fixed, pinpoint pupils are most commonly linked to drug overdose – for example, opioid use. Also linked with iritis, pilocarpine drops used for glaucoma and damage to the pons.

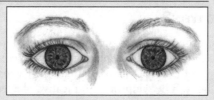

Unilateral, small. Linked with Horner's syndrome (patient also has a ptosis) – a disease affecting the sympathetic nerve supply to the head.

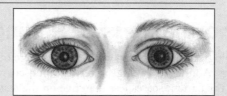

Based on Jarvis (2008) and Patient UK (2007c).

Dysphagia

Dysphagia (difficulty swallowing) commonly occurs after a stroke but can also result from a lesion affecting cranial nerves IX and X.

Speech impairment

Aphasia is a speech disorder caused by injury to the cerebral cortex. Several types of aphasia exist, including:

• expressive or Broca's aphasia – impaired fluency and difficulty finding words; this is impairment located in the frontal lobe, the anterior speech area

• receptive or Wernicke's aphasia – inability to understand written words or speech, and the use of made-up words; this is impairment located in the posterior speech cortex, which involves the temporal and parietal lobes

• global aphasia – lack of both expressive and receptive language; this is impairment of both speech areas.

Constructional impairment

Apraxia and agnosia are two types of constructional disorders.

What's the purpose of this?

Apraxia is the inability to perform purposeful movements and make proper use of objects. It's commonly associated with parietal lobe dysfunction and includes the inability to perform various simple activities on command, and/or the inability to perform the required action appropriately or in the correct sequence.

What did you say this was?

Agnosia is the inability to identify common objects (for example, household objects or body parts) or identify common sounds. Some patients – for example, stroke patients – may lose awareness of half of their body. The symptom is indicative of a lesion in the sensory cortex.

Abnormal muscle findings

Neurological disorders can cause a wide range of abnormal muscular findings. Abnormal findings in terms of muscle weakness are noted where the patient scores less than five on the tests of resisted movement. Weakness can be caused by a neurological or a muscular problem; further testing will be needed to establish which. Other abnormal muscular findings include tics, tremors and fasciculations. Findings may or may not indicate serious neurological disease.

It's a tic . . .

Sudden, uncontrolled movements of the face, shoulders and extremities, called tics, are caused by abnormal neural stimuli. Tics are normal movements which appear repetitively and inappropriately. They include blinking, shoulder shrugging and facial twitching.

. . . no, a tremor . . .

Like tics, tremors are involuntary, repetitive movements usually seen in the fingers, wrist, eyelids, tongue and legs. They can occur when the affected body part is at rest or with voluntary movement. For example, the patient with Parkinson's disease has a characteristic pill-rolling (rubbing finger and thumb together) resting tremor, and the patient with cerebellar disease has an intention tremor when reaching for an object.

. . . no, a fasciculation!

Fasciculations, which are fine twitchings in small muscle groups, are most commonly associated with lower motor neurone dysfunctions.

Abnormal sensation

Abnormal sensation findings vary in their causes and effects. Local areas of lost sensation such as crude touch or pain may be caused by peripheral nerve damage, whereas larger areas of lost sensation may indicate spinal or cerebral damage.

What a strange sensation!

The problem can range from extremely temporary (for example, pins and needles) to permanent (as in spinal resection in an accident). Common problems leading to altered sensation include shingles, trauma and back problems.

Abnormal reflexes and tone

Abnormality of the reflexes (and tone) may suggest an upper or lower motor neurone problem. In upper motor neurone problems (brain or spinal cord), reflexes are likely to be exaggerated (3+ or 4+), and tone increased. In contrast, a lower motor neurone (peripheral nerve problem) is likely to cause diminished reflexes (0 or 1+) and diminished tone.

A careful balancing act

The reason for the difference is because of the balancing act between the central and peripheral nervous systems. This is a balance between inhibition from the brain/spinal cord, and excitement from the peripheral nervous system.

The cautious owl and the excited mouse

Think of a wise cautious old owl (the brain) trying to calm down an excited little mouse (the peripheral nerves) running around his feet. If something happens to the owl (an upper motor neurone problem), the calming influence is gone and the excited mouse (peripheral nerves) can run riot! Whereas if something happens to the mouse (a lower motor neurone problem), all the excitement is gone and the wise old owl just has a snooze – so nothing much happens!

Abnormal gaits

During your assessment, you may identify gait abnormalities. (See *Identifying gait abnormalities*, below.)

Identifying gait abnormalities

The illustrations below identify five gait abnormalities.

Spastic gait	Scissors gait	Propulsive/shuffling gait	Steppage gait	Waddling gait

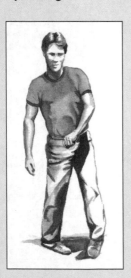 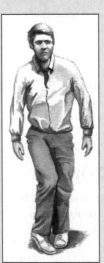 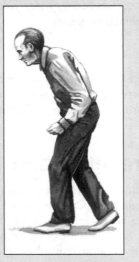 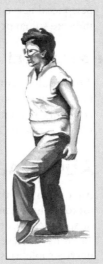 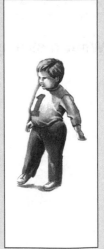

Spastic gait

Spastic gait – sometimes referred to as paretic or weak gait – is a stiff, foot-dragging walk caused by unilateral leg muscle hypertonicity linked to damage of the motor spinal tracts.

Scissors gait

Effectively results from a bilateral spastic gait affecting both legs.

Propulsive/shuffling gait

Propulsive gait is characterised by a stooped, rigid posture – the patient's head and neck are bent forward and the knees and hips are stiffly bent. The patient shuffles forward. This is a classic sign of advanced Parkinson's disease.

Steppage gait

Steppage gait typically results from footdrop caused by muscle weakness or paralysis in the lower limbs. The toes tend to scrape the ground during walking and hit the ground first on the next step. The patient uses exaggerated hip movement to compensate.

Waddling gait

Waddling gait, a distinctive duck-like walk, suggests muscular dystrophy or spinal muscular atrophy. The gait results from deterioration of the pelvic girdle muscles.

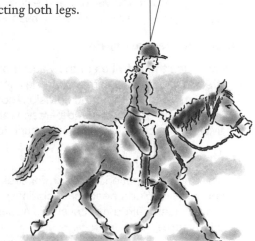

An abnormal gait may indicate a neurological abnormality.

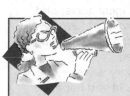

That's a wrap!

Neurologic system review

Central nervous system

Brain

- Cerebrum (cerebral cortex) – enables thinking and reasoning
- Brainstem – acts as a major sensory and motor pathway for impulses to and from the cerebral cortex; regulates automatic body functions, such as heart rate and breathing

- Diencephalon – contains thalamus, hypothalamus and epithalamus
- Cerebellum – facilitates coordinated muscle movement and maintains equilibrium.

Spinal cord

- Contains the primary pathways for messages travelling between the peripheral areas of the body and the brain
- Mediates the reflex arc.

(continued)

Neurologic system review (continued)

Peripheral nervous system

- Peripheral nerves – serve the skin, muscles, sensory organs and viscera of the body and limbs
- Cranial nerves – serve the brain, head and neck.

Autonomic nervous system

- Regulates the activities of the visceral organs
- Affects smooth and cardiac muscles and glands
- Consists of the sympathetic division (controls fight-or-flight reactions) and parasympathetic division (maintains baseline body functions).

The health history

- Determine the patient's reason for seeking care, which may include headache, dizziness, faintness, confusion, impaired mental status or balance or gait disturbances.
- Ask the patient about current health, including memory and ability to concentrate as well as current medications.
- Ask about past health/chronic illness, including illnesses such as diabetes and epilepsy, accidents or injuries (particularly head injuries), surgeries and allergies.
- Inquire about a family history of neurological disorders which may have a genetic component, such as seizures and migraine headaches.

Assessment of consciousness, mental health and cognitive status

- Observe for ABC and any changes in level of consciousness.
- Assess and reassess vital signs.
- Note the patient's appearance and behaviour.
- Listen to how well the patient speaks and expresses themselves.
- Assess cognitive function by tests such as the Mini-Mental Examination if indicated.
- Observe the patient's ability to perform simple tasks and use various objects.

Assessment of cranial nerves

- Cranial nerve I (olfactory nerve) – if indicated, assess the patient's ability to identify at least two smells, or ask about sense of smell.
- Cranial nerve II (optic nerve) – test visual acuity and visual fields with confrontation; examine the fundus and the optic nerve with the ophthalmoscope.
- Cranial nerves III (oculomotor nerve), IV (trochlear nerve), and VI (abducens nerve) – test pupil constriction and consensual reaction, light reflection and near – far. Test extraocular movement using the six cardinal positions of gaze.
- Cranial nerve V (trigeminal nerve) – check the patient's ability to feel crude touch and pain perception over the face; test temporal and masseter muscles.
- Cranial nerve VII (facial nerve) – observe the patient's face for symmetry at rest and when smiling, frowning and raising eyebrows. Test eye scrunch and cheek puff. Test taste if indicated.
- Cranial nerve VIII (acoustic nerve) – test hearing using whisper, Weber and Rinne tests, and check balance.
- Cranial nerves IX (glossopharyngeal nerve) and X (vagus nerve) – soft palate, uvula and swallow. Note phonation (speech) during the examination. Check the gag reflex if indicated.
- Cranial nerve XI (spinal accessory nerve) – check the strength of the sternomastoid and trapezius muscles.
- Cranial nerve XII (hypoglossal nerve) – assess tongue position, movement and strength; observe for tongue symmetry and speech using the tongue.

Assess tone

- Assess tone by passively moving the arms at wrist, elbow and shoulder joints.
- Assess the legs by testing foot lag, knee flip and ankle movement.

Neurologic system review *(continued)*

Assessment of motor function

- Assess muscle strength by asking the patient to move muscles and muscle groups against resistance. Assessment can include hands, wrists, elbows, shoulders, hips, knees and ankles.

Assessment of sensory function

- Test crude touch sensation in all relevant dermatomes.
- Test sharp/dull perception in all relevant dermatomes.
- Test vibratory sense with a tuning fork over bony prominences.
- Assess position sense if required by asking the patient to identify whether their toe or finger is positioned up or down as you move it.
- Assess discrimination by testing stereognosis, point localisation and extinction.

Assessment of coordination

- Assess cerebellar function by observing the patient's coordination and general balance.
- Assess point-to-point, rapid alternating movement and heel to shin.
- Perform Romberg test, and test pronator drift.
- Assess normal gait and heel-to-toe walking; test heel walking, toe walking and balance on one leg if feasible/indicated.

Assessment of reflexes

- Test deep tendon reflexes:
  - biceps reflex
  - triceps reflex
  - brachioradialis reflex
  - patellar reflex
  - Achilles reflex.
- Test superficial reflexes:
  - Babinski's reflex (normally absent)
  - cremasteric reflex (in males)
  - abdominal reflexes.

- Check for primitive reflexes if indicated (shouldn't be present in an adult but are normal in infants):
  - grasp reflex
  - snout reflex
  - suck reflex
  - glabella response.

Abnormal findings

Abnormal cranial nerve findings

- Olfactory impairment – inability to detect odours
- Visual impairment – visual field defects, pupillary changes and eye muscle impairment
- Auditory problems – difficulty hearing high-pitched sounds or total hearing loss
- Dysphagia – difficulty swallowing, typically occurring after a stroke.

Speech disorders

- Impaired fluency or expression.

Constructional problems

- Apraxia – inability to perform purposeful movement
- Agnosia – inability to identify common objects.

Abnormal muscle findings

Scores of less than 5 on muscle strength tests are abnormal and need further investigation to determine the cause.

- Tics – sudden uncontrolled movements of the face, shoulders and extremities
- Tremors – involuntary, repetitive movements in the fingers, wrists, eyelids, tongue and legs
- Fasciculations – fine twitchings in small muscle groups.

Abnormal reflexes and tone

- Increased reflexes and tone from an upper motor neurone lesion

(continued)

Neurologic system review (continued)

- Decreased reflexes and tone from a lower motor neurone lesion.

Abnormal sensation and coordination

- Sensory abnormality can indicate peripheral nerve, spinal or cerebral damage

- Coordination problems often indicate cerebellar abnormality.

Abnormal gaits

- Spastic, scissoring, propulsive, steppage and waddling.

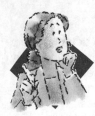

Quick quiz

1. If a patient can't recognise the sound of a ringing phone, he probably has:
   A. agnosia.
   B. apraxia.
   C. aphasia.
   D. ataxia.

2. The fifth cranial nerve is the:
   A. facial nerve.
   B. trigeminal nerve.
   C. trochlear nerve.
   D. abducens nerve.

3. Normal findings in the assessment of coordination include:
   A. downward drift of the arm when it's outstretched.
   B. positive Romberg's test result.
   C. ability to distinguish odours.
   D. smooth, coordinated gait.

4. One of the primitive reflexes is the:
   A. patella reflex.
   B. grasping reflex.
   C. brachial reflex.
   D. triceps reflex.

5. When assessing the patient's pain sensation, it is particularly important to:
   A. keep the patient's eyes open.
   B. test dull in all areas.
   C. test sharp in all areas.
   D. test both sharp and dull in all areas.

For answers see page 402.

Appendices and index

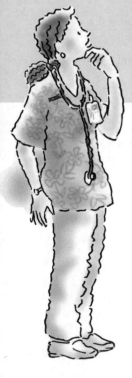

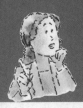

Answers to quick quizzes

Chapter 1

1. Answer B. 'How can I help you today?' is an example of an open question which allows the patient to elaborate more fully in the answer they give.

2. Answer D. Take care of the biographic data first; otherwise, you might get involved in the patient history and forget to ask basic questions.

3. Answer C. Silence allows the patient to collect his/her thoughts and continue to answer your questions.

4. Answer A. The patient's own words form subjective data.

5. Answer D. The last question on CAGE refers to whether the patient ever feels they need an eye opener.

Chapter 2

1. Answer C. The assessment of each body system begins with inspection. It's the most commonly used technique, and it can reveal more than any other technique can.

2. Answer B. The normal systolic blood pressure in an adult sits between 100 and 140 mmHg.

3. Answer A. The normal sound when percussing the lungs is resonance.

4. Answer B. The diaphragm is best at eliciting high-pitched sounds.

5. Answer D. The respiratory examination is a system-specific examination and is not part of the general survey.

Chapter 3

1. Answer A. The six main vitamin groups are A, B, C, D, E and K.

2. Answer A. A serum albumin test assesses protein levels in the body.

3. Answer B. A BMI of 27 falls into the overweight category of 25 to 29.9.

4. Answer C. The haemotocrit is the proportion of red blood cells in the full blood sample.

Chapter 4

1. Answer A. The Mini Mental State Examination measures orientation, short-term memory, calculation and language.

2. Answer A. When a patient jumps from topic to topic this is referred to as flight of ideas.

3. Answer C. Repeating a list of objects is a good test of short-term memory and one in which you can immediately know if their answers are correct or incorrect.

4. Answer D. Phobia is an irrational and disproportionate fear of objects or situations.

Chapter 5

1. Answer B. Asymmetric borders are significant and typically signal malignancy.

2. Answer D. The dorsal surface (back) of the hand is the most sensitive to temperature changes.

3. Answer B. Hirsuitism refers to excessive hair growth, particularly in women.

4. Answer C. A small, blister-like, raised fluid-filled lesion, less than 1 cm in diameter, is known as a vesicle.

5. Answer B. Clubbed fingers are typically a sign of cardiovascular or respiratory disease. Clubbing may also be found in patients with thyroid dysfunction, colitis or cirrhosis. Its causes are poorly understood.

Chapter 6

1. Answer C. The middle layer of the eyeball is called the choroid.

2. Answer B. A drooping eyelid is called a ptosis.

3. Answer B. Cones, which are located in the fovea centralis, aid in colour recognition.

4. Answer A. The Snellen chart tests visual acuity by asking the patient to read a series of letters.

5. Answer C. The red reflex results from light reflecting off the choroid.

6. Answer D. The red negative numbers are used for focusing the ophthalmoscope to examine the eyes of a patient who is short-sighted (needs visual correction to see distant objects).

Chapter 7

1.   Answer B. The light reflection should be at 5 o'clock when looking in the right ear (and 7 o'clock when looking in the left).

2.   Answer A. In the adult patient, the superior posterior auricle should be pulled up and back to straighten the ear canal.

3.   Answer A. The frontal sinuses are located in the forehead, the site of palpation for those structures.

4.   Answer B. Conductive hearing loss occurs from abnormal function of the external or middle ear, resulting in impaired sound transmission.

5.   Answer A. The olfactory nerve (cranial nerve I) is tested by asking the patient to identify an aroma.

6.   Answer B. Clear, thin nasal drainage may indicate a cerebrospinal fluid leak; therefore, you should evaluate this finding closely.

Chapter 8

1.   Answer A. Tactile vocal fremitus should always be felt equally on both sides of the chest. It is normally felt more strongly in the apices than the bases, is harder to feel in obese people and is more easily felt in thinner people.

2.   Answer B. The lungs, made up of tissue and air, make a resonant percussion sound. Solid tissue is flat or dull; air-filled spaces are hyperresonant or tympanic.

3.   Answer C. Vesicular breath sounds are soft, low-pitched and prolonged during inspiration and can be heard over the lower lobes.

4.   Answer A. The normal percussion sound in an infant is hyperresonance.

5.   Answer D. The anterior–posterior diameter of the chest in an adult is normally less than the transverse diameter.

Chapter 9

1.   Answer B. S_1 is best heard at the apex of the heart.

2.   Answer A. S_3 is a normal finding in a child. This sound can indicate heart failure in an adult.

3.   Answer A. Capillary refill time is normally less than 3 seconds. Delay indicates decreased perfusion.

4.   Answer C. S_2, the second heart sound, is made by the closing of the aortic and pulmonary valves.

5.   Answer D. The apical impulse is normally less than 2.5 cm in diameter, visible on inspection in about 50% of patients and located at the fifth intercostal space in the midclavicular line.

Chapter 10

1. Answer D. The brachial (or lateral) lymph nodes drain the arm – the ulnar side travelling via the epitrochlear nodes in the elbow, the radial side directly to the brachial nodes.

2. Answer C. In the week before a woman's menstrual period, both breasts are frequently tender.

3. Answer A. Only long-standing nipple retraction can be regarded as a normal finding. All the other findings require referral for triple assessment.

4. Answer B. The tail of Spence is a small triangle of tissue located in the upper outer quadrant of the breast, towards the axilla.

Chapter 11

1. Answer B. The epiglottis, a thin flap of tissue over the larynx, closes during swallowing to prevent aspiration.

2. Answer A. The liver has a key role in metabolising carbohydrates, fats and proteins.

3. Answer C. Hyperactive bowel sounds are a sign of constipation, diarrhoea, early intestinal obstruction or laxative use.

4. Answer A. Percussing over a solid organ, such as the liver, should create a dull sound.

5. Answer C. Choosing a site away from the painful area, position your hand at a 90-degree angle to the abdomen. Push down slowly and deeply into the abdomen, and then withdraw your hand quickly.

Chapter 12

1. Answer C. A monthly testicular self-examination can help detect testicular cancer early. Examining too frequently will lead to subtle changes being missed.

2. Answer A. The bladder is usually not percussable unless it's distended. The feeling of pressure is usually relieved with urination.

3. Answer C. To check for an inguinal hernia, ask the patient to stand and then hold their breath and bear down, or cough, while you inspect and palpate the area.

4. Answer A. The menstrual cycle varies from woman to woman, so a 32-day cycle is quite normal for some women.

5. Answer B. Although definitive diagnosis is impossible without swabbing, the symptom is most characteristic of Candida albicans, or yeast infection, which causes pruritus and a thick, white, curd-like discharge.

6. Answer D. Because a man's urethra passes through the erectile tissue of the penis, it's 10 to 15 cm longer than a woman's urethra.

Chapter 13

1. Answer A. Crepitus occurs when roughened articular surfaces of bone or bone fragments rub together. Thus it can only occur in joints which are freely movable, such as the synovial joints.

2. Answer A. Tingling of the wrist on percussion (Tinel's sign) is characteristic of carpal tunnel syndrome. The patient is also likely to have a positive Phalen's sign.

3. Answer B. Kyphosis causes a rounded back in the thoracic region.

4. Answer B. Abduction is the ability to move a limb away from the midline. In adduction, the limb is moved towards the midline.

5. Answer A. A swollen knee suggests excess fluid in the joint. The bulge sign occurs when you apply pressure to the medial or lateral side of the patella and a bulge of fluid appears on the opposite side.

Chapter 14

1. Answer A. Agnosia, or the inability to identify common objects, occurs in three forms: visual, auditory or body image.

2. Answer B. The fifth cranial nerve is the trigeminal nerve.

3. Answer D. A smooth, coordinated gait is a normal gross motor finding, as is a negative Romberg's test result.

4. Answer B. The grip, snout, sucking and glabella reflexes occur normally in infants, whose neurological systems are immature. These reflexes are abnormal in adults.

5. Answer C. Sharp must be tested in all areas as it is a pain test. Dull is a control, so testing in all areas is not necessary.

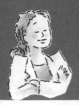

1. An 82-year-old patient is admitted with pneumonia. What's your first priority as you perform their admission assessment?
   A. Asking the patient to sign the admission forms.
   B. Assessment of the patient's airway, breathing and circulation.
   C. Percussing the patient's chest.
   D. Taking the patient's blood pressure.

2. You are taking a history from a 50-year-old patient. You ask 'Can you tell me why you have come to see me today?' This is an example of:
   A. an open question.
   B. a leading question.
   C. a closed question.
   D. a rhetorical question.

3. You are examining the abdomen of a 50-year-old woman with a 2-day history of right-sided abdominal pain. Which should you do first?
   A. Listen with a stethoscope for bowel sounds.
   B. Palpate the area that is painful.
   C. Palpate all the areas that aren't painful.
   D. Inspect the abdomen.

4. You are assessing a 52-year-old patient with angina. When you assess the pulse, you note an irregular rhythm. To further assess the irregular pulse, you decide to assess the patient's pulse deficit. Which combination would help identify the pulse deficit?
   A. Carotid and brachial.
   B. Apical and radial.
   C. Radial and brachial.
   D. Carotid and radial.

5. You're assessing the blood pressure of a patient with diabetic ketoacidosis. How high should you inflate the blood pressure cuff before releasing the valve and listening for the blood pressure?
   A. Inflate the cuff until the radial pulse disappears, and then inflate it by an additional 30 mmHg.
   B. Inflate the cuff to 200 mmHg; if you hear the sound immediately, inflate it to 220 mmHg.
   C. Inflate the cuff until the needle on the manometer stops bouncing.
   D. Inflate the cuff until the patient reports feeling a tingling sensation in their hand.

6. A 52-year-old patient complains of abdominal distention. You perform an abdominal assessment. Which sound should you hear when percussing over an air-filled bowel?
A. Tympany.
B. Dullness.
C. Flatness.
D. Resonance.

7. A 73-year-old female patient is admitted to the hospital for a hip replacement. She previously had a BMI of 36 and was told she was obese and must lose weight prior to the surgery. You measure weight and height and calculate her BMI as 29. How is the result classified?
A. The patient is a now a normal weight.
B. The patient is now underweight.
C. The patient is now overweight but not clinically obese.
D. The patient is still obese.

8. Your patient has been diagnosed with bacterial endocarditis. What might you expect to find when assessing the nails?
A. Dark, yellowish nails.
B. Transverse bands of white covering the nails.
C. Red splinter-like marks on the nails.
D. Clubbing.

9. A 23-year-old female patient is admitted to the inpatient psychiatric unit. You are concerned that excessive alcohol consumption may be contributing to her problem. You decide to assess her using the CAGE tool. Which of the following is NOT a part of the CAGE scoring system:
A. Feeling more courageous when having had a few drinks.
B. Feeling annoyed at other people's views about your drinking.
C. Feeling guilty about what you drink or things that have happened after you had been drinking.
D. Feeling in need of an 'eye opener'.

10. You assess a 13-year-old patient's visual acuity using the Snellen chart. Your finding is 6/4 on the test with both eyes. The result means that:
A. the patient can see from 6 metres away what an average person can only see from 4 metres away.
B. the patient can see from 4 metres away what an average person can only see from 6 metres away.
C. the patient's eyesight is worse than average.
D. the patient's eyesight is two-thirds of what it should be.

11. During an assessment, an 18-year-old patient states that they use an addictive substance. What's the most appropriate nursing response?
A. 'How do you obtain the substance?'
B. 'What substance do you use?'
C. 'Does your employer know about this?'
D. 'You really shouldn't do that.'

12. During an interview, your patient has episodes in which they jump abruptly from topic to topic. Which term identifies this type of speech?
    A. Neologisms.
    B. Echolalia.
    C. Pressured speech.
    D. Flight of ideas.

13. A male patient tells you he is worried about a mole that he has become more aware of recently. It is itchy and seems to have increased in size. You tell him:
    A. it is probably nothing to worry about – get your general practitioner to have a look next time you are there.
    B. moles are normally itchy and sometimes get bigger so don't worry.
    C. the mole could be malignant and needs assessing urgently.
    D. you are sorry but the mole is definitely malignant.

14. A 20-year-old male patient is suffering with severe vomiting after eating at a buffet. You need to assess his skin turgor for signs of dehydration. How should you do this?
    A. Pinch a fold skin on his forearm, back of hand or abdomen.
    B. Palpate the skin on the back of his hand.
    C. Press on his nail beds to cause blanching and assess the time taken for colour to return.
    D. Inspect the skin of the abdomen for signs of dryness.

15. As you assess your patient's skin, you notice several tiny, solid, round, raised lesions on their body. You would chart these findings as:
    A. macules.
    B. bullae.
    C. papules.
    D. plaques.

16. A 49-year-old male patient with a history of alcohol abuse is admitted with bleeding oesophageal varices. When you assess him you note several small red lesions on his trunk. They appear to be red dots with 'legs'. You would chart these findings as:
    A. purpura.
    B. spider naevi.
    C. cherry angiomas.
    D. petechiae.

17. You are assessing a 65-year-old patient who has been concerned about some loss of peripheral vision in their left eye. Although all may be relevant, the most important test to include in your assessment would be:
    A. the Snellen test.
    B. fields by confrontation.
    C. near–far test.
    D. examination with the ophthalmoscope.

18. A child presents with a sore eye that has a mucoid discharge. When you examine their eye, it appears red. Which eye abnormality do these signs and symptoms most suggest?
    A. Cataracts.
    B. Ptosis.
    C. Glaucoma.
    D. Conjunctivitis.

19. You're inspecting a child's pupils as part of a routine examination. You shine indirect light into their right eye. What is the normal response?
    A. Both pupils dilate.
    B. Both pupils constrict.
    C. The right pupil constricts, and the left dilates.
    D. The right pupil constricts and the left stays the same.

20. Where in your patient would you expect to find the inferior turbinates?
    A. In the ear.
    B. In the throat.
    C. In the eye.
    D. In the nose.

21. You examine the eardrum of an 11-year-old child with an earache and a sore throat using an auroscope. Which colour suggests a normal eardrum?
    A. Pink.
    B. White.
    C. Grey.
    D. Red.

22. You are examining the ear of a 1-year-old. In order to view the tympanic membrane with an auroscope it is most likely that you will need to:
    A. pull the pinna upwards and backwards
    B. pull the pinna downwards
    C. pull the pinna straight up
    D. not manipulate the pinna at all.

23. A mother states that her daughter has been complaining for 3 days of a cold sore, which has increased in severity. You palpate the girl's lymph nodes and identify a swollen lymph node directly under the chin. Which lymph node is this?
    A. Preauricular.
    B. Submandibular.
    C. Submental.
    D. Supraclavicular.

24. A 19-year-old college student has fallen down a flight of steps at a party. Chest X-ray shows right-sided pneumothorax. During inspection, what other characteristic of pneumothorax might you observe?
    A. Funnel chest.
    B. Barrel chest.
    C. Intercostal bulging.
    D. Tracheal deviation.

25. A 56-year-old cancer patient has been diagnosed with a pleural effusion. What sign of pleural effusion might you hear when percussing the lungs?
    A. Tympany.
    B. Dullness.
    C. Hyperresonance.
    D. Resonance.

26. You're performing the admission assessment of a 63-year-old male patient with pneumonia. While feeling his chest with the bony part of your hands, you ask him to repeatedly say 'ninety-nine'. What are you checking for?
    A. Bronchophony.
    B. Egophony.
    C. Whispered pectoriloquy.
    D. Tactile vocal fremitus.

27. Your patient develops pneumonia. What *abnormal* breath sounds might you hear when you auscultate the affected lung?
    A. Crackles.
    B. Dullness.
    C. Vesicular breath sounds.
    D. Stridor.

28. You're percussing the lungs of an 85-year-old man with chronic obstructive airways disease. What abnormal sound do you think you would be most likely to hear?
    A. Resonance.
    B. Hyperresonance.
    C. Dullness.
    D. Flatness.

29. A 63-year-old man requires a full vascular assessment. As you perform your initial assessment, you palpate the pulses on top of his feet. What are these pulses?
    A. Popliteal pulses.
    B. Dorsalis pedis pulses.
    C. Posterior tibial pulses.
    D. Anterior tibial pulses.

30. A 57-year-old obese man complains of central chest pain. Which of the following associated factors would cause you the greatest concern?
    A. The pain is intermittent and occurs with eating.
    B. The patient has recently been digging a garden pond.
    C. The pain radiated up into his jaw.
    D. The patient has recently been taking regular nurofen.

31. When auscultating heart sounds, you expect to hear a 'lub-dub' sound. What mechanical event in the heart is associated with the 'lub' sound?
    A. Closure of the mitral and aortic valves.
    B. Closure of the tricuspid and aortic valves.
    C. Closure of the aortic and pulmonic valves.
    D. Closure of the mitral and tricuspid valves.

32. You're inspecting a 58-year-old patient's chest wall to locate the apical impulse. Where should you look?
    A. At the fifth intercostal space in the left midclavicular line.
    B. Over the base of the heart.
    C. Over the aortic area.
    D. At the third intercostal space to the left of the sternum.

33. Which of the following breast findings is *not* normally a cause for concern?
    A. Nipple inversion that has been present since childhood.
    B. Unilateral breast pain at varying points in the menstrual cycle.
    C. Bilateral nipple discharge.
    D. An area of eczema that isn't healing.

34. To auscultate the pulmonary valve area, you should position the stethoscope in the:
    A. third intercostal space, right sternal border.
    B. second intercostal space, right sternal border.
    C. second intercostal space, left sternal border.
    D. fourth intercostal space, right sternal border.

35. A bluish bruise-like area around the umbilicus is a possible indication of:
    A. cholecystitis.
    B. appendicitis.
    C. gastric ulcer.
    D. pancreatitis.

36. A patient comes to the emergency department complaining of right lower quadrant abdominal pain and nausea. Which of these methods is the best way to proceed with the abdominal assessment?
    A. Palpation, percussion, inspection, auscultation.
    B. Inspection, auscultation, percussion, palpation.
    C. Auscultation, inspection, palpation, percussion.
    D. Auscultation, palpation, percussion, inspection.

37. You measure the liver span of a 50-year-old male patient. He is of below average height. The liver span is 16 cm. This finding:
    A. is well within normal limits.
    B. is fractionally over normal limits.
    C. suggests the liver is small.
    D. suggests the liver is abnormally large.

38. The normal position of the spleen is:
    A. just behind the left midaxillary line.
    B. under the left midclavicular line.
    C. anterior to the left midaxillary line.
    D. between the left midaxillary line and the left anterior axillary line.

39. A female patient with a urinary tract infection reports pain when you percuss her back at the costovertebral angle. This suggests:
   A. a ureteral stone.
   B. an ovarian cyst.
   C. kidney inflammation.
   D. bladder cancer.

40. To assess for scoliosis, you should:
   A. palpate for crepitus.
   B. measure the length of the spine from neck to waist.
   C. ask the patient to bend forwards at the waist.
   D. assess the patient lying supine.

41. A 28-year-old man tells you he is worried about a group of red, painful vesicles on his genitalia. You realise this is most likely to be:
   A. cancer.
   B. heat rash.
   C. genital herpes.
   D. syphillis.

42. You want to assess blood flow in the renal arteries. You should auscultate:
   A. just below the costal margin in both midclavicular lines.
   B. just above the umbilicus in both midclavicular lines.
   C. in the midsternal line in the epigastric area.
   D. just below the umbilicus in both midclavicular lines.

43. You examine an 80-year-old patient who cannot move their left hip outwards from the midline without extreme pain. You document this as pain on:
   A. flexion.
   B. extension.
   C. abduction.
   D. adduction.

44. A 34-year-old female patient is complaining of pain and tingling in her right wrist. During your examination, the patient reports tingling when you percuss over the inner aspect of the wrist. This finding indicates:
   A. a fractured wrist.
   B. carpal tunnel syndrome.
   C. scaphoid fracture.
   D. infection of the wrist.

45. A 58-year-old man gives you a urine specimen with a reddish brown appearance. What does this finding suggest?
   A. Hypervolemia.
   B. Benign prostatic hyperplasia.
   C. Urinary tract infection.
   D. Haematuria.

46. Which of the following is not one of the 5 Ps typically used in musculoskeletal assessment?
    A. Pain.
    B. Pressure.
    C. Pallor.
    D. Pulses.

47. A 30-year-old is brought to the emergency department with head injuries from a motorcycle accident. During your neurological assessment, the patient displays Babinski's reflex. This is characterised by:
    A. plantar flexion and fanning of the toes.
    B. dorsi flexion and fanning of the toes.
    C. vibration in the big toe.
    D. fasciculation of the foot.

48. During a physical examination, a 68-year-old patient can't identify a key or a coin when manipulating the objects with either hand, keeping his eyes closed. This abnormal finding indicates impaired:
    A. apraxia.
    B. aphasia.
    C. graphaesthesia.
    D. stereognosis.

49. You're assessing the cranial nerves of a 62-year-old male patient who has had a stroke. How should you assess the function of cranial nerve VII?
    A. Test the patient's hearing and ask him if he ever experiences dizziness or vertigo.
    B. Test the patient's ability to feel crude touch on his face as well as his ability to differentiate sharp and dull sensations on his face.
    C. Observe his face for symmetry at rest and while making facial expressions, such as smiling or frowning.
    D. Test the patient's gag reflex and his ability to swallow.

50. A patient's muscle strength is assessed by performing:
    A. deep tendon reflex testing.
    B. passive range-of-movement exercises.
    C. Romberg's test.
    D. resisted movement exercises.

Answers

1. B. The first priority is ABC – airway, breathing and circulation.

2. A. This is an example of an open question.

3. D. Inspection should always be the first part of your assessment.

4. B. When determining a pulse deficit, you normally palpate the radial pulse while auscultating the apical pulse. The apical pulse rate minus the radial pulse rate equals the pulse deficit.

5. A. You should neither underinflate nor overinflate the cuff. The ideal method is to palpate the radial pulse while inflating the cuff. When the radial pulse disappears, inflate the cuff an additional 30 mmHg and then close the valve.

6. A. When percussing over an air-filled bowel, you would expect to hear tympany.

7. C. A BMI of 25 to 29.9 is categorised as overweight; 30 or over is obese.

8. C. Splinter haemorrhages are linked to bacterial endocarditis.

9. A. The C of CAGE stands for whether the patient has ever felt they should Cut Down on their alcohol intake.

10. A. The Snellen chart measures visual acuity and provides readings such as 6/4. A person with 6/4 vision can see things from 6 m away which an average person with normal vision can only see from 4 m away.

11. B. When a patient identifies a history of substance abuse, it's important for you to assess the risks, which include determining the substance being used.

12. D. A continuous flow of speech in which the patient jumps abruptly from topic to topic is called 'flight of ideas'.

13. C. These are worrying signs which are suggestive of malignancy. Urgent review is required, but further investigation will be needed for a definite diagnosis.

14. A. To evaluate skin turgor, gently squeeze the skin on the forearm, back of hand or abdomen. If the skin quickly returns to its original shape, the patient's skin turgor is normal. If it returns to its original shape slowly or maintains a tented position, the skin has poor turgor, which is a sign of dehydration.

15. C. Papules are small, raised, solid lesions.

16. B. Spider naevi are small, spider-like leisons. They're commonly seen on the face, arms, and trunk of patients with liver disease.

17. B. All tests could be of use, but the test designed specifically to assess peripheral vision is fields by confrontation.

18. D. Conjunctivitis causes redness of the eye as well as discharge.

19. B. Shining a light in the right eye should cause right eye constriction (direct) and left eye constriction (consensual).

20. D. The inferior turbinates are in the nose.

21. C. The normal eardrum (tympanic membrane) is grey.

22. B. To perform an auroscopic examination in a 1-year-old, you will probably need to pull down on the pinna by holding and pulling down the earlobe in order to straighten the ear canal.

23. C. The submental lymph node is located directly under the chin.

24. D. With a pneumothorax, tracheal deviation may be present.

25. B. Pleural effusion characteriscally produces dullness on percussion.

26. D. Feeling vibration with the hands is tactile vocal fremitus.

27. A. With pneumonia, crackles in the affected area of the lung may be heard on auscultation. Bronchial or bronchovesicular breath sounds may also be heard. Vesicular sounds may be heard but are not abnormal.

28. B. Chronic obstructive airways disease causes air trapping, so the most likely abnormal percussion sound is hyperresonance.

29. B. The pulses on the tops of the feet are the dorsalis pedis pulses.

30. C. Central chest pain radiating to the jaw is a worrying sign, indicative of myocardial infarction. The other factors don't exclude myocardial infarction but this factor is the most worrying.

31. D. The first heart sound, S_1, which produces the 'lub' sound, is associated with closure of the mitral and tricuspid valves.

32. A. The apical impulse, also usually the point of maximum impulse, can be found at the fifth intercostal space in, or just medial to, the left midclavicular line.

33. A. Long-standing nipple inversion is normal in some women. Nipple retraction that is new, be it unilateral or bilateral, is a worrying finding, as are B, C and D.

34. C. The pulmonary valve is best heard at the second intercostal space, just left of the sternum.

35. D. This is Cullen's sign, indicative of pancreatitis or bleeding.

36. B. The proper order for abdominal assessment is inspection, auscultation, percussion and palpation. Inspection, palpation, percussion and auscultation is an acceptable alternative but inspection always comes first.

37. D. Normal liver span is 6 to 12 cm in the midclavicular line, so 16 cm indicates an enlarged liver.

38. A. The spleen normally sits wholly behind the midaxillary line.

39. C. Pain during percussion over the costovertebral angle suggests kidney inflammation.

40. C. To assess for scoliosis, inspect the spine for abnormalities while the patient is bending forwards at the waist, and as they move back into an upright position. This position can make spinal deformities more apparent.

41. C. Although the other options are feasible and cannot be excluded on inspection alone, the presentation is strongly characteristic of genital herpes.

42. A. The renal arteries sit horizontally, running from the aorta to the pelvis of the kidneys, typically at a level just below the costal margin. Another way to remember the position is midway between the nipples and umbilicus.

43. C. Moving a limb away from the midline is abduction.

44. B. Pain or tingling in the hand or fingers which occurs when the patient's wrist is percussed is called Tinel's sign. This finding, like Phalen's sign, is indicative of carpal tunnel syndrome.

45. D. A patient with haematuria may have brown or bright red urine.

46. B. Remember the 5 Ps are pain, paresthesia, paralysis, pallor and pulses.

47. B. Dorsiflexion and fanning of the toes is characteristic of Babinski's reflex. It can be normal in children of up to 2 years of age, but is always abnormal in an adult.

48. D. The ability to identify a common object by touching and manipulating it is called stereognosis.

49. C. Cranial nerve VII is the facial nerve so is tested by assessing facial symmetry and movement.

50. D. Resisted movement assesses muscle strength. Normal muscle strength is graded 5/5.

Glossary

abduction: movement away from the midline

accommodation: a change in the shape of the lens which allows the eye to focus on a nearby object; accompanied by constriction of the pupils and convergence of the eyes

adduction: movement towards the midline

alert: term used to describe a patient who can follow commands, comprehend verbal and written language, express ideas freely and is orientated to time, place and person

alopecia: hair loss

amplitude: strength of a pulse or other force; recorded by terms such as bounding, normal or weak

anisocoria: unequal pupils

ankylosis: fixation of a joint due to fibrous or bony union; results from a disease process

anorexia: loss of appetite

anthropometric measurements: measurements of the human body taken as part of a comprehensive nutritional assessment;

aphasia: language disorder characterised by difficulty expressing or comprehending speech

apraxia: inability to perform coordinated movements, even though no motor deficit is present

ascites: accumulation of fluid in the abdominal cavity

ataxia: uncoordinated actions when voluntary muscle movements are attempted

auscultation: physical assessment technique by which the examiner listens (usually with a stethoscope) for sounds coming from the heart, lungs, abdomen or other organs

bimanual palpation: method of palpation involving the use of two hands to locate body structures and assess their texture, size, consistency, mobility and tenderness

borborygmus: loud, gurgling, splashing sounds caused by gas passing through the intestine; normally heard over the large intestine

bruit: abnormal 'whooshing' sound heard over peripheral vessels that indicates turbulent blood flow

cardiac cycle: the period from the beginning of one heartbeat to the beginning of the next; includes two phases, systole and diastole

cataract: opacity of the lens of the eye

cerumen: wax-like secretion in the external ear

closed questions: questions that elicit 'yes or no' answers

coma: unconscious state in which the patient appears to be asleep, doesn't speak and responds to neither body nor environmental stimuli

consensual light reflex: reflex constriction of the pupil of one eye when the other eye is illuminated

contralateral: pertaining to the opposite side of the body

coronal: vertical lateral division through the body; that is, dissection down through the ears, shoulders, hips, etc.

crackles: intermittent, non-musical, crackling breath sounds which are caused by collapsed or fluid-filled alveoli popping open

cremasteric reflex: superficial reflex in men; elicited by stroking the upper inner thigh, which causes brisk retraction of the testis on the side of the stimulus

crepitus: noise or vibration produced by rubbing together irregular cartilage surfaces or broken ends of a bone; also the sound heard when air in subcutaneous tissue is palpated

dimpling: puckering or depression of the skin of the breast possibly caused by underlying growth

diplopia: double vision

distal: anatomically located further from the attachment of a limb to the trunk, or from a point of attachment.

dorsal: pertaining to the back or posterior surface

dysarthria: speech defect commonly related to a motor deficit of the tongue or speech muscles

dysphagia: difficulty swallowing

Erb's point: auscultatory point on the precordium at the third intercostal space to the left of the sternum; here the 'lub' and the 'dub' are normally similar in loudness

exophthalmos: abnormal protrusion of the eyeball

expressive aphasia: inability to express words or thoughts

extension: straightening or hyperextending a joint

far-sightedness: also called long-sightedness; problems seeing near objects

flaccidity: decreased muscle tone, which may cause muscle to become weak or flabby

flexion: bending a joint

fluid wave: rippling across the abdomen during the ballotment test; indicative of the presence of ascites

fremitus: palpable vibration which results from air passing through the bronchopulmonary system and transmitting vibrations to the chest wall

gynaecomastia: enlargement of breast tissue in a male

haematuria: presence of blood in the urine

hernia: abnormal protrusion of a structure through an opening; for example, the protrusion of a loop of bowel through a muscle wall

hirsutism: excessive hair growth; may be hereditary, a sign of an endocrine disorder or an effect of certain drugs

hordeolum: inflammation of the sebaceous gland of the eyelid; also called stye

hydrocele: accumulation of serous fluid in a sac-like structure such as the testis

hyperresonance: increased resonance produced by percussion

inspection: observation of the patient during which the examiner may use sight, hearing or smell to make informed observations

intensity: degree of strength; for example, the loudness of a heart murmur, recorded as soft, medium or loud

ipsalateral: pertaining to the same side of the body

jaundice: yellowish discoloration of the skin caused by the accumulation of bilirubin

lateral: position away from the midline

leading question: a question which strongly suggests a particular answer, such as 'You don't have any pain, do you?'

lethargy: slowed responses, sluggish speech and slowed mental and motor

processes in a person who is orientated to time, place and person

lichenification: thickening of the skin related to eczema which occurs especially in the antecubital and popliteal fossae

ligament: joins a bone to a bone

mammogram: X-ray of the breast used to detect tumours and other abnormalities

meatus: opening or passageway in the body, most commonly used to describe the opening of the urethra in the penis

medial: position closer to the midline

menarche: first menstrual period

menopause: cessation of the menstrual periods

murmur: abnormal sound heard on auscultation of the heart; caused by abnormal blood flow through a valve

mydriasis: dilation of the pupil due to paralysis of the oculomotor nerve or the effects of drugs

myopia: defect in vision that allows a person to see objects clearly at close range but not at a distance; also called near-sightedness

near-sightednes: also called short-sightedness; difficulty seeing distant objects

nipple inversion: inwards turning or depression of the central portion of the nipple

nystagmus: involuntary, rhythmic movement of the eye

objective data: information verifiable through direct observation, laboratory tests, screening procedures or physical examination

occult blood: blood hidden in stool or urine that can't be seen with the naked eye

open-ended question: question which requires an answer in a sentence form rather than a 'yes or no' form

palpation: physical assessment technique by which the examiner uses the sense of touch to feel pulsations and vibrations or to locate body structures and assess their texture, size, consistency, mobility and tenderness

parietal: the outer wall or lining of a body cavity

peau d'orange: orange-peel appearance of breast skin associated with breast cancer

percussion: physical assessment technique by which the examiner taps on the skin surface with their fingers to assess the size, border and consistency of internal organs and to detect and evaluate fluid in a body cavity

periosteum: the membrane which covers a bone

peristalsis: sequence of muscle contractions which propels food through the gastrointestinal tract

pitch: frequency of a sound, measured in the number of sound waves generated per second

plantar: ventral surface of the foot; downwards direction of foot movement (plantar flexion)

point of maximum impulse: point at which the upwards thrust of the heart against the chest wall is greatest, usually over the apex of the heart; also called the apical impulse

precordium: area of the chest over the heart

presbyopia: far-sightedness which occurs as a normal part of the ageing process

prone: lying on the front

proprioception: awareness of the position of the body or body parts in space

protraction: moving forwards

proximal: anatomically located nearer to the attachment of a limb to the trunk, or to a point of attachment

pruritus: severe itching

ptosis: drooping of the eyelid

rebound tenderness: sharp, stabbing pain which occurs when the abdomen is pushed in deeply and then suddenly released; usually associated with peritoneal inflammation

receptive aphasia: inability to understand spoken word

resonance: clear, hollow, low-pitched sound produced by percussion; typically heard over normal lungs

retraction: moving backwards

sagittal: vertical anterior – posterior line through the body; that is, dividing line through the nose, spine, sternum, perineum, etc.

shock: an insufficient suppy of oxygen and nutrients to the body to meet its metabolic needs

spider naevi: dilated small blood vessels which form a spider-like pattern; may be indicative of liver disease – should be investigated if the patient has more than five or six

strabismus: lack of coordination of eye muscles

striae: stripes or lines of tissue which differ in colour and texture from the surrounding tissue

stridor: loud, high-pitched crowing sound usually heard during inspiration without the need for a stethoscope

stupor: state in which a patient lies quietly with minimal spontaneous movement and is unresponsive except to vigorous and repeated stimuli

subjective data: information that the patient, family or friends give about the patient's current healthcare status during the health history; reflects the personal perspective of the patient, family and friends

supine: lying on the back

synovial joint: type of freely movable joint lined with a synovial membrane that secretes synovial fluid for lubrication

tail of Spence: extension of breast tissue which projects from the upper outer quadrant of the breast toward the axilla

tendon: joins a bone to a muscle

thrill: palpable vibration felt over the heart or vessel which results from turbulent blood flow

tinnitus: ringing sound in one or both ears

tone: normal degree of vigour and tension; in muscle, the normal degree of tension

tympany: musical, drum-like sound heard during percussion over a hollow organ such as the stomach; a normal sound

ventral: the front or anterior surface

vertigo: illusion that one's body or surroundings is moving

visceral: referring to an organ, or the outer covering of an organ

vitiligo: areas of complete absence of melanin pigment leading to patchy areas of white or light skin

wheezes: high-pitched breath sounds heard first on exhalation which occur when airflow is blocked

References and websites

Anderson, E., Gebbie, A., Smith, N. and Berrey, P. (2005) The reproductive system. In Douglas, G., Nicol, F. and Robertson, C. (eds). *Macleod's Clinical Examination*, chapter 7. 11th edn. Edinburgh: Churchill Livingstone.

Baines, E. and Kanagasundaram, N. (2008) Early warning scores. *Student BMJ*. http://student.bmj.com/issues/08/09/education/320.php

BAPEN (2003) *Malnutrition Universal Screening Tool*. Reddich, Worcs.: The British Association of Parentral and Enteral Nutrition. http://www.bapen.org.uk/must_tool.html

Beck, A., Steer, R. and Brown G. (1996) *The Beck Depression Inventory BD II Manual*. Oxford: Pearson.

Bevan, J. and Gawkrodger, D. (2005) General examination. Iin Douglas, G., Nicol, F. and Robertson, C. (eds), *Macleod's Clinical Examination*, chapter 2. 11th edn. Edinburgh: Churchill Livingstone.

Bickley, L. and Szilagyi, P. (2007) *Bates Guide to Physical Examination*, 9th edn. Philadelphia: Lippincott, Williams and Williams.

Blows, W. (2007) What are neurological observations? *Nursing Times.net*, 13 August 2007. http://www.nursingtimes.net/ntclinical/neurological_observations_1.html

BMA (2006a) *The Law and Ethics of Male Circumcision – Guidance for Doctors*. http://www.bma.org.uk/ap.nsf/Content/malecircumcision2006

BMA (2006b) *Female Genital Mutilation – Caring for Patients and Child Protection*. http://www.bma.org.uk/ap.nsf/Content/FGM

Breath Sounds Made Incredibly Easy (2005) Philadelphia: Lippincott, Williams and Wilkins.

Callaghan, P. and Waldock, H (2006) *The Oxford Handbook of Mental Health Nursing*. Oxford: Oxford University Press.

Cancer Backup (2008a) *Breast Screening*. http://www.cancerbackup.org.uk/Aboutcancer/Screening/Breastscreening

Cancer Backup (2008b) *Bowel Cancer Screening*. http://www.cancerbackup.org.uk/Aboutcancer/Screening/Bowelscreening

Cancer Backup (2008c) *Cervical Screening*. http://www.cancerbackup.org.uk/Aboutcancer/Screening/Cervicalscreening

Cancer Research (2005) *Testicular Cancer: Spot the Symptoms Early (Leaflet)*. http://info.cancerresearchuk.org/images/publicationspdfs/leaflet_testicular.pdf

Cancer Research UK (2006a) *Preventing Melanoma*. http://www.cancerhelp.org.uk/help/default.asp?page=3007

Cancer Research UK (2006b) *Testicular Self Examination*.http://www.cancerhelp.org.uk/help/default.asp?page=3570

Cancer Research UK (2007a) *Breast Cancer Symptoms*. http://www.cancerhelp.org.uk/help/default.asp?page=3284

Cancer Research UK (2007b) *Breast Cancer in Men*. http://www.cancerhelp.org.uk/help/default.asp?page=5075

Cancer Research UK (2008a) *Breast Cancer Section Overview*. http://www.cancerhelp.org.uk/help/default.asp?page=3270

Cancer Research UK (2008b) *Breast Cancer Risk Factors*. http://info.cancerresearchuk.org/cancerstats/types/breast/riskfactors/

Cancer Research UK (2008c) *UK Testicular Cancer Incidence Statistics*. http://info.cancerresearchuk.org/cancerstats/types/testis/incidence/

Department of Children, Schools and Families (2008) *Every Child Matters: Child and Adolescent Mental Health Services*. London: DCSF. http://www.everychildmatters.gov.uk/health/camhs/

DH (2001) *National Service Framework for Diabetes: Standards.* London: Department of Health.

DH (2003) *Essence of Care: Benchmarks for Food and Nutrition.* London: NHS Modernisation Agency, Department of Health. http://www.dh.gov.uk/en/Publicationsandstatistics/Publications/PublicationsPolicyAndGuidance/DH_4005475

DH (2007) *Mental Capacity Act 2005 – Summary.* http://www.dh.gov.uk/en/Publicationsandstatistics/Bulletins/theweek/Chiefexecutivebulletin/DH_4108436

DH (2008) *Healthy Weight, Healthy Lives.* London: Department of Health. http://www.dh.gov.uk/en/Publichealth/Healthimprovement/Obesity/DH_082383.

Diabetes UK (2006) *Am I Overweight?* London: Diabetes UK. http://www.diabetes.org.uk/Guide-to-diabetes/Treatment_your_health/Managing_your_weight/Am_I_overweight/

Diabetes UK (2008) *Diabetes and Blood Glucose Monitoring.* http://www.diabetes.co.uk/diabetes_care/Diabetes_and_blood_glucose.html

Dimond, B. (2007) *Legal Aspects of Mental Capacity.* Harlow: Longman.

Dimond, B. (2008) *Legal Aspects of Nursing*, 8th edn. Harlow: Longman.

Dimond, B. (2009) *Legal Aspects of Consent*, 2nd edn. Harlow: Longman

Dougherty, L. and Lister, S. (2004a) Guideline 25: observations. *The Royal Marsden Hospital Manual of Clinical Nursing Procuedures*, 6th edn. Oxford: Blackwell.

Dougherty, L. and Lister, S. (2004b) Guideline 26: observations – neurological. *The Royal Marsden Hospital Manual of Clinical Nursing Procuedures*. 6th edn. Oxford: Blackwell.

ECG Interpretation Made Incredibly Easy (2007) Philadelphia: Lippincott, Williams and Wilkins.

Egan, G. (2001) *The Skilled Helper: A Problem Management and Opportunity Development Approach to Helping*. 7th edn. Kentucky: Wadsworth Publishing Company.

Enoch, S (2006) ABC of wound healing: wound assessment. *Student British Medical Journal On-Line*, March. http://student.bmj.com/issues/06/03/education/98.php

Epstein, O., Perkin, G., Cookson, J. and de Bono, D. (2003) *Clinical Examination*, 3rd edn. Edinburgh: Mosby.

Ewing, J.A. (1984) Detecting alcoholism – the CAGE questionnaire. *Journal of the Americal Medical Association* 252: 1905.

Hastings, M. (2008) *Clinical Skills Made Incredibly Easy*. 1st UK edn. London: Lippincott, Williams and Wilkins.

Health Assessment Made Incredibly Visual (2007) Philadelphia: Lippincott, Williams and Wilkins.

Heart Sounds Made Incredibly Easy (2005) Philadelphia: Lippincott, Williams and Wilkins.

Jarvis, C. (2008) *Physical Examination and Health Assessment*. 5th edn. St Louis: Saunders.

Knott, L. (2007) *Clubbing*. http://www.patient.co.uk/showdoc/40000072/

Kumar, P. and Clark, M. (2002) *Clinical Medicine*. 5th edn. Edinburgh: W.B. Saunders.

Lederle, F. and Simel, D. (1999) Does this patient have abdominal aortic aneurysm? *Journal of the American Medical Association* 281(1):77–82.

Lumley, J.S. (2008) *Surface Anatomy*. 4th edn. Edinburgh: Churchill Livingstone.

Mackway-Jones, K., Molyneux, E., Philips, B. and Wieteska, S. (2005) *Advanced Paediatric Life Support: The Practical Approach*. 4th edn. Oxford: Blackwell Publishing.

Malviya, S., Voepel-Lewis, T., Burke, C, Merkel, S. and Tait, A. (2006) *Paediatric Anaesthesia* 16(3):258–265.

McGee, S. (2007) *Evidence Based Physical Diagnosis*. 2nd edn. St Louis: Saunders.

Meningitis Trust (2007) *Meningitis Information: Signs and Symptoms*. http://www.meningitis-trust.org/Signs-Symptoms.html

Morton, P. (1993) *Health Assessment in Nursing.* 2nd edn. Pennsylvania: Springhouse.

NHS Cancer Screening Programme (2006) *Being Breast Aware.* London: Department of Health. http://www.cancerscreening.nhs.uk/breastscreen/publications/be-breast-aware.html

NHS Direct (2008a) *What is the Body Mass Index (BMI)?* http://www.nhsdirect.nhs.uk/articles/article.aspx?articleId=850

NHS Direct (2008b) *Hormone Replacement Therapy.* http://www.nhsdirect.nhs.uk/articles/article.aspx?articleId=198#

NHS Direct (2008c) *Sexually Transmitted Infections.* http://www.nhsdirect.nhs.uk/articles/article.aspx?articleId=436&sectionId=10

NHS Scotland (2006) *Best Practice Statement: Ear Care.* Edinburgh: NHS Quality Improvement. http://www.nhshealthquality.org/nhsqis/files/Best%20Practice%20Statement%20%20Ear%20Care.pdf

NICE (2002) *Improving Outcomes in Breast Cancer: Manual Update.* London: National Institute of Clinical Excellence. http://www.nice.org.uk/Guidance/CSGBC/Guidance/pdf/English

NICE (2004) *National Clinical Guidance on Management of Adults with Chronic Obstructive Pulmonary Disease in Primary and Secondary Care. Clinical Guideline 12.* London: National Institute for Health and Clinical Excellence. http://www.nice.org.uk/guidance/CG12

NICE (2006) *Guidance on the Prevention, Identification, Assessment and Management of Overweight and Obesity in Adults and Children,* Clinical Guideline 43. London: National Institute for Health and Clinical Excellence. http://www.nice.org.uk/nicemedia/pdf/word/CG43FullGuideline2v.doc#null

NICE (2007a) *Feverish Illness in Children: Assessment and Initial Management in Children Under 5 Years,* Clinical Guideline 47. London: National Institute for Health and Clinical Excellence. http://www.nice.org.uk/CG47

NICE (2007b) *Acutely Ill Patients in Hospital,* Clinical Guideline 50. London: National Institute for Health and Clinical Excellence. http://www.nice.org.uk/CG50

NICE (2007c) *Medical Research Council (MRC) Dyspnoea Scale.* London: National Institute for Clinical Excellence.

NICE (2007d) *Triage, Assessment, Investigation and Early Management of Head Injury in Infants, Children and Adults,* Clinical Guideline 56. London: National Institute of Clinical Excellence. http://www.nice.org.uk/CG56

NMC (2007) *Record Keeping.* http://www.nmc-uk.org/aFrameDisplay.aspx?DocumentID=4008

Northridge, D., Grubb, N. and Bradbury, A. (2005) The cardiovascular system. In Douglas, G., Nicol, F. and Robertson, C. (eds), *Macleod's Clinical Examination,* chapter 3. 11th edn. Edinburgh: Churchill Livingstone.

O'Carrol, M. and Park, A. (2007) *Essential Mental Health Nursing Skills.* Mosby: London.

Overfield, T. (1995) *Biological Variation in Health and Illness: Race, Age and Sex.* 2nd edn. New York: CRC Press.

Patient UK (2006) *Advanced Directives (Living Wills).* http://www.patient.co.uk/showdoc/40025325/

Patient UK (2007a) *Consent to Treatment in Children.* http://www.patient.co.uk/showdoc/40002288/

Patient UK (2007b) *Mini Mental State Exam.* http://www.patient.co.uk/showdoc/40000152/

Patient UK (2007c) *Pupillary Abnormalities.* http://www.patient.co.uk/showdoc/40000839/

Patient UK (2008) *Squint (Strabismus) in Children.* http://www.patient.co.uk/showdoc/23068827/

Pentland, B., Stratham, B. and Olson, L. (2005) The nervous system including the eye. In Douglas, G., Nicol, F. and Robertson, C. (eds) *Macleod's Clinical Examination,* chapter 8. 11th edn. Edinburgh: Churchill Livingstone.

Powell, C. (2007) *Safeguarding Children and Young People: A Guide for Nurses and Midwives.* Maidenhead: The Open University Press.

Price, G., Uauy, R., Breeze, E. Bulpitt, C. and Fletcher, A. (2006) Weight, shape, and mortality risk in older persons: elevated waist-hip ratio, not high body mass index, is associated with a greater risk of death. *American Journal of Clinical Nutrition* 84:449.

Royal College of Nursing (2002) *Breast Palpation and Breast Awareness: The Role of the Nurse*. London: Royal College of Nursing. http://www.rcn. org.uk/__data/assets/pdf_ file/0011/78536/001754.pdf

Rennie, J. (2005) Examination of the newborn. In Rennie, J. (ed.) *Robertson's Textbook of Neonatology*, chapter 14. Edinburgh: Elsevier.

Resuscitation Council UK (2006) *Advanced Life Support*. 5th edn. London: Resuscitation Council UK. http://www.resus.org.uk/ SiteIndx.htm

Rotherham Primary Ear Care Centre (2008) *Guidance Document in Ear Care*. Rotherham: Primary Ear Care Centre.

Royal National Institute for the Blind (2007) *Understanding Glaucoma*. http://www.rnib. org.uk/xpedio/groups/public/ documents/PublicWebsite/ public_rnib003655.hcsp

Scottish Parliament (2006) *Adults with Incapacity (Scotland) Act 2000: General Information*. http://www.scotland.gov.uk/ Publications/2006/03/07090322/0

Second Task Force on BP in Children (1987) Cited in Neil, S. and Knowles, H. (2004) *The Biology of Child Health*. Basingstoke: Palgrave MacMillan.

Seidel, H., Ball, J., Dains, J. and Benedict, G.W. (2003) *Mosby's Guide to Physical Examination*. 5th edn. St Louis: Mosby.

SIGN (2003) *Management of Obesity in Children and Young People*, National Clinical Guideline 69. Edinburgh: Scottish Intercollegiate Guidelines Network. http://www. sign.ac.uk/pdf/sign69.pdf

Snadden, D., Lang, R., Masterson, G. and College, N (2005) History taking. In Douglas, G., Nicol, F. and Robertson, C. (eds) *Macleod's Clinical Examination*, Chapter 1. 11th edn. Edinburgh: Churchill Livingstone.

Tortora, J. (2005) *Principles of Human Anatomy*. 10th edn. Hoboken, NJ: John Wiley and sons.

Tywcross, A. and Smith, J. (2006) The management of acute pain in children. In Glasper, E.A. and Richardson, J (eds), *A Textbook of Children's and Young People's Nursing*, chapter 17. Edinburgh: Churchill Livingstone.

UCL Institute of Child Health (2007) *Head Circumference: Measuring a Child*, Clinical Guideline. http://www.ich.ucl. ac.uk/clinical_information/ clinical_guidelines/cpg_ guideline_00066/

Whooley, M, Avins, L., Miranda, J. and Browner, W. (1997) Case-finding instruments for depression. Two questions are as good as many. *Journal of General Internal Medicine* 12(7):439–445.

World Health Organisation (2006) *Global Database on Body Mass Index* http://www.who.int/ bmi/index.jsp?introPage=intro_ 3.html

Wound Care Made Incredibly Easy (2006) Philadelphia: Lippincott, Williams and Wilkins.

Zigmond, A. and Snaith, R. (1983) The hospital anxiety and depression scale. *Acta Psychiatrica Scandinavica* 67:361–370.

Websites

Alcohol unit calculator http://www.units.nhs.uk/

Body mass index calculator http:// www.nhsdirect.nhs.uk/magazine/ interactive/bmi/index.aspx

Breakthrough Breast Cancer: patient support and breast cancer research http://www.breakthrough. org.uk

British Heart Foundation patient support http://www.bhf.org.uk/ living_with_heart_conditions/ default.aspx

NHS immunisation schedule (regularly updated) http:// www.immunisations.nhs.uk/

Smoking pack years: calculator http://www.smokingpackyears. com/

Many references include a web address/URL. All of these were correct at the time of writing. However, the nature of web addresses is such that they are prone to change. If you cannot find the reference you are looking for via the given web address, enter the author and title as search terms into the search engine of your choice (e.g. Google), and on most occasions this should lead you to the required document or its updated version.

Index

t refers to a table; i refers to an illustration; **bold type** indicates colour pages.

t refers to a table; i refers to an illustration; **bold type** indicates colour pages.

t refers to a table; i refers to an illustration; **bold type** indicates colour pages.

t refers to a table; i refers to an illustration; **bold type** indicates colour pages.

t refers to a table; i refers to an illustration; **bold type** indicates colour pages.

t refers to a table; i refers to an illustration; **bold type** indicates colour pages.